PROGRESS IN CLINICAL AND BIOLOGICAL RESEARCH

MODELS
FOR
PROSTATE CANCER

MODELS
FOR
PROSTATE CANCER

Editor

GERALD P. MURPHY, MD, DSc

National Prostatic Cancer Project

and

Roswell Park Memorial Institute
Buffalo, New York

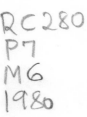
ALAN R. LISS, INC. ● NEW YORK

Address all inquiries to the publisher:

Alan R. Liss, Inc., 150 Fifth Avenue, New York, NY 10011

Copyright © 1980 Alan R. Liss, Inc.

Printed in the United States of America

Library of Congress Cataloging in Publication Data
Main entry under title:

Models for prostate cancer.

(Progress in clinical and biological research: v. 37)
Bibliography: p.
Includes index.
1. Prostate gland — Cancer — Congresses. 2. Cell culture — Congresses. I. Murphy, Gerald Patrick.
II. Series.
RC280.P7M6   616.9'94'63   79-23916
ISBN 0-8451-0037-8

MODELS FOR PROSTATE CANCER

A Planning Meeting Organized by the
National Prostatic Cancer Project
Buffalo, New York

May 7–8, 1979

ORGANIZING COMMITTEE

Chairmen

Dr. Donald S. Coffey

Dr. Donald J. Merchant

Dr. Gerald P. Murphy

Host

Roswell Park Memorial Institute

Buffalo, New York

Executive Secretary

Dr. James P. Karr

Contents

Participants

Arthur E. Bogden, Worcester Foundation, Worcester, Massachusetts 01608 [303]

Andrew Chiarodo, National Organ Site Programs Branch, National Cancer Institute, Bethesda, Maryland 20205

Alice J. Claflin, Department of Surgery, University of Miami School of Medicine, Miami, Florida 33101 [111, 161, 365]

Donald S. Coffey, Department of Pharmacology and Experimental Therapeutics, Johns Hopkins University School of Medicine, Baltimore, Maryland 21205 [311, 379]

Joseph R. Drago, Department of Urology, Hershey Medical Center, Pennsylvania State University, Hershey, Pennsylvania 17033 [265, 325]

Ruben F. Gittes, Division of Urology, Peter Bent Brigham Hospital, Boston, Massachusetts 02115 [31, 393]

Julius Horoszewicz, Department of Medical Viral Oncology, Roswell Park Memorial Institute, Buffalo, New York 14263 [115]

M. Edward Kaighn, Pasadena Foundation for Medical Research, Pasadena, California 91101 [85, 217]

James P. Karr, National Prostatic Cancer Project, Buffalo, New York 14263

Ronald W. Lewis, Department of Urology, Tulane University School of Medicine, New Orleans, Louisiana 70433 [39]

David M. Lubaroff, Department of Urology, University of Iowa Hospitals and Clinics, Iowa City, Iowa 52242 [243]

Theodore I. Malinin, Department of Surgery, University of Miami School of Medicine, Miami, Florida 33101 [111, 161]

John E. McNeal, Department of Pathology, Herrick Memorial Institute, Berkeley, California 94704 [149]

Donald J. Merchant, Department of Microbiology and Immunology, Eastern Virginia Medical School, Norfolk, Virginia 23501 [3, 233]

Don D. Mickey, Division of Urology, Department of Surgery, Duke University Medical Center, Durham, North Carolina 27710 [67]

Gerald P. Murphy, National Prostatic Cancer Project, Roswell Park Memorial Institute, Buffalo, New York 14263 [1]

The number in bold type following a participant's affiliation is the opening page number of that author's chapter.

Morris Pollard, Lobund Laboratory, University of Notre Dame, Notre Dame, Indiana 46556 [293]

Betty Rosoff, Stern College for Women, Yeshiva University, New York, New York 10016 [239]

Avery A. Sandberg, Medicine C Department, Roswell Park Memorial Institute, Buffalo, New York 14263 [9, 115]

Mukta M. Webber, Division of Urology, University of Colorado Medical Center, Denver, Colorado 80262 [133, 181]

Introduction

Gerald P. Murphy

This program on model systems in prostate cancer is devoted to an update of in vitro and in vivo systems as they relate to our understanding of prostate cancer. In 1972 a national review with scientific and clinical input from diverse areas, identified a need for model systems, both in vitro and in vivo, for fundamental research in prostate cancer. In reality, at that time no such systems were available. With sustained national funding in an investigator-initiated peer reviewed system called the National Prostatic Cancer Project, an extramural organ site program of the National Cancer Institute, such a program with its resources was able to target in on this necessary area. As one can see by the review of the data, materials and discussion from these proceedings, a great deal of additional material has been developed. Moreover, we have today not one but several model systems both in vivo and in vitro that do, indeed, fulfill all criteria of so-called animal models, or in vitro cellular models. Prostate cancer progress, in terms of diagnosis, detection, and treatment, will unquestionably be further benefited and accelerated in many new aspects as a results of the consistent and sustained multidisciplinary research utilizing these resources. We are, indeed, indebted to all who have contributed so widely to this success.

Requirements of In Vitro Model Systems

Donald J. Merchant, PhD

The ideal model system for study of prostatic cancer would reproduce the pathology seen in the human disease, demonstrate metastasis, be capable of reproducible replication by serial transfer or by initiation with defined carcinogens, be sensitive to hormonal manipulation, show responses to chemotherapeutic agents and radiation analogous to those seen in the natural disease, and be amenable to quantitative analysis. This list does not exhaust the parameters but serves as a reminder that any model system is limited in the answers it can provide, and the multiplicity of questions to be asked dictates the need for multiple model systems. These often must be relatively simple in order to provide precise answers. It is imperative, however, that we remember the complexity of the natural disease and that we are continually on guard against drawing erroneous conclusions from the use of what may be oversimplified or inadequately characterized systems.

The current need for model systems in the study of prostatic cancer and the relative roles of animal and in vitro models were discussed briefly at an earlier meeting sponsored by the National Prostatic Cancer Project [1]. Since that meeting considerable progress has been made, both in the establishment of cell lines from prostatic tissue and in the use of in vitro systems. It, therefore, is appropriate that we further define the requirements for such systems and apply the criteria to the developing models.

NEEDS FOR IN VITRO MODELS

From the initial report on the culture of human prostatic carcinoma and benign prostate hyperplasia (BPH) in 1917 [2] there have been repeated references to the need for in vitro model systems to elucidate a variety of problems. Using the unsophisticated method of culture of explants in plasma clots or soft agar in slide culture systems and conventional optics to examine and describe the outgrowth, Burrows and his collaborators asked general questions regarding factors initiating and controlling outgrowth. In part, this reflected the limited knowledge of the neoplastic state which existed at that time.

Models for Prostate Cancer, pages 3—7
© 1980 Alan R. Liss, Inc., 150 Fifth Ave., New York, NY 10011

With the extension of our knowledge concerning prostatic neoplasia and re-cognition of the limitations of animal models, more and more workers have pro-posed the use of in vitro models to explore a range of experimental problems. In the first major effort after the initial report of Burrows et al [2] Röhl used pri-mary cultures of prostatic carcinoma and BPH in an attempt to evaluate andro-gen dependency of prostatic tumors [3]. Within the past few years several groups have applied in vitro models to studies of hormone action and dependence [4–6].

Other specific aspects of prostate cancer biology that have been considered ap-propriate to in vitro analysis are etiology, including both viruses and chemical car-cinogens [7, 8] evaluation of chemotherapeutic agents [6–9], and tumor immun-ology [10, 11]. In addition, the importance of in vitro model systems has been discussed in more general terms by a number of investigators [12–17].

Analysis of these general areas of interest suggests a very broad range of rather sophisticated questions. For example, in relation to chemical carcinogenesis there are questions of identifying potential carcinogens, of the molecular basis of car-cinogenesis, and of the role of co-carcinogens, to name only a few. Likewise in the field of tumor immunology there are questions to be asked regarding the existence of tumor-specific antigens, evidence for host resistance to prostatic tumors, the rel-ative roles of humoral and cellular immune systems, immunologic enhancement, and serologic methods of diagnosis, surveillance, and prognosis. In the field of en-docrinology we are interested in hormone receptors, methods for monitoring hormone dependence or sensitivity, and the molecular basis for shifts in hormone sensitivity.

This list could be expanded significantly. However, the point to be made is re-emphasis of the fact that there is a need for multiple model systems. A review of the papers published to date on in vitro models suggests a variety as great as the number of investigators who have published, each having a specific question in mind and attempting to devise a model to meet that specific need. Once again, let me emphasize the necessity for keeping this diversity in mind in attempting to relate one system to another and, particularly, in attempting to relate the re-sults obtained from any particular system back to the natural disease.

THE RELATIONSHIP OF PROSTATE BIOLOGY TO MODEL SYSTEMS

One of the greatest weaknesses in our efforts to establish suitable model sys-tems for prostatic cancer, either animal or in vitro, is our serious lack of know-ledge of the biology of the human prostate, either normal or neoplastic. A con-siderable amount of information has been derived since the NCI sponsored con-ference on prostate biology held in 1962 [18]. It is most important to use this information in developing in vitro models. Moreover, the vast amount of in-formation that has been developed concerning the biology of eukaryotic cells in vitro must be applied.

Because of the diversity of questions to be asked and therefore the variety of models required to approach these questions, it is not feasible to discuss the requirements of specific model systems in this presentation. However, since the models tend to be modification of one of three basic systems, it will be worthwhile to discuss these in relation to prostate biology.

As Dr. McNeal will discuss in a later chapter [19], BPH and carcinoma both are believed to originate in the prostate from the acinar epithelial cells or a basal cell, though the former arises almost exclusively in the central or periurethral area and the latter arises from the outer portions of the gland. This makes the choice of normal control tissue for these two conditions to be of prime importance. Moreover, the normal variability in stromal vs acinar tissue and the variability in involvement of the glandular tissue, particularly in carcinoma makes the acquistion of uniform tissue specimens very difficult, particularly if the primary source is chips taken by transurethral resection. These problems are of particular significance for studies employing either organ culture or primary culture methods.

To add to these problems, it is quite likely that a tumor that has reached a size to be detectable will already have undergone considerable variation and selection. A common figure given for the mass of a solid tumor at the time it first becomes detectable is $10^8 - 10^9$ cells. With the relatively small size of the prostate and its architecture, it is likely that varying parts of the tumor mass might already be experiencing relatively major differences in environmental conditions. Assuming that the tumor cell population shows the degree of plasticity and susceptibility to selection pressures exhibited by other eukaryotic cells, it already may have several subpopulations with varying biological properties.

It generally is assumed that culture of a "homogeneous" population of cells that can be serially maintained will avoid many of the pitfalls of the explant or primary culture. The ultimate goal often is a cloned population to assure homogeneity. This type of system may be required, or at least be desirable, for certain types of studies such as the isolation and identification of tumor-specific antigens, studies of hormone receptors, viral studies, etc. It must be kept in mind, however, that a single cell type, and particularly a clonal line, may not be representative of the original tumor. At best it will represent only one cell type of the original tumor. It may represent only one variant within the original population, and it certainly represents only that particular tumor in that particular host. Because of the importance and utility of such models, it becomes imperative to have many such models available for comparative purposes.

Finally, we must address the question of metastatic tumors as a source of tissue for model systems. In a recent review Fidler has emphasized the heterogeneity of primary tumors and the probability of existence of subpopulations with differing metastatic potentials [20]. Evidence is presented that strongly suggests a specificity in localization of different variants within certain tissues. Thus, in the case of prostatic carcinoma, there may be metastatic cells capable of localization in the lymph nodes and others that can colonize the bone only. This suggests that cell lines derived from metastatic lesions may accurately represent only those cells capable of growing in vitro from a highly selected subpopulation of a specific tumor in a single host.

It would be quite inappropriate to use a passaged cell line derived by clonal selection from a metastatic tumor to assay potential chemotherapeutic agents as a guide to therapy in a patient who had developed resistance. Several such cell lines might be of great value, however, in the general screening of potential chemotherapeutic agents if the the models have been derived from subpopulations of metastatic cells that have resulted in rapid patient death, as suggested by Fidler [20].

SUMMARY

In summary I would encourage the continued development of a variety of model systems with maximum characterization and with careful definition of questions to be asked. At the same time it is imperative that the biology of the prostate, and of BPH and prostatic carcinoma in particular, be kept clearly in mind so that appropriate questions can be asked and valid conclusions drawn.

ACKNOWLEDGMENTS

This work was supported by NIH grants 5-R26-CA 16540-03 and DRGI-R26-CA 23699-01.

REFERENCES

1. Merchant DJ: Model systems for the study of prostatic cancer. Oncology 34:100–101, 1977.
2. Burrows MT, Burns JE, Suzuki Y: The cultivation of bladder and prostate tumors outside the body. J Urol 1:3–15, 1917.
3. Röhl L: Prostatic hyperplasia and carcinoma studied with tissue culture technique. Acta Chir Scand Suppl 240:1–88, 1959.
4. Brehmer B, Marguardt H, Madsen PO: Growth and hormonal response of cells derived from carcinoma and hyperplasia of the prostate in monolayer cell culture. A possible in vitro model for clinical chemotherapy. J Urol 108:890–896, 1972.
5. Schroeder FH, Mackensen SJ: Human prostatic adenoma and carcinoma in cell culture. Invest Urol 12:176–181, 1974.
6. Varkarakis MJ, Gaeta JF, Mirand EA, Murphy GP: Morphological responses of benign human prostatic hypertrophic tissue to chemotherapeutic agents in an in vitro culture system. J Med 6:65–71, 1975.
7. Bregman RU, Bregman ET: Tissue culture of benign and malignant human genitourinary tumors. J Urol 86:642–649, 1961.
8. Kaighn ME, Babcock MS: Monolayer cultures of human prostatic cells. Cancer Chemother Rep 59:59–63, 1975.

9. Stonington OG, Szwec N, Webber M: Isolation and identification of the human malignant prostatic epithelial cell in pure monolayer culture. J Urol 114:903–908, 1975.
10. Stonington OG, Hemmingsen H: Culture of cells as a monolayer derived from the epithelium of the human prostate: A new cell growth technique. J Urol 106:393–400, 1971.
11. Rose NR, Choe B-K, Pontes JE: Cultivation of epithelial cells from the prostate. Cancer Chemother Rep 59:147–149, 1975.
12. Schroeder FH, Sato G, Gittes RF: Human prostatic adenocarcinoma: Growth in monolayer tissue culture. J Urol 106:734–739, (1971).
13. Webber M, Stonington OG, Poché PA: Epithelial outgrowth from suspension cultures of human prostatic tissue. In Vitro 10:196–205, 1974.
14. Webber M: Ultrastructural changes in human prostatic epithelium grown in vitro. J Ultrastruct Res 50:89–102, 1975.
15. Merchant DJ: Prostatic cell growth and assessment. Semin Oncol 3:131–140, 1976.
16. Kaighn ME: Characteristics of human prostatic cell cultures. Cancer Treat Rep 61:147–151, 1977.
17. Franks LM: Tissue culture in the investigation of prostatic cancer. Urol Res 5:159–162, 1977.
18. Vollmer EP (ed): "Biology of the Prostate and Related Tissues." NCI Monograph 12, 1963.
19. McNeal JE (this volume).
20. Fidler IJ: Tumor heterogeneity and the biology of cancer invasion and metastasis. Cancer Res 38:2651–2660, 1978.

Regulation of Prostate Growth in Organ Culture

Avery A. Sandberg, MD, and N. Kadohama, PhD

The use of animal prostates or human prostatic tissues in organ culture as a means of establishing regulatory parameters affecting and/or controlling the growth, physiology, and pathology of this gland has a number of advantages as well as shortcomings vis-à-vis in vivo conditions. The interpretation of results must take these factors into consideration (Table I). Most important, in organ culture the various tissue components, their anatomical relationship and function, and their histologic structure are essentially preserved and can be readily followed for prolonged periods in vitro. For the purposes of this discussion, whose primary focus is cancer of the prostate in the human, the outstanding advantage of organ culture are that human prostatic tissue can be studied under in vitro conditions and that the effects of hormones or drugs can be determined. Data obtained in animals or with their tissues, however, often cannot be extrapolated to the human condition. Though complex and difficult even under in vivo conditions, the putative shortcoming of organ culture is the inability to monitor the exocrine activity of the prostate, probably the gland's most essential function.

The use of organ culture environment for growth and differentiation of embryonic organs or fragments of adult tissues and some of the basic techniques for this approach were applied more than 50 years ago by Strangeways and Fell [48]. The application of organ culture to prostatic tissue has found wide use in the past two decades or so. During the initial stages of application of organ culture techniques to the in vitro growth of prostatic tissues much effort was spent in defining the medium and various substances, particularly hormones, necessary for the maintenance of anatomic and functional integrity in vitro. The

Abbreviations: T = testosterone; DHT = dihydrotestosterone; VP = ventral prostate; CA = cyproterone acetate; E_2 = estradiol-17β; MCA = methyl cholanthrine; BPH = benign prostatic hyperplasia (or hypertrophy); ER = endoplasmic reticulum; DES = diethylstilbestrol; TeBG = testosterone binding globulin; EBP = estrogen binding protein; PBP = progesterone binding protein.

Models for Prostate Cancer, pages 9–29

TABLE I. Shortcomings and Advantages of Organ Culture of Prostatic Tissues

Shortcomings

1. Tissues in organ culture can only be maintained for relatively short periods (usually not more than several weeks).
2. Complications resulting from infected tissues are rather common, particularly human tissues.
3. Removal from systemic effects (eg, pituitary, testes, circulation, etc).
4. In the case of the human, infrequent availability of prostatic tissue and untoward effects of the surgery (eg, coagulated tissue during transurethral resection).
5. Lack of control for ingress or egress of substances to and from the cells, respectively.
6. In the case of cancer, parameters such as spread and metastases cannot be observed vs events studied in vivo.
7. Inability to monitor exocrine activity of the gland vs studies in vivo.
8. Lack of systemic metabolism of a drug to its active form.

Advantages

1. Lack of systemic effects.
2. Maintenance of stromal/epithelial ratio and other anatomic relationships vs lack of these in cell culture.
3. Events can be observed.
4. Ready manipulation of environment.
5. Ease of sampling.
6. Tissues can be divided into a number of specimens affording a means of studying events chronologically or concomitantly.
7. Testing of drugs at various concentrations *and* combinations of drugs directly on prostatic tissues.
8. Only way in which *human* prostatic tissue can be studied repeatedly.

ultimate application of organ culture has been in the field of carcinogenesis of the prostate and the testing of drugs potentially useful in prostatic disease. In this presentation no attempt will be made to give the details of the various methodologies used, since they can be found in other publications [11, 23–26, 35]. The use of prostatic organ culture has led to a clarification of testosterone (T) metabolism in this gland and the key role played by its reduction product (DHT) in the maintenance of epithelial anatomy and control of mitosis.

STUDIES OF ANIMAL PROSTATES IN ORGAN CULTURE

The Crucial Role of T, DHT, and Other Androgenic Substances

Prostatic tissue in organ culture rapidly deteriorates in solutions not containing additives, the most crucial of which is T. The presence of T in the serum or plasma in certain media probably accounts for the survival of prostatic tissue in organ culture. The conversion of T to DHT by 5α-reductase is an essential step for the survival of prostatic tissue, since the 5α-reduced product is the active androgen in all mammalian prostates studied to date.

When prostatic tissue (rat ventral prostate; VP) is grown in organ culture without hormones the epithelial cells undergo changes resembling those seen in vivo after castration. Large autophagic vacuoles, residual bodies, and dilations of rough endoplasmic reticulum (ER) were noted in two days of culture, and by four days the ER was markedly decreased and no secretory vacuoles were visible. The treatment of explants with T results in an apparent intensification of the morphologic equivalents of secretion. Besides the well-developed rough ER and Golgi complex, numerous large secretory vesicles with flocculent content are observed. These observations are compatible with the concept that T promotes the formation and probably also the excretion of the secretin in the epithelial cells and that it also prevents partially the appearance of signs of cellular degeneration.

It has also been shown that, in the absence of T, the epithelium of the rat VP in organ culture becomes flattened, the acini unfolded, and the stroma more cellular. These changes can be prevented or reversed by the addition of T to the culture medium, but it may be important that they are more marked in organs from immature animals [22].

Studies on the metabolism and effects of T in organ culture primarily of the rat VP, have led to the following observations [3, 4, 36]: 1) Only the 5α metabolites of T and not the 5β ones are physiologically active; 2) DHT controls cellular division in the prostatic epithelium; 3) T maintains epithelial height and secretory activity and keeps stroma at a minimum; 4) DHT is more active than T in provoking epithelial hyperplasia, which is seen only after high doses of T; 5) 3β-androstanediol fully maintains epithelial height and stimulates secretory activity but does not cause hyperplasia; and 6) T action in the prostate may be related to its conversion to different active metabolites.

These findings confirm in organ culture what has been described in vivo, though the levels of T or DHT necessary for these effects are somewhat more optimally defined by organ culture systems than in vivo (10^{-6} to 10^{-9} M concentrations of T and DHT). The ability of prostatic tissue to convert T to DHT with subsequent binding of the DHT by receptors keeps the activity of intracellular T low and promotes passive diffusion down an arbitrary gradient from blood, particularly in bloods containing binding proteins for these androgens [28]. The activity of androstenedione in rat VP may be attributed to the formation of active 5α-reduced metabolites inside the cells [37]. Cyproterone acetate (CA) appears to counteract the action of T in organ culture [7, 43].

The presence or absence of human or animal serum in the incubation medium has led to differences in the response of the prostatic tissue to endogenous and/or exogenous T or DHT. The most likely explanation resides in the ability of testosterone binding globulin (TeBG) present in such serum to "tie up" the androgen, with the result that in the presence of serum much less free or unbound T is available to the prostatic gland than when serum is not present [27]. Of course, the influence of the serum will depend on its source, since some animals do not contain TeBG whereas others do, the level of the TeBG varying considerably such as its greatly increased concentrations during pregnancy [39] and, also on the concentration of T, DHT and possibly other androgens in the culture medium. Both in vivo and in vitro the presence in serum of binding proteins for corticosteroids (transcortin), estrogens (TeBG, EBP), and progesterone (transcortin, PBG) may seriously influence not only the activity of these steroids but also that of T and/or DHT.

It has been reported that the 17α- rather than the 17β-DHT is the active androgen in the dog prostate [46, 47]. Epitestosterone and DHT were partially successful in maintaining epithelial height of the dog prostate in organ culture. The only substance that sustained epithelial height and secretory activity while keeping stromal cells at a minimum was 5α-androstane-3α, 17α-diol (17α-DHT) [46, 47]. It should be pointed out, however, that the preponderant metabolic pathway taken by T in the dog is in the 17β direction [50]; and that the role of 17α-DHT in the dog prostate is still unclear.

Fischer et al [10] showed that dog prostatic explants cultivated in organ culture for a minimum of nine days showed decreased viability in the presence of high concentrations of T, whereas those cultivated at lower levels of T appeared similar to control explants in T free medium.

Estrogens

In explants derived from six-week-old rats, E_2 suppressed the growth of columnar cells completely. Combined with T, E_2 reduced the T effect from 70% to 15% columnar cells. The remainder consisted of flat or cuboidal cells with little or no secretory activity. The response of glands from nine-month-old rats differed strikingly. E_2 was less effective than in the young organ and did not increase the regression seen in controls kept in nonsupplemented medium. If combined with T, E_2 did not inhibit the T effect and the proportion of columnar cells in T-treated explants equalled that in explants exposed to both steroids [25].

Prolactin

Apparently prolactin enhances the effects of T; eg, epithelial cell size is augmented with a marked enlargement of the supranuclear area resulting in the appearance of very tall columnar cells; cell proliferation is promoted, leading to increased formation of new alveoli.

It was found that doses of prolactin that augmented T effect did not increase the uptake of T or the formation of DHT. It is possible that the prolactin effect is mediated via an increased adenyl cyclase activity.

The enhancing effect of prolactin on T is more pronounced in the glands of older animals [24, 25].

Polyamines

Edwards et al [9], using the ventral and dorsal prostates of mice maintained as explants in organ culture, showed regressive changes with complete necrosis by the fifth day, if the explants were cultured in a control medium (embryo extract in chicken plasma). When cultured in the presence of T plus the control medium, the explants continued to maintain their epithelial height and stromal characteristics after five days; however, by the seventh day regressive changes similar to those seen in explants cultured in the absence of T were observed. With spermine and spermidine in the medium along with insulin and T, the stromal and epithelial integrity of the explants was kept intact for 14 days. When either T or spermine was omitted from the list of additives, survival and maintenance of normal morphology were not greatly impaired. Omission of spermidine did not affect the results if the other substances were added.

Spermine and spermidine are present in extremely high concentrations in rat prostate explants when compared to numerous other tissues from rodents and other animals. When rat prostatic fluid is analyzed, similar high concentrations of these polyamines are present. Though some evidence exists that these polyamines promote clonal growth of cells in culture, that these factors can replace others in the culture medium (eg, fetuin), and that they can stimulate DNA synthesis and cell growth in human fibroblast cultures, their exact role in prostatic physiology remains to be elucidated. Polyamines have been reported to stimulate protein and polypeptide synthesis in vitro; possibly, one of their actions in the prostate may be related to that area. In some other studies, inhibition of cells with spermine and spermidine in culture has been also demonstrated, indicating the rather conflicting nature of the possible effects of these polyamines on cellular growth.

Vitamin A

Vitamin A is an important factor for the maintenance of secretory epithelia, including that of the prostate, and though the in vivo induction of a deficiency of this vitamin in animals takes a prolonged period, changes can be very readily observed in organ culture. Thus, VP glands of mice grown in media composed of plasma and serum which contained physiological amounts of the vitamin did not alter their growth pattern or increase secretory activity when the vitamin A was added [24]. Cultivation in completely defined media not containing the vitamin resulted in the appearance of widespread, irregularly distributed foci of squamous metaplasia after ten days in vitro. Excessive keratin formation and the mingling of squamous and normal secretory epithelium, considered typical of vitamin A deficiency, were observed. Addition of vitamin A to the defined medium completely prevented the squamous changes and fully preserved the secretory character of the epithelium.

TABLE II. Summary of the Main Effects of Hydrocortisone and Testosterone on the Ventral Prostate Gland of the Rat Grown in Vitro

	Height epithelium	Folding	Secretory activity	Number of alveoli	Stroma
Before explantation	Cuboidal, columnar	Present	Present	− −	Scanty
Natural medium					
Controls	Flat	Absent	Absent	Severely reduced	Markedly increased
Hydrocortisone	Cuboidal, columnar	Absent	Present	Unchanged	Absent
Testosterone	Flat (center) cuboidal, columnar (periphery)	− −	Present (periphery)	Slightly reduced	Slightly increased
Semi-defined medium					
Controls	Flat cuboidal	Absent	Reduced absent	Unchanged	Absent
Hydrocortisone	Cuboidal, columnar	Absent	Present	Unchanged	Absent
Testosterone	Cuboidal	Slight	Present	Unchanged	Slightly increased

From Lashitzki [21].

Adrenal Steroids

The role of adrenal secretory products in prostatic anatomy and physiology is difficult to establish in vivo, though their overall effects may be studied under such conditions. Studies in organ culture have shown that cortisol counteracts the prostatic regression in all cultures to which it was added. Some details of the action of adrenal steroids in organ culture are shown in Table II [21].

Cortisol, and to a lesser extent prednisolone, caused an increased incorporation of labeled precursors into the DNA and protein of the rat VP and an augmentation of the effects of T exceeding a simple summation of the responses to individual hormones [43]. The most characteristic feature of cortisol-treated epithelial cells was the copious supply of rough ER. Of some interest was the formation of endoplastic reticulum whorls, which could not be observed in control and T treated tissues. Cortisol was shown to promote the formation of juvenile secretory vesicles.

Insulin

The stimulatory effects of insulin on the prostate in organ culture are probably a reflection of an enhance uptake by and possibly effects of T or DHT in prostatic epithelial cells (Table III). It is doubtful whether insulin has a prostatic

TABLE III. Effects of Insulin in Organ Culture of Prostatic Tissues

Prostate source	Effects	Reference
Mouse VP	Irregular hyperplasia in 5−7 days in the absence or presence of serum	Franks, 1961 [11]
Mouse VP (castrated)	T and insulin necessary to restore gland and to cause increase in secretory epithelium Uptake of T influenced by insulin Augmentation of citric acid Production related to synthesis of an enzyme (?) for which insulin must be present	Lostroh, 1971 [30]
Rat VP	Insulin caused incorporation of labeled precursors into RNA and protein Caused an augmented effect in the presence of T	Santti and Johansson, 1973 [43]
Rat VP	Delayed the onset of degeneration	Ichihara et al, 1973 [16]
BPH tissue	Insulin plus placental lactogen plus T stimulatory; some stimulation with insulin plus E_2	Dilley and Birkhoff, 1977 [8]

effect in the absence of T or DHT. The presence of these steroid hormones in the explants and/or serum appears to be sufficient for the stimulatory effects of of insulin [11, 30]. Insulin delayed the onset of degeneration of the epithelial cells, but marked degenerated changes were noted on day 6. There were no specific ultrastructural characteristics that could be interpreted as specific for insulin action in the epithelial cells [16].

STUDIES WITH HUMAN PROSTATIC TISSUES

Studies With BPH Tissues

The use of organ culture for studying parameters of human noncancerous and cancerous prostatic tissues is of relatively recent vintage.

Schrodt and Foreman [44] were apparently the first to explant human prostatic tissue (BPH) in organ culture. The tissue was grown in Trowell medium [49] on agar rafts supported on grids of tantalum mesh. In most explants the morphology of the epithelium and stroma was well maintained during the first three days, and in some explants up to nine days. In older cultures the secretory epithelium was often low columnar and occasionally underwent squamous metaplasia. The fine structure resembled that of fresh tissue, including abundant rough ER and secretory vesicles and granules. Exposure to T-propionate (50 μg/ml of medium) caused severe epithelial necrosis.

In another study [32], in which BPH slices were cultured for a period of a week in Eagle's basal medium supplemented with insulin and bovine serum, no morphological responses to T or DES were observed. The authors drew attention to a possible source of a misinterpretation of results based on the uptake of labeled thymidine into the DNA of organ culture tissues — ie, the possibility that reduplication of the DNA at the explant surface may be balanced by necrosis deep in the explant, with the result that the total amount of DNA in explants may remain relatively stable.

Harbitz et al [13] extended the above studies to several other hormones and examined the effects of T, DHT, E_2, progesterone, and CA on BPH tissue grown in Trowell medium. They found that the epithelium and its enzymes were well maintained in androgen-free medium and, furthermore, that none of the hormones altered epithelial morphology, the normal enzyme pattern, or DNA synthesis.

When explants of BPH tissues were grown in a chemically defined medium (Trowell T8) for periods of two to 12 days, the fibromuscular stroma survived less well than the acinar epithelium [12]. This author also showed that, in a chemically defined medium, DNA synthesis in acinar epithelium and edge cells, shown autoradiographically by the incorporation of ^{3}H-thymidine into cell nuclei, was regularly present in explants cultured for four days. The incorporation of ^{3}H-uridine was demonstrable in acinar epithelium as well as in stromal cells after six days in vitro. In these short-term experiments the glandular epithelium retained the histologic features of BPH and the ability to synthesize DNA and RNA, despite diffuse degeneration of the fibromuscular stroma. The author indicated that the organ culture technique using chemically defined medium should have considerable value for the study of the diseased human prostate and its responses to defined external influences.

Shipman et al [45] showed that BPH tissue grown in organ culture appeared to be less sensitive than rat VP to withdrawal of hormonal support, in that the changes that occur during culture of BPH were more typical of a repair mechanism of injury than of a castration effect. Cell kinetics were investigated using labeled deoxyuridine and vincristine; both approaches demonstrated a spontaneous surge in proliferative activity of BPH, reaching a peak at about day 4. In contrast, proliferative activity in rat prostate tended to fall off over the period of two to eight days of culture.

McRae et al [33] have indicated that the failure of T to influence BPH tissue in organ culture may be attributed to three possible causes. First, the tissue in organ culture may not behave as it does in vivo, even though it has been shown in organ culture that the BPH tissue does take up and metabolize T in a way similar to normal animal tissues, both quantitatively and qualitatively. Second, BPH tissue may not be hormone dependent at all and, hence, may not be susceptible to influences by T. Third, the length of time that the cultures have been maintained may be insufficient to demonstrate morphological changes under the influences of T. It may be that more appropriate biochemical measurements are needed to demonstrate dependence of BPH tissues over these relatively short periods. These same authors [33], in developing an organ culture method for human prostatic tissue, suggested, on the basis of results in preliminary investigations, that T does influence DNA and acid phosphatase production even in the absence of a morphologic change of BPH tissue in organ culture.

The findings on BPH tissues in organ culture and the relative independence of such tissues of hormonal controlling factors are of relevance to the problem of cancer of the prostate, for, under suitable conditions, satisfactory growth or maintenance of human BPH can be achieved in vitro. Although the tissue is derived from different patients and cultivated by different techniques, the findings nevertheless reveal a generally consistent pattern. In contrast to the rodent prostate, tissue from benign BPH grows or is relatively well maintained in androgen free medium. It is unlikely that this property has been acquired during cell transformation or cell selection or is due to a loss of steroid receptors, since it occurs in organ cultures explanted shortly after removal from the patients [26].

Other Considerations of BPH Tissue in Organ Culture

In androgen-deprived target tissues one of the first consequences of T treatment is an increase in RNA synthesis that precedes the increase in DNA synthesis and the restoration of normal morphology. RNA synthesis is, therefore, a sensitive criterion of hormonal effects, and attempts were made to correlate the action of T, DHT, 3β-androstanediol, and E_2 on epithelial structure with that on RNA synthesis [26]. In nonsupplemented medium and in the presence of hormones, the BPH epithelium multiplied to form several layers projecting into the lumen. In the controls, the cells showed some evidence of squamous metaplasia. Testosterone and DHT prevented the latter and preserved the secretory character of the epithelium; in addition, DHT increased the proliferation of the epithelium beyond that seen in controls and in the other experimental explants. In contrast to the androgens, E_2 caused much cellular breakdown, including the loss of the secretory cells lining the alveolar lumen.

The cytologic changes were reflected in variations of RNA synthesis. The incorporation of labeled uridine into RNA was determined by autoradiography separately in epithelium and smooth muscle and expressed as the percentage of labeled cells in the average number of grains per cell. In the epithelium the uptake was increased by T and DHT, reduced by E_2, and not affected by 3β-androstanediol. In smooth muscle the number of labeled cells was similar to that in controls and androgen-treated explants and decreased by E_2, but the grain counts per cell were raised by the androgens and again reduced by E_2. Thus, although the growth of the tissue in organ culture appeared independent of androgens, the explants continue to exhibit hormone responsiveness under the conditions of these experiments with human BPH tissue.

The hormonal study of BPH in organ culture is based not only on cell growth but also includes maintenance of epithelium and its function as important criteria of hormonal action. While the data relating to androgen independence of growth and epithelium maintenance are in good agreement, those concerned with hormonal response of BPH in organ culture are still controversial. MacMahon and Thomas [32] and Harbitz et al [13] reported a failure of steroid hormones to modify the morphology of the epithelium or its enzymes. In contrast, alteration of epithelial growth or morphology and changes in RNA synthesis by T, DHT, and E_2 were demonstrated by Lasnitzki [26]. In this context, two points deserve special attention. First, unlike DHT, which seems to play a similar role in the human tissue as in the rat prostate, 3β-androstanediol is ineffective and may, therefore, have no function in the maintenance of the human hyperplastic epithelium. Second, the changes of RNA synthesis induced by the steroid hormones in smooth muscle cells suggest that, like the epithelium, they are also hormone responsive. Since the muscle forms a substantial part of the stroma, the finding is important and should be considered in the evaluation of hormonal effects and their application to the clinical state.

When BPH prostates were maintained in organ culture for periods of up to eight days, there was an increased number of cells with histochemically demonstrable acid phosphatase for a short time in culture (4—6 days); however, by eight days such cells decreased in number [19].

Dilley and Birkhoff [8] studied the effect of various combinations of insulin and other hormones on glandular BPH tissue maintained in organ culture for four days. Six of nine specimens were stimulated 80% or more by insulin plus placental lactogen plus T, but only one was stimulated by insulin plus T. Four of the ten were stimulated by insulin plus E_2. Histologic and autoradiographic results indicated that all growth occurred in the epithelium.

Chung and Coffey [7] demonstrated the formation of androgen glucuronides by normal human prostatic and BPH tissue minces when incubated with labeled T. Apparently, the normal gland tends to synthesize T-glucuronide, whereas the hypertrophic one appears to make mostly DHT-glucuronide. The total amount of steroid glucuronides formed in the two types of tissues was similar — ie, 1.5% of the total androgen accumulated in the tissues. However, the ratio of total DHT- to T-glucuronide found in BPH was 15, which is about 20 times as much as observed in the normal prostatic tissue. The anti-androgen CA markedly inhibited the formation of the androgen glucuronide by the BPH tissue, with only slightly decreased accumulation of the steroids in the tissue.

Studies with Prostatic Cancers

McMahon et al [31] studied tissues from cancers of the prostate in organ culture. In the presence of T, differentiation of the cells occurred accompanied by an increased mitotic index. DES produced no changes.

Bard and Lasnitzki [2] studied the uptake and metabolism of T, androstenedione and DHT by BPH and prostatic carcinomas in organ culture. DHT was a major metabolite of both T and androstenedione in the benign tissue and androstanediols of DHT. Over half of the carcinomas produced less DHT from T than did the BPH tissue. Carcinomas from the older patients showed an enhancement of 17β-hydroxysteroid dehydrogenation. There was no relationship between these differences in metabolism of T and the degree of differentiation of the carcinomas. Estradiol decreased the production of DHT, both from T and from androstenedione, and at lower androgen concentrations increased the production of androstanediols from T, androstenedione, and DHT. The uptake of DHT but not of the other two androgens was stimulated by E_2.

Some of the carcinomas were still hormone responsive in vitro [32]. One tumor from a patient treated with DES was relatively differentiated and showed alveoli lined with crowded small cells. In DES-treated explants the cells were larger and less basophilic and the interalveolar stroma was increased. Additions of T to the medium strikingly increased the differentiation of the tissue. The epithelial cells were much taller than in the tumor in vivo owing to a striking increase in cytoplasmic height; there were fewer but larger alveoli per unit area. The second carcinoma from an untreated patient was anaplastic and consisted of densely packed cells separated by fine strands of fibers. Treatment of the cultures with DES for four days did not change this growth pattern, but T produced effects that could be interpreted as attempts at differentiation. The cells were larger and in some regions became arranged in a pattern suggesting alveolar formation. The promotion of differentiation by T in the carcinomas was unexpected but highly interesting and awaits further corroboration.

EFFECTS OF CARCINOGENS AND OTHER AGENTS ON PROSTATIC TISSUES IN ORGAN CULTURE

The advantages offered by prostatic tissue in organ culture as a means of studying the effects of carcinogens and/or the changes involved in the genesis of malignant transformation are obvious. The ease of observation and sampling of the tissue to ascertain the effects of carcinogens, the ability to add substances to the medium with possible anticarcinogenic activity, and the readiness with which concentrations and combinations of various substances can be manipulated are but a few of these advantages. Major disadvantages are the inability to study metastatic spread or to ascertain whether the transformed tissue has the ability to grow as a tumor in vivo.

Noyes [34] indicated that in long-term organ culture of normal (?) human prostatic tissue, functional and morphologic normality of the glandular epithelium is essentially maintained. MCA at a level of 4 μg/ml in the culture fluid apparently induced morphologic changes that were not observed in untreated cultures. The changes observed after exposure to the carcinogen for the 15—20 days included hyperplasia and anaplasia of the glandular epithelial cells, with large variations in nuclear size and shape. Even though the author suggested that the changes have a neoplastic potential, it should be indicated that in the past when such preparations were injected into animals, tumors did not develop.

Vitamin A is necessary for the maintenance of normal differentiation and function of secretory epithelium, and this applies to the prostate. Thus, in organ cultures of mouse prostates grown in vitamin A-deficient medium the epithelium underwent squamous metaplasia; the addition of the vitamin to the culture medium prevented this change [23—26]. In one study [29] the authors tested the effects of vitamin A and its analogues on MCA-induced changes in the mouse prostate in organ culture. The compounds studied included retinol, retinoic acid, and two analogues of retinoic acid, with virtually no growth-promoting vitamin A activity. When the prostates of mice were grown in organ culture for seven to nine days and then MCA was added to the culture medium, the latter stimulated the alveolar epithelium to become hyperplastic, such epithelium frequently displaying the first stages of squamous metaplasia or undergoing parakeratosis. All vitamin A-related compounds were highly active in inhibiting the effects of MCA. When added together with the carcinogen, the vitamin A compounds inhibited epithelial cell multiplication and maintained normal differentiation, thus counteracting the hyperplastic and metaplastic changes induced by MCA. Since all four compounds were highly active in antagonizing the effects of MCA, it is apparent that the anticarcinogenic activity of vitamin A is not correlated with the growh-promoting activity of the vitamin. Apparently, the vitamin A effects are not due to their surface active properties.

Chopra and Wilkoff [5, 6] determined the effect of β-retinoic acid (RA) on carcinogen-induced hyperplasia of mouse prostate glands in organ culture resulting from the addition of MCA or its analogue MNNG, the latter not requiring activation. The development of hyperplasia was inhibited when RA was added simultaneously with MCA or MNNG. However, RA had no significant effect on cell proliferation in untreated control cultures. The elimination of the carcinogen from the hyperplastic cultures after eight days of treatment did not reverse hyperplasia of the alveolar epithelium. When the withdrawal of MCA or MNNG was followed by treatment of the cultures with RA, hyperplasia was markedly reversed within 96 hours. Thus, RA actively inhibited and reversed the effect of MCA and MNNG, two carcinogens that may have different mechanisms of action. Ascorbic acid had no effect on prostate carcinogenesis in organ culture [1].

Lasnitzki [20] has carried out extensive research on the morphological effects produced by polycyclic hydrocarbons and hormones in organ cultures of mouse and rat prostate glands. Those pieces of prostate cultivated in plasma clots and not treated with the test compounds, maintained for periods up to two weeks a differentiated appearance consisting of a single layer of epithelial cells surrounding the alveoli. When these prostate fragments were treated with microgram quantities of oncogenic hydrocarbons, the epithelial cells underwent hyperplasia and squamous metaplasia, which the author considered to be preneoplastic changes.

In order to ascertain whether the above morphological effects were associated with malignancy, the organ culture technique of Lasnitzki was adapted to liquid media using the VP from inbred C3H mice [4]. In addition to the hyperplasia and squamous metaplasia following exposure to MCA, pleomorphism of the epithelial cells and invasion through the basement membrane were observed. Some of the slides were read as malignant by pathologists. Disappointingly, however, when nearly 900 of these hydrocarbon-treated pieces from the organ cultures were implanted into isologous mice under a variety of conditions, no tumors were produced. Thus, these profound morphologic alterations were not associated with detectable malignancy. Therefore, it was concluded that morphologic transformation cannot be seriously considered as being malignant unless tumor formation can be consistently detected in suitable hosts. However, when established cell lines were obtained from some of the morphologically altered hydrocarbon-treated organ cultures they did give rise to sarcomas on inoculation into C3H mice [14].

Despite the fact that the morphologic changes produced by chemical oncogens in organ culture cannot be equated with malignancy, studies of these sort are considered useful. The changes seen histologically in these cultures often parallel premalignant changes seen in vivo. Thus, observation of organ cultures is particularly valuable in the case of epithelial tissues, since when chemical oncogenesis in cell culture has been successful, the tumors ultimately produced in animals have almost invariably been in sarcomas.

A profound inhibitory effect on growth of rat VP explants was shown to be produced by Estracyt, which was more pronounced than that seen after E_2. When the nitrogen mustard was linked to position-17 of DHT no inhibition of the parameters, including incorporation of ^{3}H-thymidine into the explants of the rat VP, was observed [15].

ORGAN CULTURE AS A TEST SYSTEM FOR DRUGS POTENTIALLY USEFUL IN HUMAN PROSTATIC CANCER: OUR EXPERIENCE

In an attempt to develop test systems for drugs potentially useful in human cancer of the prostate a number of in vivo and in vitro preparations and systems have been used by us [38–42], including organ culture [17–18]. The latter

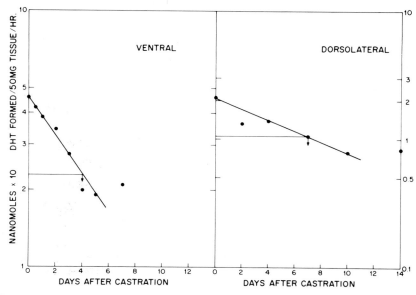

Fig. 1. Rate of loss of 5α-reductase activity in rat prostate following castration. Groups of three 400-gm adult Wistar rats were orchiectomized. Ventral and dorsolateral lobes of the prostate were removed at various times after surgery, and triplicate determiniations of the enzyme activity were performed using homogenates equivalent to 50 mg of tissue. The decrease in 5α-reductase activity, particularly in the VP, indicates dependence of the enzyme on testicular secretion, primarily T.

approach offers the advantage in that human prostatic cancer tissues can be used and the drugs tested directly on such tissues. The advantages of this approach are limited, however, by the fact that even though a positive result in organ culture probably indicates that a drug might be useful under clinical conditions, the ineffectiveness of a drug does not necessarily imply that such an agent will not be effective in vivo. Such an ineffective drug may have to undergo metabolic conversion in vivo to a more active form — eg, flutamide [38, 39]. Primary reliance in this organ culture system has been placed on two indices: The histology of the glandular tissue and the relative level of 5α-reductase activity. The activity of the latter enzyme has been used as an index of drug effect both in vivo and in vitro [38–42], and though some human cancers of the prostate may not contain much 5α-reductase activity, most of the cancers studied have had such enzymatic activity, though the levels vary from one tumor to another. A distinct advantage of the organ culture system is the fact that very small amounts of tissue are required and that a combination of various drugs can be tested in a relatively short time.

Examples of the use of prostatic organ culture to study a number of parameters, including the effects of drugs, are shown in Figures 1–7.

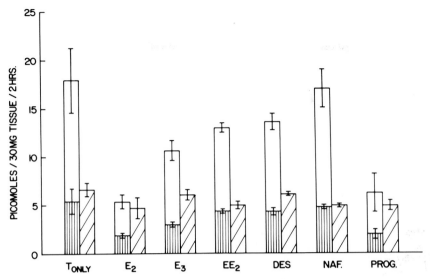

Fig. 2. Effect of estrogenic agents on T metabolism in human prostate in organ culture. After one day in control medium, explants prepared from a specimen of human prostate (BPH) were maintained for two days in medium containing 0.5 μM T or T plus an estrogenic agent (1 μg/ml). On the final day tissues were exposed to ^{3}H-labeled T for two hours. Metabolites of T were extracted and analyzed. E_2, estradiol-17B; E_3, estriol; EE_2: ethynl estradiol; DES, diethylstilbestrol; NAF., nafoxidine; PROG., progesterone. In this and the following figures the ordinates show the picomoles of DHT formed from T. E_2 and progesterone were particularly effective in inhibiting 5α-reductase. In this and in Figures 3, 4, and 7 the 5α-reductase activity is indicated by a summution of the open bars (DHT formation) plus the striped bars (A-diol). The oxidative pathway is indicated by the hatched bars (Δ^4-A-dione). Valves are means $\pm$ SE for triplicate determinations.

The importance of using human prostatic cancerous tissue for testing drugs potentially useful in this condition vs results obtained with animal tissues, even with a tumor resembling the human in many respects (eg, the R3327 adeno-carcinoma of the rat, which has androgen receptors and responds to endocrine manipulation) is illustrated in Figure 7. Based on the 5α-reductase activity in organ culture, the rat tumor was sensitive both to Estracyt and cis-platinum and, particularly, to the combination of both drugs. On the other hand, the human prostatic tumor was only affected, as far as the 5α-reductase activity is concerned, by Estracyt and not by cis-platinum. A combination of both drugs was essentially no more effective than Estracyt alone. Thus, the results, indicate that data obtained with animal tissues, including prostatic tumors, cannot always be extrapolated to the human condition, and it would appear to us that the most direct and fruitful approach is to test various agents against human prostatic cancers under organ culture conditions.

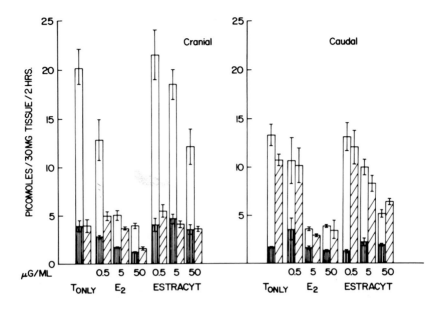

Fig. 3. Comparison of the effect of E_2 and Estracyt on T metabolism in baboon prostate in organ culture. After one day in control medium, explants prepared from cranial and caudal lobes were maintained in medium containing 0.5 μM T or T plus 0.5, 5 and 50 μg/ml of E_2, or Estracyt. On the final day, tissues were exposed to ^{3}H-T for two hours. Values are means ± SE for triplicate determinations. E_2 was more effective in inhibiting 5α-reductase.

CONCLUSIONS

From a review of the behavior of prostatic tissue in organ culture it is apparent that such an approach can be used to study parameters controlling histologic and functional integrity of such tissue, particularly of normal constituency. The essential independence of hormonal control, or for that matter, of other controls by BPH and possibly cancerous tissue, might be due either to the presence of large amounts of DHT and possibly other active androgens within such tissue or to the attainment of some independent status by such tissue outside the body. The somewhat variable effects of T on BPH and prostatic cancer tissues remain to be ascertained and clarified. Certainly, the response of such tissues is minimal when compared to that of normal animal prostates under similar conditions. It is possible that the human tissues reflect an advanced stage of independence from direct hormonal control, as evidenced by the minimal effects of T and other agents in organ culture conditions. However, organ culture offers the distinct advantages of using human prostatic cancer tissues in vitro and the ability to test various

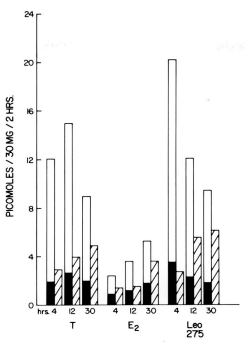

PICOMOLES / 30 MG / 2 HRS.

Fig. 4. Comparison of the effect of E_2 and Leo 275 on T metabolism in human prostate in organ culture. All media contained 0.5 μM T. E_2 concentration was 6 μg/ml. Leo 275 concentration was 10 μg/ml (equivalent to 6 μg/ml of E_2). Explants in duplicate dishes were exposed to media containing 1.2 nM ^{3}H-labeled T for the following periods: 2–4 hours, 10–12 hours, and 28–30 hours. Metabolites were extracted and analyzed by TLG. Open bar, DHT; closed bar, A-diol; hatched bar, Δ^4-A-dione. As in the case of baboon prostate (Figs. 1 and 2), E_2 was a more effective inhibitor of 5α-reductase than Leo 275.

drugs either singly or in combination against such tissues and establishing the sensitivity of such tissue to these drugs. Since in all probability human prostatic tissues, particularly cancerous ones, differ morphologically and/or biochemically from one case to another, such a system offers an important avenue of ascertaining the effects of drugs directly on each cancer, with the amount of tissue required for such testing being rather small. Hence, one can envision the ultimate testing of each cancer with a battery of drugs under organ culture conditions in order to ascertain the agent most likely to be effective against a particular cancer.

ACKNOWLEDGMENTS

This work was supported in part by a grant (CA-15436) from the National Cancer Institute.

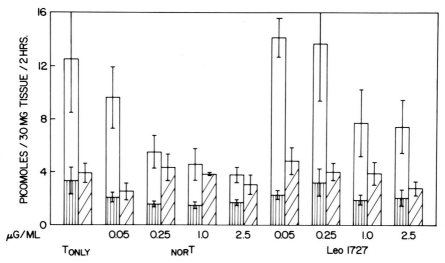

Fig. 5. Effect of nor-T and Leo 1727 on T metabolism in human prostate in organ culture. After one day in control medium, explants prepared from a specimen of human prostate (BPH) were exposed to media containing 0.5 μM T or T plus 0.05, 0.25, and 1.0 μg/ml of nor-T or Leo 1727. Experiment was performed as described in Figure 2. Values are means ± SE for triplicate determinations. Nor-T appeared to be a more effective inhibitor of 5α-reductase than Leo 1727.

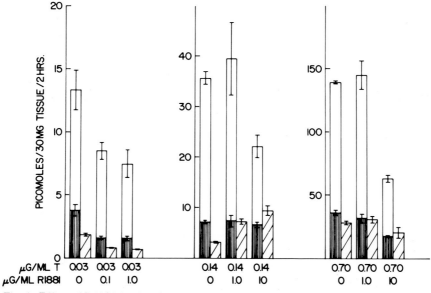

Fig. 6. Effect of R1881 (anti-androgen) on T metabolism in baboon ventral prostate in organ culture. After one day in control medium, explants were maintained for two days in medium containing varying concentrations of R1881 at three different concentrations of T.

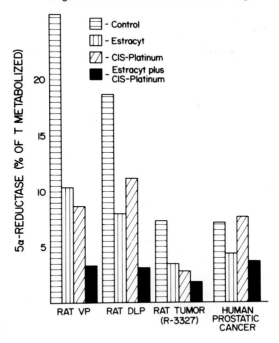

Fig. 7. The effects in organ culture of Estracyt (50 μg/ml) and cis-platinum (54 μg/ml) on 5α-reductase activity of rat ventral and dorsolateral prostate and on the rat prostatic tumor R3327. The effects on a human prostatic cancer are also shown. In the normal prostate both drugs reduced the 5α-reductase activity significantly, particularly the combination of the two drugs. Even though the 5α-reductase activity in the rat tumor was significantly more than that of the normal glands, the activity was definitely reduced by both drugs and, again, particularly by a combination of the drugs. In the case of the human prostatic cancer, Estracyt definitely reduced the activity of the 5α-reductase under organ culture conditions, similar to that in the rat tumor, but cis-platinum either alone or in combination with Estracyt failed to show any evidence of activity.

REFERENCES

1. Bal E, De Lustig ES: Prostate carcinogenesis in vitro. Unresponsiveness to ascorbic acid. Medicina 36:23–28, 1976.
2. Bard DR, Lasnitzki I: The influence of oestradiol on the metabolism of androgens by human prostatic tissue. J Endrocrinol 74:1–9, 1977.
3. Baulieu EE, Lasnitzki I, Robel P: Metabolism of testosterone and action of metabolites on prostate glands grown in organ culture. Nature 219:1155–1156, 1968.
4. Baulieu EE, Lasnitzki I, Robel P: Testosterone, prostate gland and hormone action. Biochem Biophys Res Commun 32:575–577, 1968.
5. Chopra DP, Wilkoff LJ: Inhibition and reversal by β-retinoic acid of hyperplasia induced in cultured mouse prostate tissue by 3-methylcholanthrene of n-methyl-n'-nitro-nitrosoguanidine. J Natl Cancer Inst 56:583–589, 1976.
6. Chopra DP, Wolkoff LJ: Reversal by vitamin A analogues (retinoids) of hyperplasia

induced by n-methyl-n'-nitro-n-nitrosoguanidine in mouse prostate organ cultures. J Natl Cancer Inst 58:923–930, 1977.

7. Chung LWK, Coffey DS: Androgen glucuronide II. Differences in its formation by human normal and benign hyperplastic prostates. Invest Urol 15:385–388, 1978.

8. Dilley WG, Birkhoff JD: Hormone response of benign hyperplastic prostate tissue in organ culture. Invest Urol 15:83–86, 1977.

9. Edwards WD, Bates RR, Yuspa SH: Organ culture of rodent prostate. Effects of polyamines and testosterone. Invest Urol 14:1–5, 1976.

10. Fischer TV, Burkel WE, Kahn RH, Herwig KR: Effect of testosterone on long-term organ cultures of canine prostate. In Vitro 12:382–392, 1976.

11. Franks LM: The growth of mouse prostate during culture in vitro in chemically defined and natural media, and after transplantation in vivo. The effects of insulin and normal human serum. Exp Cell Res 22:56–72, 1961.

12. Harbitz TB: Organ culture of benign nodular hyperplasia of human prostate in chemically-defined medium. Scand J Urol Nephrol 7:6–13, 1973.

13. Harbitz TB, Falkanger B, Sander B: Benign prostatic hyperplasia of the human prostate exposed to steroid hormones in organ culture. Arch Pathol Microbiol Scand Sect A Suppl 248:89–93, 1974.

14. Heidelberger C: Chemical oncogenesis in culture. Adv Cancer Res 18:317–366, 1973.

15. Høisaeter PA: Incorporation of ^{3}H-thymidine into rat ventral prostate in organ culture. Influence of hormone-cytostatic complexes. Invest Urol 12:479–489, 1975.

16. Ichihara I, Santti RS, Pelliniemi LJ: Effects of testosterone, hydrocortisone and insulin on the fine structure of the epithelium of rat ventral prostate in organ culture. Z Zellforsch 143:425–438, 1973.

17. Kadohama N, Kirdani RY, Murphy GP, Sandberg AA: 5α-reductase as a target enzyme for anti-prostatic drugs in organ culture. Oncology 34:123–128, 1977.

18. Kadohama N, Kirdani RY, Murphy GP, Sandberg AA: Estramustine phosphate: Metabolic aspects related to its action in prostatic cancer. Urology 119:235–238, 1978.

19. Kreisberg JI, Brattain MG, Pretlow TG II: Studies on human hyperplastic prostates maintained in organ culture. Invest Urol 15:252–255, 1977.

20. Lasnitzki I: Growth pattern of the mouse prostate gland in organ culture and its response to sex hormones, vitamin A and 3-methylcholanthreme. In: "Biology of the Prostate and Related Tissues." NCI Monograph 12, 1963, pp 381–403.

21. Lasnitzki I: The effect of hydrocortisone on the ventral and anterior prostate gland of the rat grown in culture. Endocrinology 30:255–233, 1964.

22. Lasnitzki I: Action and interaction of hormones and 3-methycholanthrene on the ventral prostate gland of the rat in vitro. I. Testosterone and methylcholanthrene. J Natl Cancer Inst 35:339–348, 1965.

23. Lasnitzki I: The rat prostate gland in organ culture. In Griffiths K, Pierrepoint CC (eds): "Some Aspects of the Aetiology and Biochemistry of Prostatic Cancer." Third Tenovus Workshop, Cardiff, Wales, 1970, pp 68–73.

24. Lasnitzki I: The prostate gland in organ culture. In Brandes D (ed): "Male Accessory Sex Organs. Structure and Function in Mammals." New York: Academic Press, 1974, pp 348–382.

25. Lasnitzki I: The effect of hormones on rat prostatic epithelium in organ culture. In Goland M (ed): "Normal and Abnormal Growth of the Prostate." Springfield, Illinois: Charles C Thomas, 1975, pp 29–54.

26. Lasnitzki I: Human benign prostatic hyperplasia in cell and organ culture. In Grayback JT, Wilson JD, Scherbenske MJ (eds): DHEW Publication No. (NIH) 76–1113, 1075, 235–248.

27. Lasnitzki I, Franklin HR: The influence of serum on uptake, conversion and action of

testosterone in rat prostate glands in organ culture. J Endocrinol 54:333–342, 1972.

28. Lasnitzki I, Franklin HR, Wilson JD: The mechanism of androgen uptake and concentration by rat ventral prostate in organ culture. J Endocrinol 60:81–90, 1974.

29. Lasnitzki I, Goodman DS: Inhibition of the effects of methylcholanthreme on mouse prostate in organ culture by vitamin A and its analogs. Cancer Res 34:1564–1571, 1974.

30. Lostroh AJ: Effect of testosterone and insulin in vitro on maintenance and repair of the secretory epithelium of the mouse prostate. Endocrinology 88:500–503, 1971.

31. McMahon MJ, Butler AVJ, Thomas GB: Morphological responses of prostatic carcinoma to testosterone in organ culture. Br J Cancer 26:388–394, 1972.

32. McMahon MJ, Thomas GH: Morphological changes of benign prostatic hyperplasia in culture. Br J Cancer 27:323, 1973.

33. McRae CU, Ghanadian R, Fotherby K, Chisholm GD: The effect of testosterone on the human prostate in organ culture. Br J Urol 45:156–162, 1973.

34. Noyes WF: Effect of 3-methycholanthrene (NSC-21970) on human prostate in organ culture. Cancer Chemother Rep 59:67–71, 1975.

35. Robel P, Baulieu EE: Biologie expérimentale – Irrigation continue appliquée à la culture organotypique. C R Acad Sci Paris 274:3295–3298, 1971.

36. Robel P, Lasnitzki H, Baulieu EE: Hormone metabolism and action: Testosterone and metabolites in prostate organ culture. Biochimie 53:81–96, 1971.

37. Roy AK, Baulieu EE, Feyel-Cabanes T, Le Goascogne C, Robel P: Hormone metabolism and action: II. Androstenedione in prostate organ culture. Endocrinology 91:396–403, 1972.

38. Sandberg AA: Potential test systems for chemotherapeutic agents against prostatic cancer. Vit Horm 33:155–188, 1975.

39. Sandberg AA: Regulation of plasma steroid binding proteins. In James VHT (ed): "Endocrinology," Proceeding of the Fifth International Congress of Endocrinology, Hamburg, July 18–24, 1976. Amsterdam: Excerpta Medica, 1:452–457, 1977.

40. Sandberg AA, Gaunt R: Model systems for studies of prostatic cancer. Semin Oncol 3:177–187, 1976.

41. Sandberg AA, Kirdani RY, Yamanaka H, Varkarakis MJ, Murphy GP: Potential test systems for drugs against prostatic cancer. Cancer Chemother Rep 59:175–184, 1975.

42. Sandberg AA, Müntzing J, Kadohama N, Karr JP, Sufrin G, Kirdani RY, Murphy GP: Some new approaches to potential test systems for drugs against prostatic cancer. Cancer Treat Rep 61:289–295, 1977.

43. Santti RS, Johansson R: Some biochemical effects of insulin and steroid hormones on the rat prostate in organ culture. Exp Cell Res 77:111–120, 1973.

44. Schrodt GR, Foreman CD: In vitro maintenance of human hyperplastic prostate tissue. Invest Urol 9:85–94, 1971.

45. Shipman PAM, Littlewood V, Riches AC, Thomas GH: Differences in proliferative activity of rat and human prostate in culture. Br J Cancer 31:570–580, 1975.

46. Sinowatz F, Pierrepoint CG: Hormonal effects on canine prostatic explants in organ culture. J Endocrinol 72:53–58, 1977.

47. Sinowatz F, Chandler JA, Pierrepoint CG: Ultrastructural studies on the effect of testosterone, 5α-dihydrotestosterone, and 5α-androstane-3α, 17α-diol on the canine prostate cultured in vitro. J Ultrastruct Res 60:1–11, 1977.

48. Strangeways TSP, Fell HB: Experimental studies on the differentiation of embryonic tissues growing in vivo and in vitro. Proc R Soc B 100:273, 1926.

49. Trowell OA: The culture of mature organs in a synthetic medium. Exp Cell Res 16:118–147, 1959.

50. Yamamoto Y, Osawa R, Kirdani RY, Sandberg AA: Testosterone metabolites in dog bile. Steroids 31:233–247, 1978.

The Nude Mouse—Its Use as Tumor-Bearing Model of the Prostate

Ruben F. Gittes

The athymic nude mouse was shown years ago to accept certain xenografts of human tissue and was quickly reported to be a useful carrier for heterologous tumor transplants [1—7]. In the decade that has elapsed, several different laboratories have attempted a spectrum of tumor transplantation with variable results. We review here the experience with the athymic nude mouse as an ex vivo carrier for human prostate tissue, especially prostate carcinoma.

METHODS

Nude Mouse Colonies

Since the description by Pantelouris [8] and other early investigators of the immunologic deficiency in nude mice, it has been clear that the athymic state makes the mice particularly susceptible to environmental infections, especially the nonbacterial ones in which the T-cell defenses are particularly important. They are likely to fall prey to chronic infections that produce a wasting syndrome [9—11]. They are also sensitive to temperature changes because of their lack of hair and require special precautions in that regard.

Although some early investigators suggested that germ-free conditions be followed for these colonies [12], such facilities have not been practical or available to most laboratories [11]. The following precautions have been adopted widely and seem to be adequate in most cases to maintain a viable colony that permits transplantation experiments. The mice will live four to eight months under these conditions.

Room and cage isolation. A separate room which has an ultrafiltered laminar air flow system coupled with the use of commercially available individual cage filter tops is advisable. Ideally, procedures should be carried out on the mice in such a separate room, and they should not be cross-contaminated with other experimental animals, especially those that are not maintained in a conventional manner. Limited access to the room by the involved investigators should be maintained.

Models for Prostate Cancer, pages 31—37

Breeding. Breeding stock should be established using a combination of one homozygous male to three or four heterozygous females in each breeding cage. Homozygous females have proven to be poor mothers, and this arrangement gives a 50% yield of homozygous offspring. These are readily culled before weaning, and the best arrangement seems to be to separate the new litters so as to give the heterozygous mothers all homozygous or all heterozygous pups, preventing litter discrimination and selective loss of the homozygous offspring.

Temperature regulation. The room should be maintained at a temperature not lower than 75°F (25°C) and with a humidity at least 50%. Their lack of hair makes them sensitive to cold, and dry air seems to cause encrustations of their eyes and respiratory passages which take a great toll. Each cage should be provided with abundant supply of tissue paper or cotton wool to provide them with an enclosure which they use for protection against temperature changes.

Sterilization of materials. All shavings, cages, food, water, bedding, and filter tops for the cages should be sterilized to avoid the introduction of pathogens. For long-term observations, we have used antibiotic-water (tetracycline).

Tumor Transplantation

The prostate tumor to be implanted has been minced into small fragments of no more than 2 mm diameter so as to permit survival of the tissue by diffusion while a new circulation is established from the transplant bed. To minimize the destruction of the cells, a number of methods have been tried, including partial digestion with enzymes and mechanical dissociation with a plunger and syringe. However, mechanical fragmentation with a sharp scapel blade or with iridectomy scissors seems to be adequate. The mincing is done in a Petri dish with cold buffered tissue culture medium.

The source of prostate cancer has been both open surgical specimens and biopsy specimens. Particularly desirable is the use of a lymph node containing an obvious focus of metastatic disease, so as to avoid the joint implantation of benign and malignant tissue. When the source is an open biopsy of the prostate, we have made a point of taking fragments from the area that is obviously carcinoma and the control fragments from the area that looks like benign tissue. Adjacent fragments have been submitted for control histology.

The site of implantation has usually been the subcutaneous vascular space of the flank. Several laboratories have also tried an intramuscular site for better vascularization. In our own laboratory we have attempted a number of transplantations into the testes of the nude mouse so as to achieve the added benefit of an immunologically privileged site that might diminish the antibody response. In addition, it has been thought that the intratesticular site would provide a beneficial added concentration of testosterone to the prostate tissue graft.

Period of Observation

The observation of the fate of such prostate cancer transplants has always been in terms of many months. The thin skin of the nude mouse allows for easier observation of the implant site, and an early nodule can easily be detected. Unfortunately, most such impants never grow to a nodule even after observations of more than six months. Longer observation is not practical because of the high rate of death among the nude mice at that age.

In most laboratories, nodules present some time after implantation have been removed for histologic confirmation, subpassage to other nude mice, and karyotype studies [13].

Endocrine Manipulation of the Host

The use of androgen supplements has been practiced in many laboratories with testosterone pellets implanted subcutaneously. Androgen deprivation has been achieved by the use of females or castrated nude mice. Very high levels of ambient androgen have been achieved in our laboratory by transplantation into the nude mouse testes.

RESULTS

The nude mouse has failed to provide a satisfactory growth environment for the vast majority of attempts at implanting prostate cancer. The incidence of "take" of prostate cancer has been close to zero. The few cases reported as accepted have been anaplastic [14–16] except for a single line established temporarily by Reid [17, 18]. But she noted that the single success resulted from implanting over 100 specimens. This has been true also with human breast tumors and human lymphomas in other laboratories.

In our own experience when we made intensive attempts to achieve successful transplantation in the standard subcutaneous or intramuscular sites, we had no takes of prostate cancer in over 50 tumors attempted, implanted in several hundred mice with or without testosterone pellets. As shown in Table I, our early tabulated experience [19] showed only the persistence of some benign prostatic hypertrophy tissue, demonstrating no progressive growth, and the coincident loss of the originally implanted prostatic carcinoma.

It should be noted that even where benign prostatic tissue has persisted, we have observed the development of squamous metaplasia and interstitial fibrosis [20]. The same change has been observed in Sato's laboratory [18] and in Schroder's laboratory [14]. The implanted tissue was clearly altered from its original state by residence in the nude mouse, even if found to be surviving.

TABLE 1. Attempts at Ex Vivo Culture of Prostatic Carcinoma*

Source	Number	Number of transplants to nude mice	Number of mice with growth	Number of tissue culture attempts	Subculture established
Radical prostatectomy	17	8	4	16	No
Positive lymph node	5	1	0	5	No
Transurethral resection chips	7	1	0	7	No
Needle biopsy	6	0	0	6	No

*Attempts made from January 1, 1974, to June 30, 1974.

DISCUSSION

The original hope of many laboratories was that the nude mouse would provide an indifferent, inert environment for the growth of human prostate cancer so as to permit the in vivo testing of endocrine dependence, chemotherapy susceptibility, etc. The negligible success of the attempts at such transplantation in the last several years leaves no doubt that this hope has been dashed. Even human tumors such as those of the colon, skin, lung, and anaplastic tumors that were first considered "easy" to establish in nude mice have yielded a take of little more than 25% [15, 20].

It is more and more apparent that the nude mouse is not an inert recipient. Cytotoxic antibodies formed against xenografts may be quite effective in preventing the take or the growth of implanted tumors or skin when these come from species of great genetic diversity [2, 22–24]. In an unpublished work from our own laboratory, we have confirmed that nude mice will accept most mouse and rat tumors. They will accept allogeneic mouse skin both as a first and second set transplant. But they will reject more than half of the initial transplants of rat skin and most of the second set transplants of rat skin. And, in spite of the early reports of takes of human skin [23], nude mice that we have tested have invariably failed to support the survival of human skin for more than a couple of weeks and, in most cases, prevented its take right from the start [24].

It has been increasingly recognised that nude mice are not immunologically inert and that the non-take or rejection of xenografted tissues may very well be on an immunological basis. Natural killer lymphocytes are found in all mice, including the athymic nude mice, and these have been proved to be cytotoxic for various tumor cells [24, 26–28]. Other investigators have shown that some anaplastic xenografted tumors such as the human line HeLa, will fail to grow if viral antigens are added and present on the cell surface [29]. Similarly, the rejection of skin grafts by nude mice can be increased if rabbit complement is injected into the host [30]. Conversely, it was noted that with human breast tumors, which usually take with an incidence of only 5% in nude mice, the administration of antilymphocyte serum (ALS) increased the take up to 20–30% [31], suggesting a suppression of the lymphocytes or the natural killer cells by the ALS.

It has been suggested that the reason for the difficulty in growing these tumors might be that growth factors unique to the site of origin of the tissue are absent in the recipient site. It has been claimed that human breast tumors grew more easily in the mammary fat pad of nude mice [32]. But there is no positive evidence for such a requirement for the prostate. Indeed, the rat prostate tumor, R3327, does grow slowly but reliably in nude mice, maintaining its differentiated histology.

In all, this once hopeful model has failed to provide a reliable or even occasional growth medium for human prostate cancer. A host of experimental evidence suggests that there is a continuing immunologic barrier to xenografts in the nude mouse, mediated through antibody formation or natural cytotoxic killer cells. It appears that, at best, even if a tumor is allowed to grow by the host nude mouse, there is a necessary amount of immunologic selection of the cells allowed to grow and of the type of growth achieved in the still hostile environment.

REFERENCES

1. Rygaard J, Povlsen CO: Heterotransplantation of a human malignant tumour to "nude" mice. Acta Pathol Microbiol Scand 77:758, 1969.
2. Povlsen CO, Fialkow PJ, Klein E, Klein G, Rygaard J, Wiener F: Growth and antigenic properties of a biopsy-derived Burkitt's lymphoma in thymus-less (nude) mice. Int J Cancer 11:30, 1973.
3. Povlsen CO, Rygaard J: Heterotransplantation of human adenocarcinomas of the colon and rectum to the mouse mutant nude. A study of nine consecutive trnasplantations. Acta Pathol Microbiol Scand (Sect A) 79:159, 1971.
4. Povlsen CO, Rygaard J: Heterotransplantation of human epidermoid carcinomas to the mouse mutant nude. Acta Pathol Microbiol Scand (Sect A) 80:713, 1972.
5. Giovanella BC, Stehlin JS, Williams LJ: Heterotransplantation of human malignant tumors in "nude" thymusless mice. II. Malignant tumors induced by injection of cell culture derived from human solid tumors. J Natl Cancer Inst 52:921, 1974.
6. Giovanella BC, Stehlin JS: Assessment of the malignant potential of cultured cells by injection in "nude mice." In Rygaard J, Povlsen CO (eds): "Proceedings of the First International Workshop on Nude Mice." Stuttgart: G. Fischer Verlag, 1974, p 279.
7. Sordat B, Fritsche R, Mach J-P, Carrel S, Ozzello L, Cerottini J-C: Morphological and functional evaluation of human solid tumors serially transplanted in nude mice. In Rygaard J, Povlsen CO (eds): Stuttgart: G. Fischer Verlag, 1974, p 269.
8. Pantelouris EM: Absence of thymus in a mouse mutant. Nature 217:370, 1968.
9. Kindred B: Immunological unresponsiveness of genetically thymusless (nude) mice. Eur J Immuno 1:59, 1971.
10. Jutila JW, Reed ND: Pathogenesis of wasting disease in congenitally thymusless (nude) mice. Fed Proc (2991) 31:746, 1972.
11. Rygaard J, Povlsen CO: The nude mouse versus the hypothesis of immunological surveillance. Transplant Rev 28:43, 1976.
12. Giovanella BC, Stehlin JS: Heterotransplantation of human malignant tumors in "nude" thymusless mice. I. Breeding and maintenance of "nude" mice. J Natl Cancer Inst 51: 615, 1973.
13. Visfeldt J, Povlsen CO, Rygaard J: Chromosome analyses of human tumours following heterotransplantation of the mouse mutant nude. Acta Pathol Microbiol Scand (Sect A) 80:169, 1972.
14. Okada K, Schroeder FA, Jellinghause W, Wullstein HK, Heinemeyer HM: Human prostatic adenoma and carcinoma. Transplantation of cultured cells and primary tissue fragments in "nude" mice. Invest Urol 13:395, 1976.
15. Shimosato Y, Kameya T, Nagai K, Hirohashi S, Kodie T, Hayashi N, Nomura T: Transplantation of human tumors in nude mice. J Natl Cancer Inst 56:1251, 1976.
16. Mickey DD, Stone KR, Wunderli H, Mickey GH, Vollmer RT, Paulson DF: Heterotransplantation of a human prostatic adenocarcinoma in nude mice. Cancer Res 37: 4049, 1977.

17. Reid L, Sato G: Development of transplantable tumors of human prostate gland implanted in nude mice. J Cell Biol 70:360, 1976.

18. Reid L, Shin S: Transplantation of heterologous endocrine tumor cells in nude mice. In Fogh H, Giovanella B (eds): "The Nude Mouse in Experimental and Clinical Research." New York: Academic Press, 1978.

19. Gittes RF: Discussion of etiology and prevention of prostatic cancer. Cancer Chemother Rep 59:79, 1975.

20. Gittes RF, McLaughlin AP: Experimental approaches to BPH: Implants of BPH in immunosuppressed animals. In "Benign Prostatic Hyperplasia," NIAMDD Monograph, DHEW Publication NO (NIH) 76-1113, 1975, p 263.

21. Katsuoka Y, Baba S, Hata M, Tazaki H: Transplantation of human renal cell carcinoma to the nude mice: As an intermediate of in vivo and in vitro studies. J Urol 115:373, 1976.

22. Baldmus CA, McKenzie IFC, Winn HJ, Russell PS: Acute destruction by humoral antibody of rat skin grafted to mice. J Immunol 110:1532, 1973.

23. Reed ND, Manning DD: Long term maintenance of normal human skin on congenitally athymic (nude) mice. Proc Exp Biol Med 143:350, 1973.

24. Martin WJ, Martin SE: Naturally occurring cytotoxic anti-tumor or antibodies in sera of congenitally athymic (nude) mice. Nature 249:564, 1974.

25. Norstrand L, McDonald J, Gittes RF: Unpublished data.

26. Miller RG, Schilling RM, Phillips RA: Requirement for non T-cells in the generation of cytotoxic T lymphocytes (CTL) in vitro. II. characterization of the active cells in the spleen of nude mice. J Immunol 118:166, 1977.

27. Herberman RB, Nunn ME, Larvin DH: Natural cytotoxic reactivity of mouse lymphoid cells against syngeneic and allogeneic tumors. I. Distribution of reactivity and specificity. Int J Cancer 16:216, 1975.

28. Klein G, Klein E: Immune surveillance against virus-induced tumors and nonrejectability of spontaneous tumors: Contrasting consequences of host versus tumor evolution. Proc Natl Acad Sci USA 74:2121, 1977.

29. Reid L. Holland J, Jones C: Virus carrier state suppresses tumorigenicity of tumor cells in nude mice. J Gen Biol 42:609, 1979.

30. Koene R, Gerlag R, Jansen J, Hagemann J, Wijcleved P: Rejection of skin grafts in the nude mouse. Nature 251:69, 1974.

31. Giovanella BC, Stehlin JS, Lee SS, Shepard R, Williams LJ: Heterotransplantation of human breast carcinomas in "nude" thymus deficient mice. Proc Am Assoc Cancer Res 17:124, 1976.

32. Outzen HC, Custer RP: Growth of human normal and neoplastic mammary tissues in the cleared mammary fat pad of the nude mouse. J Natl Cancer Inst 55:1461, 1975.

Nonhuman Primate Prostate Culture

Ronald W. Lewis, MD, and Bernice Kaack, PhD

The limitations and problems of animal models of prostate disease are complex, as previously reported [1, 2]. One of the major drawbacks is inability to extrapolate animal data to human disease because of anatomical and physiological dissimilarities between the prostates of various mammalian species [2–5]. Some of these reports also point out the similarity of the nonhuman primate prostate to that of man, particularly the caudal prostate of the nonhuman primate [3, 4, 6–13]. Despite several reports of benign or malignant prostatic disease in lower mammals [2, 14–21], these models often show little similarity to either human benign prostatic hyperplasia or adenocarcinoma of the prostate [1, 2].

As stated by Handelsman, it is generally believed that models using spontaneous tumors would provide more information applicable to man than those using induced or transplantable tumor, especially with reference to metastases [1]. In the nonhuman primate such spontaneous disease of benign or malignant nature, although present, appears to be rare and is seldom diagnosed prior to death of the aged monkey [6, 22–25].

Although in vitro models of prostate disease using tissue culture also have limitations [1], such systems offer a unique approach to the development of an animal model of prostate disease [26]. We have developed a tissue culture method for growth of nonhuman primate prostate epithelial cells in monolayer. Preliminary data on the use of this in vitro system in combination with autologous forearm transplantation suggests an accessible prostatic in vivo model. Such a system allows for manipulation of the prostatic tissue without placing the animal's total body at risk. In addition, we are able to study an in vitro and in vivo system simultaneously under the same initial experimental conditions.

Models for Prostate Cancer, pages 39–65
© 1980 Alan R. Liss, Inc., 150 Fifth Ave., New York, NY 10011

METHODS

Tissue Culture Techniques

The tissue culture technique is basically that described by Webber for the culture of human prostate [27]. It is a monolayer epithelial cell culture produced after epithelial cell encapsulation of implants in suspension cultures.

Cranial and caudal prostate tissue is obtained from sacrificed animals, immediately after death, or surgically from anesthetized animals. The tissue is transferred to the laminar hood environment in sterile covered glass Petri dishes containing culture media with antibiotics. With a sterile forceps and scissors the tissue is minced into 0.5 to 1 mm explants. The explants are placed into microtest plates,* one explant per well. Media (0.3 ml) is then added to each well. The media is CMRL-1066 with L-glutamine† with 20% fetal calf serum† and the following additives: 100 units of penicillin/ml, 100 μg of streptomycin/ml, 50 μg of gentamicin/ml, 1 unit of insulin/ml, 1 international unit (IU) of vitamin A/ml (in the form of β retinoic acid),‡ and 0.1 mg amphotericin B (fungizone)/ml medium. The medium has pH of 7.3. The microtest plates are then incubated at 37°C in a humidified 5% CO_2 atmosphere. The medium is changed every three to four days under the laminar flow hood.

After being in suspension culture for seven to nine days the explants are transferred in a laminar flow hood to plastic tissue culture Petri dishes,** one to five explants per Petri dish. Three ml of the medium described above is added, taking care not to float the explants off the dish. The Petri dishes are reincubated, and the medium is carefully changed every three to four days. At each medium change the Petri dishes are examined under the inverted microscope and cell monolayer growth is observed. At various stages of monolayer growth the cultures are fixed in acetone-free methanol after being washed in warm (37°C) balanced salt solution and stained with a rapid Giemsa stain according to the method of Poché [28].

Identification Studies

Electron microscopy was also performed on the monolayer cell growths, according to the following technique. Tissue culture samples were fixed in culture dishes with Karnovsky's fixative for two hours [29]. They were washed in buffer

---

*Tissue Culture multi-well plate with cover, well capacity 0.35 ml (Catalog Number 76-003-05). Linbro Division, Flow Laboratories, Inc., Hamden, CT 06517.

†Grand Island Biological Company, Grand Island, NY 14072.

‡Pure retinol in crystalline form from Hoffmann-La Roche, Inc., Research Division, Nutley, NJ 07110.

**Tissue Culture Petri Dish, 60 × 15 mm (Catalog Number 3002-500), Falcon Plastics, Division of Bioquest, Cockeysville, MD 21030.

and post-fixed in 1% osmium tetroxide for one hour. Dehydration was done in ascending concentrations of ethanol, and cultures were embedded in Luft's epoxy resin in the culture dish [30]. Low-viscosity resin cannot be used since it reacts with the plastic culture dishes. Ultrathin sections were stained with Watson's saturated alcoholic uranyl acetate for one hour and then in Reynolds's lead citrate for 15 minutes [31, 32].

Prostatic acid phosphatase in tissue culture was demonstrated by the technique of Stonington et al [33]. Prostatic acid phosphatase will stain in the reaction after immersion of the monolayers in 10% neutral formalin for up to five hours. The cell cultures were incubated with naphthol AS-MX phosphate substrate* for four to eight hours at 37°C. As a result of the acid phosphatase activity naphthol AS is liberated, immediately couples with the diazonium salt of the Fast Violet B dye,[†] forming an insoluble and visible pigment at the sites of the phosphatase activity [33].

In fresh tissue studies prostatic acid phosphatase was demonstrated histochemically by the method of Carson [34]. In fresh tissue studies frozen sections of 6–10 μ were cut on a Cryo-cut microtome[‡] and mounted on slides subbed with gelatin. Naphthol AS-MX phosphate substrate was utilized as substrate [35] and the azodye Fast Violet B was employed for staining the acid phosphatase.

Combination Animal Model

The in vitro/in vivo animal model consisted of two phases. First, as above, explant suspension cultures, from surgically harvested cranial and caudal prostate were grown in microtest plates for seven days. After seven days in suspension culture the explants were implanted into forearm musculature of the donor animal. Explants were placed in pockets in the muscle created by a scalpel blade and suturing the overlying muscle with 6 0 monofilament suture, thereby providing marked implant sites. Tissue was harvested at one-month, three-month, and six-month intervals. Samples were fixed and stained with hemotoxylin and eosin for light microscopy and fixed and stained for scanning and transmission electron microscopy. Samples were also stained for prostatic acid phosphatase.

In two of the in vitro/in vivo animals prostatic implants were harvested from the forearm musculature at six months. They were placed in suspension culture followed by Petri dish implantation or were placed directly in Petri dish culture.

---

*Naphthol AS-MX Phosphoric Acid-Disodium Salt (Catalog Number N5000), Sigma Chemical Company, P.O. Box 14508, St. Louis, MO 63178.
[†]Fast Violet B Salt (F-4377), Sigma Chemical Company.
[‡]American Optical Instruments Company, Buffalo, NY.

RESULTS

Growth of prostatic epithelial cells was accomplished in twenty nonhuman primates, as seen in Table I. Cell monolayers were carried for as long as 60 days, although generally monolayers appeared to remain stable and did not continue to increase in radius after four weeks. Four animals have been used in the in vitro/in vivo prostate model (Table I).

Histology

Epithelial cells for the most part migrated to the surface of the explant while in suspension culture as shown in Figure 1. This encapsulation appeared to be started at three days and was well established by day 7 to 9 in suspension cultures. As reported by Webber and Stonington there was a concurrent development of hypocellularity of the central stromal and vascular tissue at the time the epithelial cell encapsulation was occurring [36]. However, as opposed to their findings in human prostate, after day 12 in suspension cultures, the epithelial cells began also to break down. Therefore Petri dish transfer was performed by day 12, preferably at days 7 to 9, to obtain the best subsequent monolayer growth. This epithelial cell encapsulation explains the predominant epithelial cell monolayers that subsequently grow out from the explant when placed in the Petri dish phase (Fig. 2). Occasionally fibroblast initial monolayer growth or overgrowth develops as shown in Figures 3 and 4. The percentage of fibroblast contamination in this series of animals varied from 5–10%.

The prostatic epithelial cells were usually uniform, tightly joined, cuboidal or polyhedral in shape, with a single nucleus and a single nucleolus (Fig. 5). At the periphery of the monolayer the cells became less tightly joined and often were

TABLE I. Nonhuman Primate Prostates Cultured

12 Rhesus (Macaca mulatta)
3 Baboons (Papio papio)
3 Stumptails (Macaca arctoides)
1 Patas (Erythrocebus patas)
1 Cyno (Macaca fasicularis)

20

In vitro/in vivo model
2 Rhesus (Macaca mulatta)
2 Cyno (Macaca fasicularis)

4

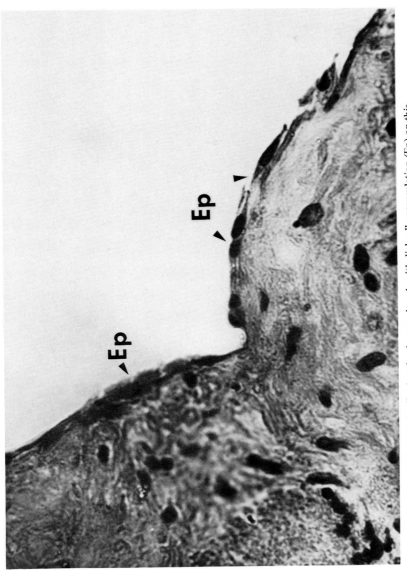

Fig. 1. Epithelial cell migration has produced epithelial cell encapsulation (Ep) on this caudal lobe prostate explant after seven days in suspension culture (magnification, × 720).

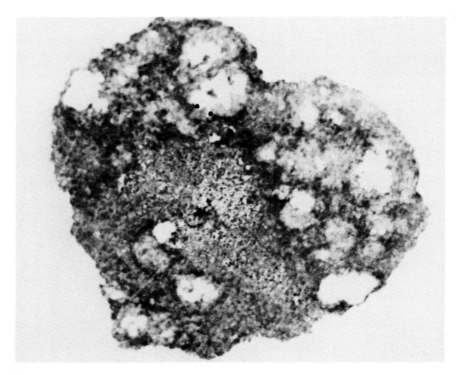

Fig. 2. Example of typical monolayer produced in approximately 10–12 days after explants taken from suspension culture and placed in plastic tissue culture Petri dish (magnification, × 10).

stellate, with long cytoplasmic bridges between adjoining cells (Fig. 6). Occasional giant cell formation was seen (Fig. 7). There did not appear to be a histologic difference between the epithelial cell type seen from the cranial or the caudal regions of the nonhuman primate prostate. In one of the tissue culture systems there was a large percentage of giant cell formation. Attempts were made to produce similar giant cell formation in a nonhuman primate kidney epithelial cell line by exposing it to the medium from the prostatic cell culture; no such giant cell formation was produced.

Electron microscopy of the monolayers showed typical epithelial cell characteristics when compared to fresh prostatic epithelial cells (Figs. 8–10). Such findings were microvilli surface, secretory granules below this surface (some associated with Golgi apparatus), normally organized mitrochondria, intact nuclei, and desmosome junctions between adjoining cells.

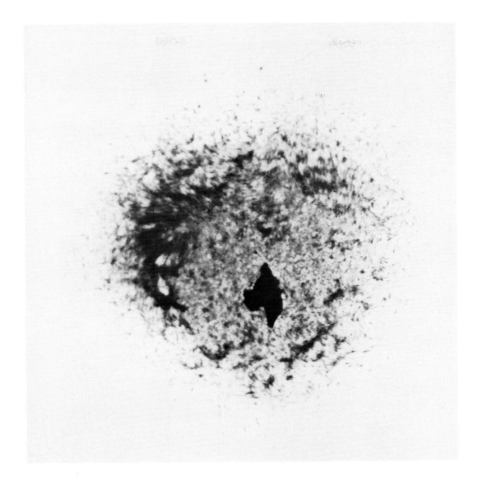

Fig. 3. Example of fibroblastic growth seen in 5–10% of Petri dish explants in this series (magnification, × 10).

Formalin-resistant prostatic acid phosphatase was demonstrated by heavily staining granular material in the monolayer cultures (Fig. 11). Prostatic acid phosphatase was found in both the cranial and caudal prostatic epithelial cell monolayers of apparently equal intensity. This was different from fresh tissue in which a heavier concentration of prostatic acid phosphatase was found in the caudal prostate tissue than in the cranial prostatic tissue.

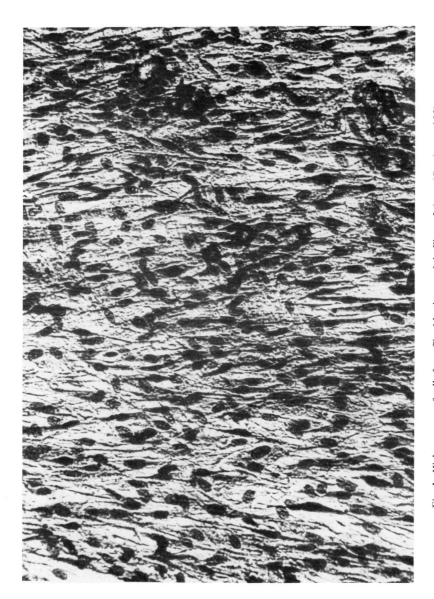

Fig. 4. Higher power of cells from fibroblastic growth in Figure 3 (magnification, × 180).

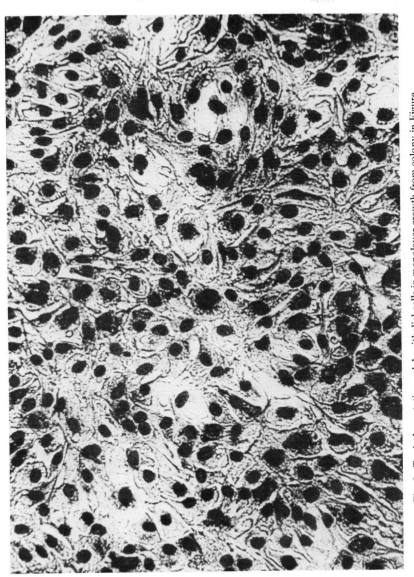

Fig. 5. Typical prostatic caudal epithelial cells in monolayer growth from colony in Figure 2 (magnification, × 180).

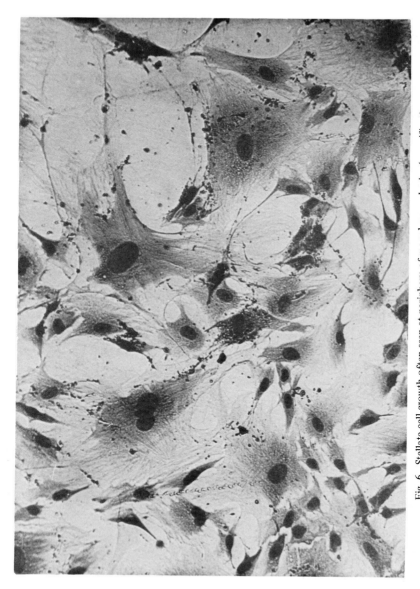

Fig. 6. Stellate cell growth often seen at periphery of monolayer colonies (magnification, × 180).

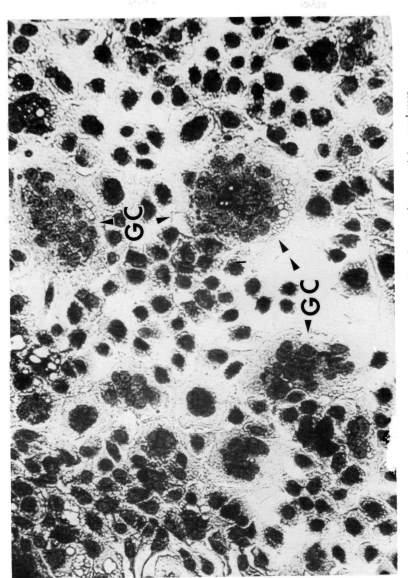

Fig. 7. Giant cell formation seen in some colonies of nonhuman primate prostate monolayers (magnification, × 180).

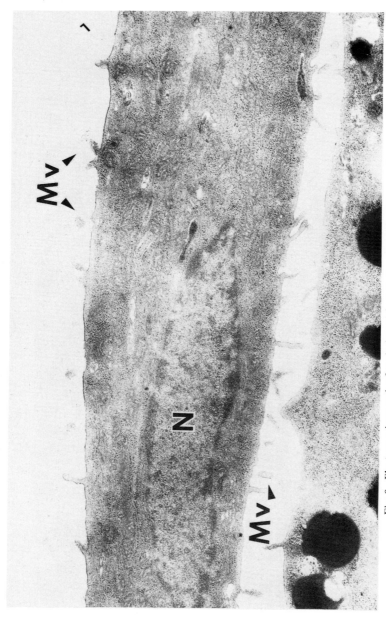

Fig. 8. Electron micrograph of typical caudal prostatic epithelial cell in monolayer growth: N = nucleus, Mv = microvilli surface (magnification, × 9,000).

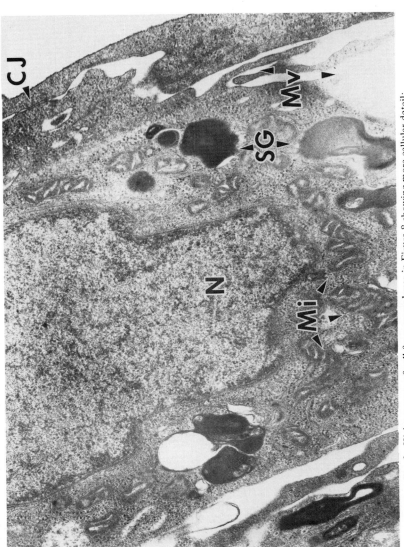

Fig. 9. Higher power of cell from monolayer in Figure 8 showing more cellular detail: N = nucleus, Mi = mitochondria, CJ = intracellular junction, Mv = microvilli border of cell, SG = secretory granules (magnification, × 16,000).

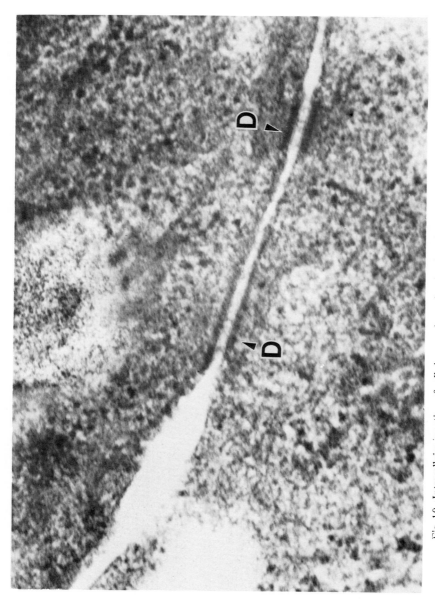

Fig. 10. Intracellular junction of cells in monolayer showing desmosomes (D) (magnification, × 30,000).

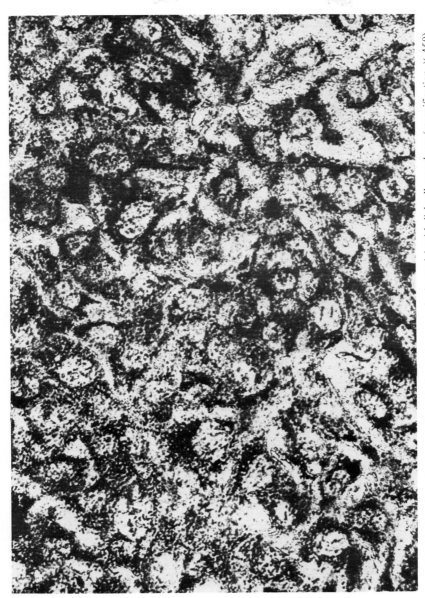

Fig. 11. Heavily stained prostatic acid phosphatase granules in caudal epithelial cell monolayer (magnification, × 450).

Effects of Additives

The presence of vitamin A in the form of β retinoic acid did deter squamous metaplasia. In three experiments comparing cell growth in medium with or without β retinoic acid, retinoic acid slowed growth determined by measurement of radius of the monolayer from edge of explant. The cells grown in media with retinoic acid were also larger than the control cells and became vacuolated earlier than the control. The cells in vitamin A became very vacuolated when compared to those without vitamin A.

In another experiment testosterone added to the medium at a concentration of 0.3 μg/cc failed to increase the number of explant monolayers produced or change the quality of the monolayer. However, all media did contain 20% fetal calf serum which was not steroid extracted.

Animal Model

The harvested implants from the forearm musculature of the in vitro/in vivo models showed good epithelial cell growth occurring commonly in sheets or clumps of cells and occasionally as encapsulated acini (Figs. 12 and 13). There was only occasional small white cell infiltration, perhaps indicating a rejection process. Prostatic acid phosphatase was found in the harvested implants. Electron microscopy showed good epithelial cells with gland formation (Figs. 14–16).

Attempts were made to reinstitute monolayer prostate epithelial cell growth; in one of the in vitro/in vivo animals this was not successful. In a second animal, caudal prostate implants, after six months in forearm musculature, were placed directly onto Petri dish culture after surgical harvesting. Epithelial cell monolayers were produced which showed histologic similarity to previous prostatic epithelial cultured cells.

DISCUSSION

This animal model of prostate disease in the nonhuman primate is desirable because of the well-established anatomic and physiologic similarities between nonhuman primates and man. The limitations of any model system, whether the model is primarily an in vitro tissue or cell culture system or an in vivo autologous or heterologous system, have been clearly stated [1].

The nonhuman primate prostate has been shown to be histologically similar to the prostate of man [3, 4, 6, 7, 9]. The ultrastructure of caudal prostate of the nonhuman primate is in all respects identical with the prostate of man [12]. In unpublished ultrastructural studies at the Tulane Delta Primate Center of nonhuman primate caudal prostatic tissue we have also found the same striking similarities. However, there are still important anatomic differences. The nonhuman primate prostate is composed of two distinct lobes, cranial and caudal.

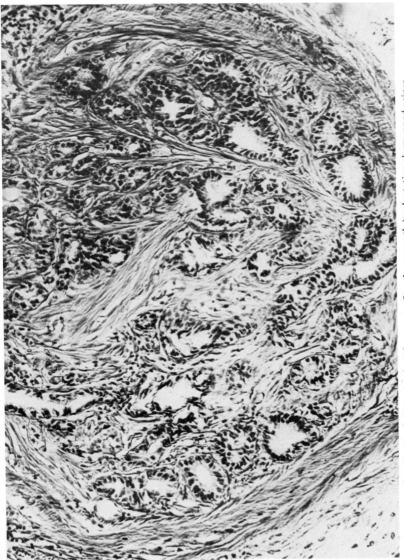

Fig. 12. Cranial lobe implant from arm after three month implantation shows good acinar formation and retained stroma with fibrous encapsulation (magnification, × 180).

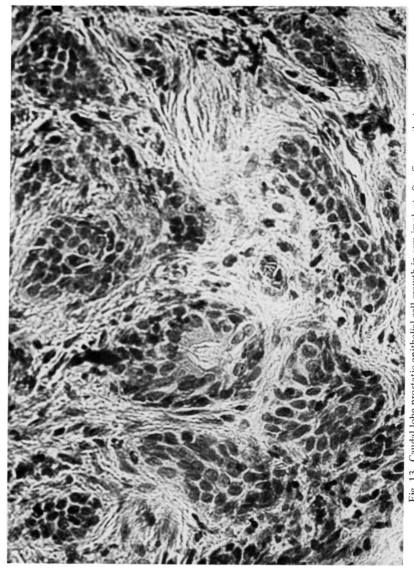

Fig. 13. Caudal lobe prostatic epithelial cell growth in arm implant after five months in arm with sheets and clumps of cells and one acinus with good stroma (magnification, × 450).

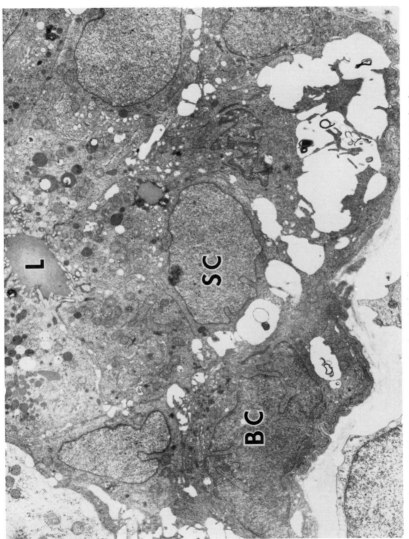

Fig. 14. Electron micrograph of secreting gland in arm implant of cranial prostate in place for six months: BC = basal cell, SC = secretory epithelial cell, L = lumen of acinus (magnification, × 6,000).

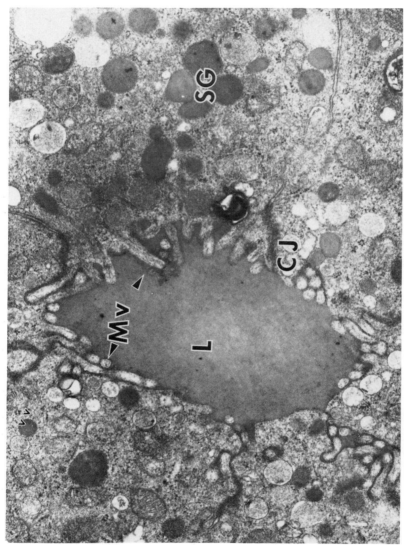

Fig. 15. Higher magnification of Figure 14 showing detail of cellular structures of actively secreting prostatic epithelial cell: L = lumen, MV = microvilli, CJ = tight intracellular junction, SG = secretory granules below microvilli surface (magnification, × 24,000).

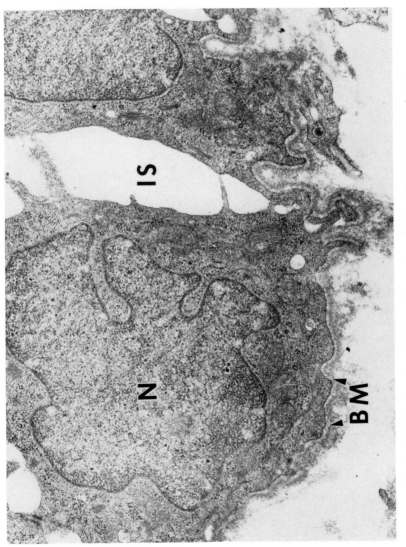

Fig. 16. Magnification of basal cell from Figure 14 showing excellent basement membrane (BM), intracellular space (IS), and nucleus of basal cell (N) (magnification, × 24,000).

Homologous relationships to the human are still theoretical [7, 25]. The cranial lobe appears to be very similar if not identical to the coagulation gland found in lower mammals [37, 38]. Neither the caudal nor cranial glands surround the urethra in the nonhuman primate. Therefore, bladder outlet obstruction, the usual first manifestation of human prostatic disease, is not evident in the nonhuman primate, even in natural disease.

Physiologic similarities between the prostate of nonhuman primates and man have been reported. These include zinc concentration under varying experimental conditions [10, 39, 40], prostatic tissue protein comparative studies by immunoelectrophoresis and agar diffusion [4], acid phosphatase content [12], effect of anti-androgenic drugs [12], radioactive-labeled androgen uptake [13], and respiration and glycolysis [5]. Two of these studies point out the greater similarity of nonhuman primate prostate to man than to other non-primate mammals [4, 5]. Five of these stress the greater similarity of the caudal lobe of the monkey prostate to man as compared to the cranial lobe [10, 12, 13, 39, 40].

In a review of caudal and cranial prostate pathology at the Delta Primate Center, consisting of 100 animals (Table II), prostatic cystic hyperplasia was found in the cranial and caudal lobes of the nonhuman primate in 13% of animals examined [25]. This resembled the cystic hyperplasia found in the dog. In this series an additional case of adenocarcinoma of the caudal prostate was found [25], the second such case reported [24]. In the caudal prostate of three other animals, changes of localized atypical cells with one case of possible neural invasion were found. These areas, however, showed normal glandular formation. The histologic findings would be consistent with well-differentiated adenocarcinoma if found in the human on needle prostate biopsy. Thus spontaneous tumors do occur in the nonhuman primate prostate, but diagnosis of such disease is rare. The rarity of reported disease may be due to the small number of primates studied, incompleteness of autopsies, and the infrequent study of aged primates.

Since such disease does occur naturally in the prostate of the nonhuman primate, yet is rarely discovered, then either of two pathways is open to developing a nonhuman primate animal model of prostate disease. The first is to try to collect aged primates for naural disease models. The second is experimental manipulation of prostatic epithelial cells in tissue culture in an attempt to produce benign or malignant disorders, and it is a viable alternative. Such has been the design of the work at the Delta Primate Center. The advantages of tissue or cell culture in the investigation of prostatic cancer has been recently well stated by Franks. He concludes that the development of basic techniques is where the future in this field lies [26].

Prostatic epithelial cells have been grown in tissue culture at our center, essentially with the techniques of Webber and Stonington and their associates [27, 28, 33, 36]. We have found that 20% fetal calf serum appeared to be a good concen-

TABLE II. Prostate Tissue Studies

Animal species	Number of prostates examined
Macaca mulatta	25
Pan tryglodytes	13
Macaca fasicularis	10
Callicebus moloch	10
Erythrocebus patas	9
Saimiri sciurea	8
Macaca arctoides	8
Cercocebus (species unknown)	2
Papio (comatus and papio)	2
Ateles geoffroyi	1
Hylobates lar	1
Macaca radiata	1
Unknown species	10
	100

tration in the medium for epithelial cell outgrowth and for deterring fibroblastic contamination. Such contamination was seen in only 5–10% of the cultures in the 20 animals in this group.

We recognize that the results in our testosterone studies may have been affected by steroids in the fetal calf serum and feel, as expressed by others, that steroid extraction of the serum is optimal [41]. Studies with steroid extraction of serum and the addition of estrogen, testosterone, and dihydrotestosterone to the medium are planned. The failure of the response to the testosterone might also be due to the fact that the epithelial cells growing in monolayer as a result of initial encapsulation may be different from the normal intact epithelial cells, as hypothesized by Franks and Barton. As expressed by the same authors, these cells may be of a form that favors growth rather than differentiation, or perhaps these cells can only function as secretory cells in the presence of normal relationships with supporting stroma and muscle [42].

We have used vitamin A additions to our medium in the form of β retionic acid at the concentration of 1 IU/cc of media. We have had very little squamous metaplasia in our culture system, which we attribute to the use of vitamin A, as have others [43]. The increased vacuolization of the epithelial cells in culture and the slower growth of colonies of cells from the explants in vitamin A-containing medium suggest that this vitamin may play a more important role in maintaining the secretory function of these cells than in their growth. It is also apparent that in studies of chemical or virus transformation the use of vitamin A may be a competitor to or inhibitor of transformation [44]. The value of this vitamin as an additive must therefore be coupled with the goal of the experiment. We plan to use this vitamin as an additive in functional and hormonal studies but to de-emphasize it in carcinogenesis studies.

In these nonhuman primate epithelial cell cultures we have relied on a single marker, that of prostatic acid phosphatase with special emphasis on its resistance to formalin [33–35], to indicate the epithelial cultured cells are of prostatic origin. We are currently involved in establishing hormone binding, particularly radioactive labeled dihydrotestosterone, as a second marker to validate these cells as prostate epithelial cells. Demonstrations of binding of sex hormones in human prostate epithelial cell culture systems has been made by autoradiography [45]. Immunofluorescent labeling is another possibility.

Although in the prostate cultures giant cell formation has been seen, cytopathic effects are not seen in other nonhuman primate epithelial cell culture systems when media from the prostate monolayers are used on these other lines. There-fore, no viral cytopathic effects can be entertained by the presence of these giant cells, as suggested in human prostate cell cultures [46].

The in vitro/in vivo model allows for experimental manipulation of the prostatic tissue while in the in vitro state. Part of the tissue can then be implanted into an area that can be surgically approached on numerous occasions with little morbidity to the animal. The implanted tissue can also be palpated for evidence of growth. Three pilot animals have demonstrated that the prostatic tissue kept in suspension culture for seven to nine days can be successfully implanted into forearm musculature with little rejection. The tissue appears to retain epithelial cell characteristics by light and electron microscopy examination and maintain prostatic acid phosphatase secretion for up to six months after arm placement. This tissue has also been harvested at six months and epithelial cell growth has been reinstituted in Petri dish culture with histologic similarity to the initial prostate epithelial cell culture monolayer.

The last animal in the in vitro/in vivo group had exposure of the tissue during the in vitro state to an oncogenic U-V inactivated Herpes virus and subsequent arm implantation. Biopsy material is to be obtained at three-month intervals. Although this is certainly preliminary data, it is mentioned to demonstrate a possible application of this in vitro/in vivo technique as an animal model of prostate disease.

Another advantage of this system is that a part of the experimentally manip-ulated implants can then be transferred to the Petri dish phase of this culture system for further studies and for pure in vitro observation of possible changes from normal growth or differentiation.

CONCLUSION

A basic nonhuman primate prostate tissue and epithelial cell culture technique has been presented with characterization of the resulting monolayer cells. The coupling of this in vitro system with in vivo forearm musculature implantation after seven to nine days in suspension culture provides a potential animal model for the study of prostate disease. The advantages of the isolated in vitro epithelial cell culture system are primarily found in basic characterization of the nonhuman primate epithelial cell and examining the response of this cell to various hormones and substances.

ACKNOWLEDGMENTS

The authors wish to acknowledge Mr. E.N. Fussell for the preparation of the photomicrographs and the electron microscopy work. Also acknowledgment is given to Jan Hardy for preparation of the manuscript.

The research was supported in part by USPHS grant 2 P40 RR 00164-17.

REFERENCES

1. Handelsman H: The limitations of model systems in prostatic cancer. Oncology 34:96–99, 1977.
2. Brendler H: Experimental prostatic cancer: Background of the problem. Natl Cancer Inst Monogr 12:343–349, 1963.
3. Price D: Comparative aspects of development and structure in the prostate. Natl Cancer Inst Monogr 12:1–25, 1963.
4. Van Camp K: Histological and biochemical studies on prostatic tissue of mammalians. Acta Zool Pathol Antverp 48:123–136, 1969.
5. Muntzing J, et al: Comparison and significance of respiration and glycolysis of prostatic tissue from various species. J Med Primatol 4:245–251, 1975.
6. Roberts JA: The male reproductive system. In Fiennes RNT-W (ed): "Pathology of Simian Primates." Basel: S Karger, 1972, pt I, pp 878–888.
7. Blacklock NJ, Bouskill V: The zonal anatomy of the prostate in man and in the rhesus monkey (Macaca mulatta). Urol Res 5:163–167, 1977.
8. Ablin RJ, et al: Clinical and experimental considerations of the immunologic response to prostate and other accessory gland tissues of reproduction. Urol Int 25:511–539, 1970.
9. Schoonees R, et al: Anatomy, radioisotopic blood flow and glandular secretory activity of the baboon prostate. S Afr Med J (Suppl)42:87–94, 1968.
10. Schoonees R, et al: Correlation of prostatic blood flow with 65 zinc activity in intact castrated and testosterone-treated baboons. Invest Urol 6:476–484, 1969.
11. Schoonees R, DeKlerk JN, Murphy GP: The effect of Depostat (SH582) on the baboon prostate. J Surg Oncol 1:317–324, 1969.
12. Muntzing J, et al: Histochemical and ultrastructural study of prostatic tissue from baboons treated with antiprostatic drug. Invest Urol 14:162–167, 1976.
13. Ghanadian R, et al: Differential androgen uptake by the lobes of the rhesus monkey prostate. Br J Urol 49:701–704, 1977.

14. Franks LM: "Biology of the Prostate and Its Tumors" In Castro JE (ed): The Treatment of Prostatic Hypertrophy and Neoplasia. Baltimore: University Park Press, 1974, pp 1–26.
15. Dunning WF, et al: Methylcholanthrene squamous cell carcinoma of the rat prostate with skeletal metastases, and failure of the rat liver to respond to the same carcinogen. Cancer Res 6:256–262, 1963.
16. Fraley EE, Ecker S: Tumor production in immune-suppressed hamsters by spontaneously transformed human prostatic epithelium. J Urol 106:95–99, 1971.
17. Paulson DF et al: Properties of prostatic cultures transformed by SV40. Cancer Chemother Rep 59:51–55, 1975.
18. Lopez DM, Voigt W: Adenocarcinoma R 3327 of the Copenhagen rat as a suitable model for immunological studies of prostate cancer. Cancer Res 37:2057–2061, 1977.
19. Dunning WF: Prostate cancer in the rat. Natl Cancer Inst Monogr 12:341–369, 1963.
20. Voigt W, Dunning WF: In vivo metabolism of testosterone-^{3}H in R-3327, an androgen-sensitive rat prostatic adenocarcinoma. Cancer Res 34:1447–1450, 1974.
21. Voight W, Feldman M, Dunning WF: 5 α-dihydrotestosterone-binding proteins and androgen sensitivity in prostatic cancers of Copenhagen rats. Cancer Res 35: 1840–1846, 1975.
22. Fox H: Diseases in Captive Wild Mammals and Birds. Philadelphia: Lippincott, 1923, p 314.
23. Zuckerman S, Sandys OC: Further observations on the effects of sex hormones on the prostate and seminal vesicle of monkeys. J Anat 73:597–616, 1939.
24. Engle ET, Stout AP: Spontaneous primary carcinoma of the prostate in a monkey (Macaca mulatta). Am J Cancer 39:334–337, 1940.
25. Lewis RW, Kim JCS, Irani D, Roberts JA: The prostate of the nonhuman primate: Normal anatomy and pathology. Submitted to Investigative Urology.
26. Franks LM: Tissue culture in the investigation of prostatic cancer. Urol Res 5:159–162, 1977.
27. Webber M, et al: Epithelial outgrowth from suspension cultures of human prostatic tissue. In Vitro 10:196–205, 1974.
28. Poché PA, Webber MM, Jankowsky L: A rapid method for in situ staining of prostatic and other tissue culture cells. Stain Technol 49:229–233, 1974.
29. Karnovsky MJ: A formaldehyde-gluteraldehyde fixative of high osmolality for use in electron microscopy. J Cell Biol 27:137A–138A, 1965.
30. Luft JH: Improvements in epoxy resin embedding methods. J Biophys Biochem Cytol 9:409–414, 1961.
31. Watson ML: Staining of tissue sections for EM with heavy metals. II. Application of solutions containing lead and barium. J Biophys Biochem Cytol 4:475–479, 1958.
32. Reynolds ES: The use of lead citrate at high pH as an electron-opaque stain in EM. J Cell Biol 17:208–212, 1963.
33. Stonington OG, et al: Isolation and identification of the human malignant prostatic epithelial cell in pure monolayer culture. J Urol 114:903–908, 1975.
34. Carson FL: Acid phosphatase staining in the histopathology laboratory. Am J Med Technol 39:333–337, 1973.
35. Burstone MS: Histochemical demonstration of acid phosphatases with naphthol AS-phosphate. J Natl Cancer Inst 21:523–539, 1958.
36. Webber MM, Stonington OG: Stromal hypocellularity and encapsulation in organ cultures of human prostate: Application in epithelial cell isolation. J Urol 114:246–248, 1975.

37. Van Wagenen G: The coagulating function of the cranial lobe of the prostate gland in the monkey. Anat Rec 66:411–421, 1936.

38. Greer WE, Roussel JD, Austin CR: Prevention of coagulation in monkey semen by surgery. J Reprod Fertil 15:153–155, 1968.

39. Schoonees R, DeKlerk JN, Mirand EA, Murphy GP: The effect of bovine growth hormone on zinc-65 metabolism and prostatic blood flow of intact, testosterone-treated, and castrated adult male chacma baboons. Invest Urol 8:103–115, 1970.

40. Schoonees R, DeKlerk JN, Murphy GP: The effect of prolactin on organ weights and zinc-65 uptake in male baboons. J Surg Oncol 2:103–106, 1970.

41. Schroeder FH, MacKensen SJ: Human prostatic adenoma and carcinoma in cell culture – The effects of androgen-free culture media. Invest Urol 12:176–181, 1974.

42. Franks LM, Barton AA: The effects of testosterone on the ultrastructure of the mouse prostate in vivo and in organ cultures. Exp Cell Res 19:35–50, 1960.

43. Lasinitzki I: Growth pattern of the mouse prostate gland in organ culture and its response to sex hormones, vitamin A, and 3-methylcholanthrene. Natl Cancer Inst Monogr 12:381–403, 1973.

44. Chopra DP, Wilkoff LJ: Inhibition and reversal by β-retinoic acid of hyperplasia induced in cultured mouse prostate tissue by 3-methylcholanthrene or N-methyl-N[1]-nitro-N-nitrosoguanidine. J Natl Cancer Inst 56:583–587, 1976.

45. Stonington OG, Szwec N: Sex hormone binding by cultured human malignant prostatic epithelial cells. Presented at annual meeting of American Urological Association, Chicago, Illinois, April 1977.

46. Webber MM: Cytopathic effects in primary epithelial cultures derived from the human prostate. Invest Urol 13:259–270, 1976.

Characterization of a Human Prostate Adenocarcinoma Cell Line (DU 145) as a Monolayer Culture and as a Solid Tumor in Athymic Mice

Don D. Mickey, PhD, Kenneth R. Stone, PhD, Heidi Wunderli, PhD, George H. Mickey, PhD, and David F. Paulson, MD

A long-term tissue culture cell line derived from a human prostatic adenocarcinoma metastatic to brain is described and designated DU 145. This cell line has been growing in vitro for a period of three years and has been passed 120 times. The cells are epithelial in appearance and form colonies in soft agar suspension culture. A karyotype analysis demonstrated an aneuploid human karyotype with a modal chromosome number of 64. Three large acrocentric marker chromosomes, a translocation on the Y chromosome, and metacentric minute chromosomes have been identified. The cell line, DU 145, also forms solid tumors in athymic nude mice. Tumors grown in nude mice reveal a strong similarity to the original patient tumor. Ultrastructural comparisons of tumor cells propagated in nude mice show no major differences when compared to the original tumor cells and to the tissue culture cells. Solid tumor can be removed from nude mice and reinitiated into in vitro tissue culture while retaining the marker chromosomes. The DU 145 cells, when injected into nude mice, form solid epithelial tumors interspersed with fibroblastic connective tissue of mouse origin and are incapsulated by mouse connective tissue. The tumors do not metastasize in the mice.

MATERIALS AND METHODS

Clinical History

A 69-year-old white male with a three-year history of lymphocytic leukemia was admitted to the Durham Veterans Administration Hospital in August 1975 with widespread metastatic carcinoma of the prostate. His symptoms included left-sided weakness, headache, and left homonymous hemianopsia. Medication included diethystilbestrol (1 mg daily). Evaluation showed central nervous system extension. He underwent bilateral orchiectomy, transurethral resection of the prostate, and parieto-occipital craniotomy for excision of a tumor mass within a period of three weeks. After transient improvement of central nervous system functions, the symptoms reappeared in October, and he died in January 1976. During the period of clinical treatment the patient had biopsy-demonstrated tumor in prostate, bone marrow, and brain. Autopsy findings revealed, in addition to these foci, multiple metastases to abdominal lymph nodes, liver, and right femoral neck associated with a pathological fracture. The lungs revealed only microscopic foci of metastatic tumor. The intestines and pancreas were free of tumor.

Tissue Culture

Tumor tissue removed from the metastatic central nervous system lesion at the time of craniotomy was taken for in vitro culture. One piece of tissue was cut into small fragments and immobilized under glass coverslips according to the procedure of Peterson et al [1]. A second portion of the tumor tissue was manipulated to loosen individual cells from the tumor bulk. Small fragments and free cells removed by this "spillout" method [2] were then seeded onto collagen-coated Petri dishes [3]. Growth medium used was medium 199 (GIBCO, Grand Island, NY) supplemented with 20% bull serum (Kansas City Biologicals, Lenexa, KS), 0.9% sodium biocarbonate, 62.5% international units (IU)/ml of penicillin G, 0.005% streptomycin sulfate, and 0.5 μg/ml of fungizone. Subcultures were performed by 7–10 minute incubation with 0.025% trypsin-1 mm EDTA and calcium- and magnesium-free phosphate-buffered saline. Cells were subcultured at 1:10 dilutions.

Microscopy

Histological analysis by light microscopy was obtained by fixing 1 mm^3 blocks of tissue in glutaraldehyde, sectioning, and staining with hematoxylin and eosin. Tissue taken for ultrastructural analysis was put directly into cold 2.5% glutaraldehyde in 0.1 M cacodylate buffer (pH 7.4) and fixed as small cubes of tissue. The samples were washed in 0.1 M cacodylate buffer containing 5% sucrose (4°C; overnight), further fixed with 1% osmium tetroxide in 0.1 M cacodylate buffer and postfixed with 1% uranyl acetate in veronal acetate buffer for two hours. The samples were dehydrated through a graded series of ethanol and embedded as described by Luft [4].

Thin sections were cut on a Porter-Blum MT-2 microtome with a diamond knife. They were collected on collodion-carbon-coated grids, stained with both 2% uranyl acetate and lead citrate [5], and viewed in a Phillips 300 transmission electron microscope. Photographs were taken on Kodalith LR film 2572 (Eastman Kodak Company, Rochester, NY).

Karyotypic Analysis

For cells excised directly from the tumor, the tissue was treated with Colcemid (GIBCO, NY) to block cellular division in metaphase and with hypotonic KCl to free the chromosomes from the spindle. Chromosomes subsequently were fixed and spread according to the method of Harnden [6]. For the analysis of cells grown in vitro, Colcemid, 0.04 μg/ml, was added to tissue culture dishes for 0.5–2.0 hours at 37°C. Cells were removed from the dish by mild trypsinization and pipetting. Suspended cells were pelleted, washed once in Hanks balanced salt solution and resuspended in warm hypotonic KCl solution (75 mM). After incubation at 37°C for eight minutes, the swollen cells were repelleted by centrifugation, and the bulk of the supernatant solution was removed by aspiration. Cells were gently suspended in 0.5 ml supernatant solution and five drops of freshly prepared glacial acetic acid–methanol at 1:3. After five minutes, additional fixative was added to a volume of 5 ml and left for 30 additional minutes. Cells were then centrifuged, resuspended in 5 ml of fixative, spun down again and suspended in 0.5 ml fixative, spread on a clean microscope slide, and flame dried. The chromosomes were stained with the aceto-orcein procedure of Mittwoch [7] and the trypsin-Giemsa stain for G-banding according to the procedure of Seabright [8].

Heterotransplantation

Cells growing in vitro from the 13th passage were scraped from tissue culture dishes and washed free of growth medium with a phosphate-buffered saline solution and injected subcutaneously into the rear flank areas of six-week-old homozygous nude mice of NIH/S background. The total number of cells per mouse in the original injections was 1×10^6. Thereafter, tumors could be passed from mouse to mouse by surgically removing tissue after anesthesia by sodium pentobarbital administered IP and transferring small sections of solid tumor tissue to additional mice.

Peroxidase Labeling Assay

Anti-mouse sera used in this assay was obtained by immunization of rabbits with a mixture of homogenized mouse heart, liver, kidney, and spleen. Absorption of the anti-mouse serum was done with human tissue homogenate three times at 37°C for two hours, ten times at room temperature for two hours, and three times at 4°C overnight. For a control, the anti-mouse serum was absorbed with mouse tissue homogenate using the same absorption schedule. Both absorbed sera were checked for specificity by immunodiffusion.

Peroxidase labeling was done according to Denk et al [9]. Incubation with pronase (Calbiochem, B grade) was for ten minutes at 37°C. Goat anti-rabbit IgG serum was used at a dilution of 1:10. Peroxidase-antiperoxidase (PAP) complex (Miles Laboratories, Elkhart, Indiana) was diluted 1:25, which gave a concentration of 0.066 mg antiperoxidase/ml. The primary antiserum was obtained from immunized rabbits as described above and used at the dilutions indicated. Azur methylene blue [10] was used as a counter-stain. Photographs of these stained slides were taken with a Nikon Microflex model AFM automatic attachment to a Wild light microscope using Panatomic film with a dark blue filter (Wratten gelatine filter 80C).

RESULTS

Origin of Cell Line DU 145

Surgical tissue was obtained from the brain tumor metastasis of the patient and from the primary prostatic adenocarcinoma. The histological appearance of both the metastatic brain lesion and the primary lesion was similar. The prostatic tissue was described as poorly differentiated adenocarcinoma, whereas the brain metastasis was identified as a moderately differentiated adenocarcinoma with foci of poorly differentiated cells.

Out of a total of eight attempts to grow the brain tumor tissue in tissue culture, three produced epithelial cultures; the other five produced a mixture of fibroblastic and epithelial cells. Only the epithelial cultures were carried in long-term tissue culture. Once the epithelial outgrowth began, there was a steady accumulation of small (approximately 15 μ diameter) polygonal cells that exhibited no mobility. Colonies developed from single cells seeded during transfer such that isolated islands of cells were produced. The morphologic appearance of these cells in monolayer culture is shown in Figure 1a. The cells grow as a tightly packed epithelial monolayer and have many small lipid inclusions present within the cytoplasm. Figure 1b is the in vitro appearance of DU 145 after growing as a solid tumor in nude mice.

Growth Properties of Cell Line DU 145

The morphology and in vitro growth properties of DU 145 have changed little during the three years the cells have been in tissue culture. The line continues to contain relatively small polygonal nonmotile cells that grow as isolated islands in culture and become tightly packed when they reach confluency. Initially, subculture was performed very conservatively and divided at a 1:2 ratio in order to maintain a high cell density in the dishes. At present, they may be subcultured at a 1:10 or a 1:15 ratio since they are now thoroughly adapted to the tissue culture environment. The bull serum additive, used in the original isolation, has now been replaced with 10% calf serum. The population doubling time is 34 hours, and this is demonstrated at the 39th passage in Figure 2.

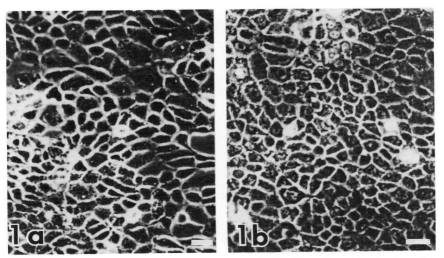

Fig. 1a. Phase-contrast micrograph of DU 145 tumor cells in vitro prior to passage in nude mouse (bar, 100 μm). b. Phase-contrast micrograph of DU 145 cells in vitro after solid tumor growth in nude mice (bar, 100 μm).

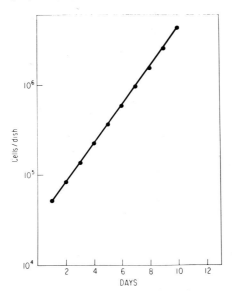

Fig. 2. Growth curve for cell line DU 145 at passage 39. A 60 mm Petri dish was seeded with 10^5 cells. At 24-hour intervals, the cells from duplicate dishes were removed by trypsin–EDTA treatment and counted in a hemocytometer. An average of four counts for each time period was used to determine each point. Least-squares analysis was used on the raw counts to refine accumulated data. The curve indicates a population doubling time of 34 hours.

DU 145 grows slowly in soft agar but will produce sizeable colonies of cells in agar layer when seeded at 10^4-10^5 cells per dish. Agar dishes containing less than 10^4 cells per dish failed to produce colonies within three weeks of observation. The inability of DU 145 cells to grow in soft agar suspension at low population densities parallels the relatively poor plating efficiency on plastic Petri dishes in liquid culture and is characteristic of this cell line. It appears that the poor plating efficiency is due to a low affinity of trypsinized cells for the plastic Petri dishes and not to the inability of the cells to survive at low population densities.

Cell line DU 145 is neither hormone-sensitive nor hormone-dependent. The cells grow equally well in media containing either fetal bovine serum or bull serum, which differ widely in their basic hormonal constitution. This is consistent with the growth characteristics of the tumor cells in the patient, as the clinical history of the patient reflects both orchiectomy and diethylstilbestrol, neither of which retarded the growth of the metastatic brain lesion.

DU 145 reflects a weakly positive staining reaction for acid phosphatase by the method of Stonington et al [11]. The intensity of the acid phosphatase reaction of DU 145 tissue culture cells was weak when compared to the intensity of staining by benign hyperplastic cell cultures. A similarily weak staining reaction was noted also on frozen sections of the original brain tumor lesion. Not all cells in the culture showed equallyd ense perinuclear staining by this qualitative procedure, reflecting either a cell-cycle-dependent reaction or a variation in cell population present. Serum acid phosphatase levels in the patient were within normal limits, even though the patient had widespread metastatic prostate carcinoma. A serum acid phosphatase value of the patient during the period of the primary prostatic tissue growth was not recorded.

Prior to the original publication of this human prostate carcinoma as a cell line [12], Flow Laboratories determined that the line was free of mycoplasma contamination, and Nelson-Rees (personal communication) confirmed that HeLa chromosomes were not present.

Karyotype Analysis

Karyotypic analyses were made on DU 145 during its development as a cell line at transfers 14, 57, and 90. The cell line is nearly triploid in chromosome number and shows evidence of extensive chromosomal rearrangements. Cells had a modal chromosome number of 64 at transfer 57 as determined by counting 50 intact metaphase spreads. The range was 46 to 163 chromosomes. Several characteristic chromosome markers were present: three long acrocentric marker chromosomes (M1, M2, and M3), several minute chromosomes, and a Y chromosome bearing a translocated fragment of other unidentified chromatin on the long arm. A G-banded karyotype of a cell with 65 chromosomes plus three minute chromosomes is shown in Figure 3. During the development of cell line DU 145, there were no other cell lines maintained in the laboratory that had similar marker chromosomes.

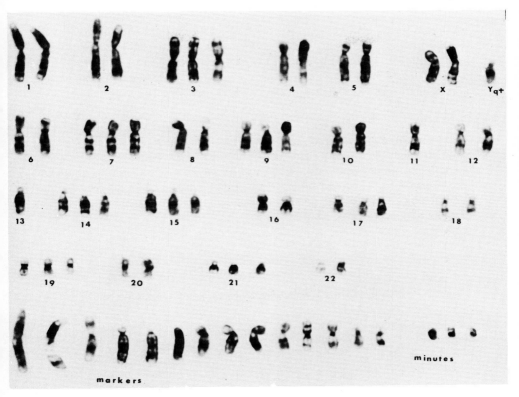

Fig. 3. A revised G-banded karyotype of a cell with 65 chromosomes plus three minute chromosomes. The Y translocation chromosome (Yq+) is shown in the upper righthand corner. A large complex of rearranged or marker chromosomes, including the minutes, is shown on the bottom line.

Heterotransplantation

After inoculation of 1×10^6 cells subcutaneously into two original weanling nude mice, one of the animals produced a palpable tumor that measured 10 mm in diameter after five weeks of growth [Mickey et al, 13]. Seven weeks after injection, a portion of this tumor was removed, with residual subcutaneous tumor remaining in situ. Separated portions were 1) fixed for light and electron microscopy, 2) prepared for karyotype analysis, 3) reintroduced into tissue culture and 4) reinjected as solid pieces of tumor into additional homozygous weanling mice by subcutaneous implantation. The secondary passage tumors were slow in growing and took 12 weeks to reach a size of 10 mm from transplant fragments 2 mm in diameter. At present, this tumor has been passed serially to more than 100 animals and can be grown in both males and females equally well. None of the animals are treated with testosterone prior to injection. In experiments to compare the effect of hormonally treated animals with untreated animals, testosterone-injected animals supported tumors but did not accelerate the rate of growth of the tumors. Tumors always have been formed only at the site of injection. No metastatic spread has been noted in any of the animals supporting tumors.

Microscopy

Histological examination of the patient's prostatic tumor (Fig. 4) revealed a typical distribution of tumor tissue in prostatic stroma with variably sized nests and with large tumor nodules almost totally composed of tumor epithelium with little stroma (Fig. 5). While glandular differentiation was present, most of the tumor revealed little glandular differentiation and in many areas the tumor exhibited striking cytological anaplastic change.

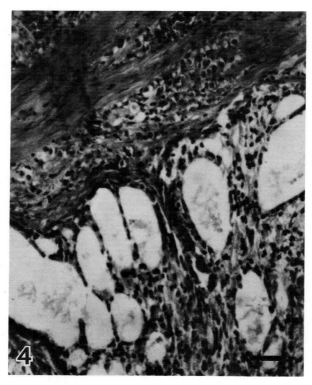

Fig. 4. Glandular differentiation in patient's prostatic tumor (bar, 25 μm; hematoxylin and eosin stain).

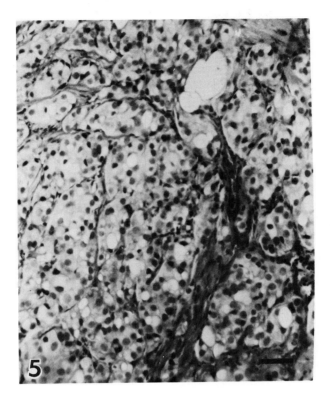

Fig. 5. Primary tumor in patient's prostate showing an area of lesser glandular differentiation (bar, 25 µm; hematoxylin and eosin stain).

The light microscopic morphologies of the patient's metastatic brain tumor and the tumor obtained from nude mice were entirely similar. The metastatic brain lesion in the patient revealed a greater tendency for glandular differentiation than in the prostate, and the tumor obtained from the mouse (Fig. 6) reflected the similar differentiation. Figure 6 demonstrates an accumulation of secretory material in the glandular spaces and is composed of large cells with cytological anaplastic change, including hyperchromatic nuclei and prominent nucleoli. Areas of solid tumor epithelial growth were noted also in the mouse-supported tumor and were similar to the growth seen in the prostate of the patient. The tumor obtained from the mouse exhibited features of rapid growth in that there were numerous areas of abundant central necrosis (not shown) and several mitotic figures (Fig. 7).

The electron microscopy of thin sections of the patient's metastatic lesions showed areas of solid tumor epithelial growth exhibiting large regions of epithelial

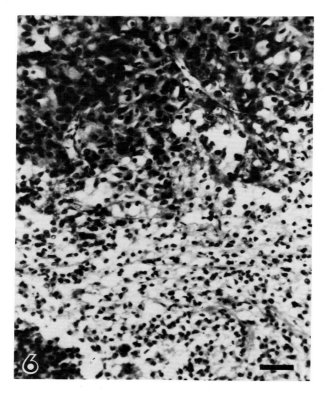

Fig. 6. Mouse-supported tumor revealing glandular area (bar, 25 μm, hematoxylin and eosin stain).

cells lined with some stromal elements (Fig. 8). Contrary to most prostatic glandular cells, few secretory granules were found in the periluminar cells. However, there were randomly distributed cells that contain many secretory granules (Fig. 9). In addition to the intercellular luminae, many intracellular luminae are present also (Figs. 8 and 9). Cells were noted to be in close apposition, forming numerous interdigitations; cell-to-cell contacts are mainly made by desmosomes, and junctional complexes in the periluminar region are frequent. The shapes of the nuclei range from regular round to highly indented. Clusters of chromatin are distributed along the nuclear membrane, the rest of the chromatin being finely dispersed. The endoplasmic reticulum is predominantly of the rough type, and many well developed Golgi complexes also are present (Fig. 9). Tonofilament bundles, regularly associated with desmosomes but also free in the cytoplasm, are frequent. Many lipid droplets, pinocytotic vesicles, and large heterogeneous

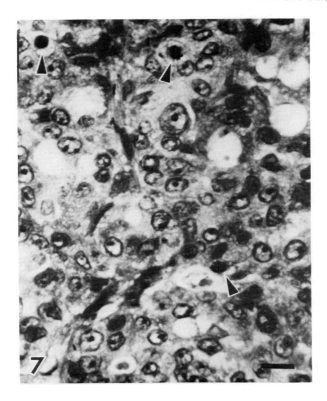

Fig. 7. Mouse-supported tumor revealing solid tumor area. Arrowheads indicate mitotic figures (bar, 15 μm; hematoxylin and eosin stain).

populations of lysosomes occur. Many of the cells contain necrotic regions.

The overall aspect of the tumor supported in nude mouse is similar to the regions of solid tumor epithelial growth found in the patient's metastatic tumor. Desmosomes and interdigitations are frequent (Fig. 10). The shape of the nuclei and the chromatin distribution are very similar in both tumors. Stretches of rough endoplasmic reticulum, many free ribosomes, many vacuoles and lipid droplets, as well as multivesicular bodies and myelin-like structures can be found. Tonofilament bundles and microtubules also occur (Fig. 11). In summary, there were no major morphologic differences between the tumor grown in nude mouse and the metastatic tumor of the patient.

The tissue culture cells originating from the tumor supported in nude mice and from the patient's metastatic tumor were similar also in ultrastructural morphologies. Cell processes of two or three cells tended to overlap and locally

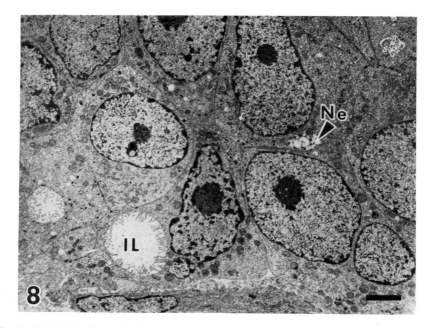

Fig. 8. Epithelial cells, patient's metastatic tumor. IL = intracellular lumen; Ne = necrotic area (bar, 4 μm).

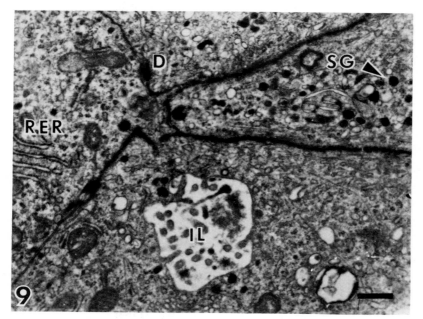

Fig. 9. Epithelial cells, patient's metastatic tumor. RER = rough endoplasmic reticulum; D = desmosomes; SG = secretory granules, IL = intracellular lumen (bar, 1 μm).

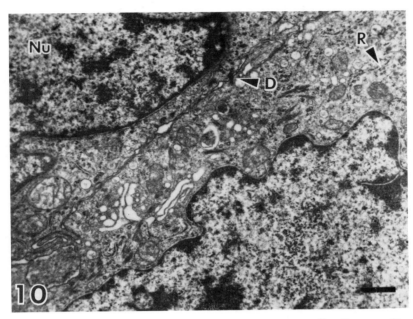

Fig. 10. Epithelial cells, mouse-supported tumor. D = desmosomes; R = ribosomes; Nu = nucleus (bar, 1 μm).

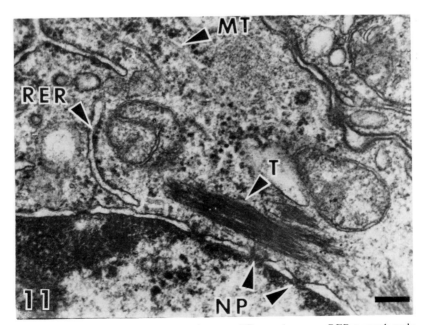

Fig. 11. Epithelial cells, mouse-supported tumor. NP = nucleopores; RER = rough endoplasmic reticulum; T = tonofilaments; MT = microtubules (bar, 0.5 μm).

form a double or triple layer (Fig. 12). Surface activity, in the form of microvilli, was was concentrated between the cells rather than on the monolayer surface (Fig. 12). Cell-to-cell contact was achieved by desmosomes. Many mitochondria, well-developed Golgi complexes, and endoplasmic reticulum of the smooth type occurred. Although lysosomes and lipid droplets were frequent, secretory granules were rare. Microtubules did occur in large numbers in both types of tissue culture cells as well as in both solid tumors. As in both solid tumors, necrotic areas were found in most tissue culture cells. No virus-like particles were found in any of the described tissues or cells. This is in contrast to the report by Webber et al [14], who found evidence of Herpes viruses in cultured prostate tissues, and from the report of Ohtsuki et al [15], who described particles resembling type C RNA viruses in one of 49 biopsy specimens of human prostate carcinoma.

Origin of Connective Tissue in Mouse-Supported DU 145

The origin of the connective tissue strands interdigitating between the human epithelial prostate tumor cells supported in nude mouse was studied in the light microscope using the unlabeled antibody enzyme technique of Denk et al [9]. Anti-mouse serum, which had been absorbed with heterologous tissue homogenate (see Materials and Methods), was used as a source of primary antibodies in the peroxidase labeling as shown in Figure 13. A very strong labeling of the tumor-surrounding capsule, the vessels, and all strands of connective tissue was observed (Fig. 13a). Labeling was performed on six mouse-supported tumors from different transfers of DU 145. The anti-mouse serum always yielded a strong labeling of all stromal elements. Labeling was seen with decreasing intensity over a range of dilutions from 1:5 to 1:75. Different controls were performed to check the specificity of the labeling: 1) no labeling was seen when either the primary antibodies or the goat anti-rabbit IgG serum were omitted (not shown); 2) labeling was abolished by homologous absorption of the anti-mouse serum with mouse tissue (Fig. 13b); 3) no labeling occurred if the anti-mouse serum was used as the source for primary antibodies on the original human surgical tissue (not shown); 4) application of anti-mouse serum after heterologous absorption with human tissue to a spontaneous mouse tumor (confirmed to be of mouse origin by karyotype analysis) produced labeling of stromal and epithelial components (not shown). This demonstrates that injected DU 145 tissue-culture-grown cells forms solid tumors of epithelial type in the mice and that these human epithelial tumor cells are surrounded by mouse-supplied stroma and interspersed by fibroblastic stroma (collagen fibers) of mouse origin.

DISCUSSION

In situ lesions of prostate carcinoma are often complex aggregates of both benign and malignant cells, and it is difficult to define origins of cells cultured

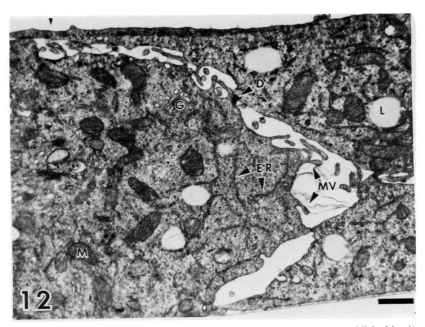

Fig. 12. Cross-section through monolayer of mouse-supported tumor reestablished in vitro. Figure shows overlapping portions of adjacent cells. M = mitochondria; ER-endoplasmic reticulum; D-desmosomes; L-lipid droplets; G-Golgi complex; MV-microvilli; arrowhead = top of monolayer (bar, 1 μm).

from these lesions. The origin of DU 145 was from a metastatic brain lesion, and therefore the probability is enhanced that the epithelial cells growing in culture from this brain lesion were prostate carcinoma cells. When in situ tissue is taken from the prostate for culture, cells of normal, benign hyperplastic, and malignant origin may be admixed and it is not possible to physically separate these cells without useful markers to identify the various cell types. In primary prostate lesions, it is not possible to define accurately the cells grown in vitro. This problem does not exist if the tissue examined and grown in vitro originates from a metastatic lesion such as the brain tissue in the patient presented here. In these studies an attempt was made to verify the prostatic origin of the metastatic brain lesion by culturing identical cells from the prostatic chips removed by transurethral resection. These cultures, however, were lost within 48 hours to fungal contamination. Bacterial and fungal contamination also prevented successful cultivation of prostate, liver, skin, bladder, and brain tissues taken at autopsy. Therefore, it was not possible to make direct comparisons between DU 145 cells grown from the brain lesion with cells cultivated from the patient's prostate.

Cell line DU 145 is not hormone-sensitive since it grows equally well in either

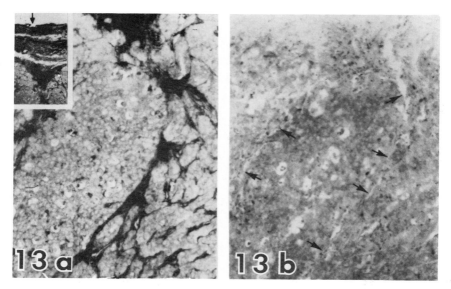

Fig. 13. Mouse-supported tumor labeled with anti-mouse serum (dilution 1:10) absorbed with human tissue homogenate. Note strong labeling of all stromal elements. 13a: Inset area of same section showing strongly labeled capsule of mouse tissue which surrounds the human tumor. Arrow indicates outside capsule. 13b: Control section, identical portion as illustrated in 13a, labeled with anti-mouse serum (dilution 1:10) and absorbed with mouse tissue homogenate. No peroxidase label can be seen in areas that are heavily labeled with peroxidase in 13a.

20% fetal bovine serum or bull serum [16]. Similar insensitivity to hormonal control has been noted by others examining prostate cells in vitro [17–19], although there are scattered reports of hormone response in vitro [20–24]. In the case of DU 145, either the cells that grew in vitro were hormone insensitive by in vitro selection or the tumor tissue removed from the patient was hormone insensitive prior to diethylstilbestrol therapy.

Several investigators have succeeded in establishing solid tumor growth of prostate material either by injecting tissue-culture-grown cells or fragments of primary tissue into nude mice [25–27]. Sato et al [26] reported the growth of human prostatic tumors in hormonally conditioned animals. Prostate cells that had been grown for short periods in culture prior to inoculation were injected beneath the splenic capsule of the nude mice and removed after periods as long as three months. After removal, the cells were reestablished in tissue culture. Recipient mice for all of these experiments were males three or four months old that had been inoculated with testosterone prior to transplantation. Sato indicated that the growth of human prostatic cells in nude mouse splenic tissue was testosterone dependent. Okada et al [25] reported the transplantation of both primary tissue fragments and cultured cells of prostate adenocarcinoma into nude mice. Castrated animals were used and were found to be more receptive for prostate tissue growth than were animals that had not been castrated. In addition, castrated mice that subsequently were treated with testosterone were the most receptive group. Serial transplants of these tumors in nude mice were not attempted with either prostate carcinoma or adenoma tissue. Metastasis was not observed. Shimosato et al [27] included two prostatic adenocarcinomas as a small portion in a series of 91 human tumors transplanted into nude mice. One of these was a poorly differentiated adenocarcinoma and was serially transplanted for three transfers. No mention of testosterone dependence was made in these studies. The prostate carcinoma cell line PC3 [28] also grows as a solid tumor in untreated male and female nude mice.

ACKNOWLEDGMENTS

We would like to thank Ms. Debra A. Kuhlman for her excellent technical assistance in all phases of this work. This work was supported in part by NIH grants CA 19840 and CA 15417 from the National Prostate Cancer Project and by the Medical Research Service of the Veterans Administration.

REFERENCES

1. Peterson LJ, Paulson DF, Bonar RA: Response of human urothelium to chemical carcinogens in vitro. J Urol 111:154–159, 1974.
2. Lasfargues EY, Ozzello L: Cultivation of human breast carcinomas. J Natl Cancer Inst 21:1131–1147, 1958.
3. Hauschka SD, Konigsberg IR: The influence of collagen on the development of muscle clones. Proc Natl Acad Sci USA 55:119–126, 1966.
4. Luft JH: Improvements in epoxy resin embedding methods. J Biophys Biochem Cytol 9:409–414, 1961.
5. Reynolds ES: The use of lead citrate at high pH as an electron-opaque stain in electron microscopy. J Cell Biol 17:208–212, 1963.
6. Harnden DG: Skin culture and solid tumor technique. In Yunis JJ (ed): "Human Chromosome Methodology," Ed 2. New York: Academic Press, 1974, pp 167–184.
7. Mittwoch U: Sex chromatin bodies. In Yunis JJ (ed): "Human Chromosome Methodology." Ed 2. New York: Academic Press, 1974, pp 73–93.
8. Seabright M: The use of proteolytic enzymes for the mapping of structural rearrangements in the chromosomes of man. Chromosoma (Berlin) 36:204–210, 1972.
9. Denk H, Radsziewicz T, Weirich E: Pronase pretreatment of tissue sections enhances sensitivity of the unlabeled antibody-enzyme (PAP) technique. J Immunol Meth 15:163–167, 1977.
10. Thomas JT: Phloxine-methylene blue staining of formalin-fixed tissue. Stain Technol 28:311–312, 1953.
11. Stonington OG, Szwec N, Webber M: Isolation and identification of the human malignant prostatic epithelial cell in pure monolayer culture. J Urol 114:903–908, 1975.
12. Stone KR, Mickey DD, Wunderli H, Mickey GH, Paulson DF: Isolation of a human

prostate carcinoma cell line (DU 145). Int J Cancer 21:274–281, 1978.

13. Mickey DD, Stone KR, Wunderli H, Mickey GH, Vollmer RT, Paulson DF: Hetero-transplantation of a human prostate adenocarcinoma cell line in nude mice. Cancer Res 37:4049–4058, 1977.
14. Webber MM: Cytopathic effects in primary epithelial cultures derived from human prostate. Invest Urol 13:259–270, 1976.
15. Ohtsuki Y, Seman G, Dmochowski L, Bowen JM, Johnson E: Brief communication: Virus-like particles in a case of human prostate carcinoma. J Natl Cancer Inst 58:1493–1496, 1977.
16. Paulson DF, Stone KR, Mickey DD, Bonar RA, Wunderli H: Development and application of basic research techniques in bladder cancer research. Cancer Res 37:2969–2973, 1977.
17. McMahon MJ, Thomas GH: Morphological changes of benign prostatic hyperplasia in culture. Br J Cancer 27:323–335, 1973.
18. Harbitz TB, Falkanger B, Sander S: Benign hyperplasia of the human prostate exposed to steroid hormones in organ culture. Acta Pathol Microbiol Scand Sect. A (Suppl) 248:80–93, 1974.
19. Schroeder FH, Mackensen SJ: Human prostatic adenoma and carcinoma in cell culture. The effects of androgen-free culture medium. Invest Urol 12:176–181, 1974.
20. Brehmer B, Marquardt H, Madsen PO: Growth and hormonal response of cells derived from carcinoma and hyperplasia of the prostate in monolayer cell culture. A possible in vitro model for clinical chemotherapy. J Urol 108:890–896, 1972.
21. McMahon MJ, Butler AVJ, Thomas GH: Morphological responses of prostatic carcinoma to testosterone in organ culture. Br J Cancer 26:388–394, 1972.
22. Okada K, Laudenbach I, Schroeder FH: Human prostatic epithelial cells in culture: Clonal selection and androgen dependence of cell line EB 33. J Urol 115:164–167, 1976.
23. Webber MM: Effects of serum on the growth of prostatic cells in vitro. J Urol 112:798–801, 1974.
24. Webber MM, Stonington OG, Poché PA: Epithelial outgrowth from suspension cultures of human prostatic tissue. In Vitro 10:196–205, 1974.
25. Okada K, Schroeder FH, Jellinghaus W, Wullstein HK, Heinemeyer HM: Human prostatic adenoma and carcinoma: Transplantation of cultured cells and primary tissue fragments in "nude mice." Invest Urol 13:395–403, 1976.
26. Sato G, Desmond W, Kelly F: Human prostatic tumors in conditioned animals and culture. Cancer Chemother Rep 59:47–49, 1975.
27. Shimosato Y, Kameya T, Nagai K, Hirohashi S, Koide T, Hayashi H, Nomura T: Transplantation of human tumors in nude mice. J Natl Cancer Inst 56:1251–1260, 1976.
28. Kaighn ME, Lechner JF, Narayan KS, Jones LW: Prostate carcinoma: Tissue culture cell lines. Natl Cancer Inst Monogr 49:17–23, 1978.

The Pasadena Cell Lines

M. E. Kaighn, PhD, J. F. Lechner, PhD, M. S. Babcock, MS,
M. Marnell, BS, Y. Ohnuki, PhD, and K. S. Narayan, PhD

Initial efforts to culture human prostatic tissue were reported more than 60 years ago in Volume 1 of the *Journal of Urology* [1]. With the exception of several articles dealing mostly with primary cultures [2–4], no further papers on the subject appeared until the early 1970s. Most cultures originated from benign prostatic hypertrophy (BPH) or prostatic carcinoma and could be maintained only briefly [5–8].

The first established line was isolated by more than 200 sequential passages of a BPH explant [9]. This line (MA 160) was thought to have arisen by "spontaneous transformation" of benign adenoma cells. Subsequent work has shown that MA 160 contains HeLa marker chromosomes as well as the rapidly migrating glucose-6-phosphodehydrogenase (G6PD) isozyme [10]. Another line, EB 33, was established in 1973 [11]. This line may also be contaminated with HeLa cells [10]. In view of this uncertainty, neither MA 160 nor EB 33 can be considered an adequate model.

In 1975 we reported the first development of clonally isolated human prostatic monolayer cultures. Of the five specimens from which cells were successfully cultured, four were diagnosed as BPH, and one was diagnosed as normal. The "normal" cells were fibroblastic [12].

In 1977 isolation of two prostatic adenocarcinoma lines metastatic to brain [13, 14] and bone [15, 16] were simultaneously reported. These appear to be the first authentic established prostatic lines available. These lines were isolated using existing methodology.

On the other hand, culture of normal prostatic epithelium presented a different problem. Primary cultures could easily be isolated [17]. However, subcultures were uniformly nonviable [18]. Development of a new, nonenzymatic method

Abbreviations: EGF = epidermal growth factor; FGF = fibroblast growth factor; HC = hydrocortisone; RPA = 12-O-tetradecanoyl-phorbol-13-acetate.

Models for Prostate Cancer, pages 85–109

made possible subculture of normal, neonatal prostatic epithelial cells capable of up to 45 population doublings [19, 20].

In this report, we will describe characteristics of human prostatic lines we have isolated and details of the procedures we have evolved.

MATERIALS AND METHODS

Human Tissues

Normal prostatic tissue was obtained from neonates who had died from respiratory failure [19, 20]. When possible, foreskin tissue was also taken for comparison. Tissue "chips" from patients with benign prostatic hypertrophy (BPH) were used to isolate these cell lines [12]. The PC-3 line was isolated from a bone metastasis of a 62-year-old Caucasian diagnosed as having undifferentiated Grade IV adenocarcinoma of the prostate [15, 16]. PC-5-PI was derived from an in situ prostatic carcinoma (Grade IV) of a 70-year-old Caucasian. PC-5-B was isolated from a bone marrow metastasis of the same patient [21]. Informed consent was obtained by established procedures. All tissue specimens were transported to the laboratory in cold nutrient medium [20] containing 10% FBS and antibiotics.

Culture Media

The nutrient media underwent a series of changes during the course of the studies reported here. Initially, we used F12K [22]. This was modified by the addition of HEPES buffer [23] and designated PFMR-1 [19]. Nutrient medium PFMR-4 was developed by further modifying F12K. PFMR-4 differs from F12K in the following components: Sodium bicarbonate and sodium chloride were reduced from 3×10^{-2} M to 1.4×10^{-2} M and 1.3×10^{-1} M to 1.0×10^{-1} M, respectively; HEPES (N-2-hydroxyethylpiperazine-N'-2-ethanesulfonic acid) buffer, 3×10^{-2} M was included; cysteine was replaced by cystine, 1.5×10^{-4} M; trace elements were included; the osmolality was reduced from 320 to 280 mOsm/kg [see Ref. 20 for details]. All nutrient media were supplemented with selected fetal bovine serum (FBS) [24, 25]. Unless otherwise specified, "growth medium" consisted of PFMR-4 containing 7% FBS. All media and other solutions were prepared in our laboratory from the purest available chemicals. Glass distilled water was used for solutions and glassware washing. All media were sterilized by membrane filtration [20].

Primary and Subcultures

Methods for the isolation and subculture of HP1-7 [12], PC-3 [15, 16], and NP-2 [19, 20] have been published. Enzymatic dispersion was used successfully with BPH and carcinoma but not with normal prostatic tissue.

Cryopreservation

Cultures were preserved in liquid nitrogen at the earliest possible passage level. This permitted repeated experiments to be carried out with the cells at similar population doubling levels. For storage in liquid nitrogen the cells were suspended in PFMR-4 medium supplemented with 20% FBS and 7.5% dimethylsulfoxide. One to three million cells were dispensed into 1.2 ml borosilicate ampoules, sealed and cooled to $-70°C$ in a Linde biological freezer at the rate of $-1°C$ per minute. The ampoules were then transferred directly to a liquid nitrogen refrigerator.

Clonal Growth Assay

Plates containing test media (4 ml/60 mm Petri dish) were equilibrated in the CO_2 incubator for one hour. Each dish was subsequently inoculated with 300 cells in 0.2 ml and incubated in an atmosphere of 2% CO_2 and 98% air at 36.5°C for seven to ten days. The colonies were fixed with 10% formalin and stained with 0.1% crystal violet. Clonal plating efficiency (PE) and the number of cells per clone were both determined. For each variable, the number of cells/clone was determined for 16 clones in four replicate dishes. The average number of population doublings/clone was calculated by dividing the $\log_{10}$ of the average number of cells/clone by $\log_{10}^2$ [20, 25, 27].

Growth in Soft Agar

Colony-forming ability in soft agar was determined at several densities ranging between 3×10^2 to 1×10^5 cells/60 mm culture dish. Serial dilutions of suspended cells were prepared in growth medium (PFMR-4, 7% FBS) containing 0.3% BactoAgar (Difco Laboratories, Detroit, MI) at 45°C. Three ml of each dilution was added as an overlay to previously prepared dishes, each containing 2 ml of 0.5% agar in growth medium. The cultures were fed after two weeks of incubation (36.5°C) with 2 ml of liquid growth medium. Colonies were scored after three weeks of growth [20].

Electron Microscopy

Cultures were fixed and processed in situ for transmission electron microscopy (TEM) as described previously [16, 19, 20]. After rinsing with HBS, the cultures were fixed at 4°C for 30–60 minutes in a mixture of 2% glutaraldehyde and 1% formaldehyde in 0.1 M sodium cacodylate buffer, pH 7.4, containing 0.1% calcium chloride. The samples were rinsed in the same buffer containing 0.25 M sucrose and fixed with 2% osmium tetroxide in 0.1 M cacodylate buffer, pH 7.4, for one to two hours at room temperature. They were then rinsed and processed either in 0.5% uranyl acetate in 50% ethanol for 15–30 minutes or in 1% tannic acid. Specimens were further processed as described previously [19].

Confluent cultures on 12 mm glass coverslips were processed for scanning electron microscopy (SEM) at room temperature using the same fixatives. Following fixation, the specimens were dehydrated in a graded series of ethanol and critical point-dried from carbon dioxide. The specimens were sputter-coated with gold-palladium prior to examination [16].

Chromosome Preparations

Four or five days after plating, the cells were treated with a final concentration of 0.05 μg/ml Colcemid (GIBCO) for two hours and then exposed to hypotonic solution (one part PFMR-4 medium: three parts distilled water) for 20–25 minutes at room temperature. The cells were fixed with freshly prepared glacial acetic acid and absolute methanol (1:3 v/v), dropped on clean slides, and allowed to air dry. Conventional Giemsa staining was used for quick surveys of ploidy and chromosome number distribution. Q-banding with quinacrine mustard [28, 29] and C-banding [30] were used routinely. Sequential staining [21] was also used to analyze cell lines with unique karyotypes with subtle chromosomal changes.

RESULTS

Cultures Derived From Benign Adenomas (BPH)

Our first attempt to isolate human prostatic cells employed enzymatic dissociation of minced tissue fragments obtained by transurethral resection (TUR). Primary cell suspensions were cloned directly. The first specimen, HP1, yielded 17 clones having both epithelial and fibroblastic morphology [12]. These cells were used mostly to work out culture conditions and in attempts to identify prostate-specific markers. All had tartrate-inhibitable acid phosphatase. However, this criterion proved of no value for cultured cells [12, 31].

All cultures derived from BPH tissues have thus far had the normal human male karyotype with some tetraploid cells. One line, HP1-7, has been studied in some detail. It is 54% diploid and 46% tetraploid. The Q-banding pattern indicates euploidy (46,XY; 92,XX,YY). Monolayers form a closely associated mosaic pattern by SEM (Fig. 1). Except for microvilli, the cell surfaces were featureless. Both the number and length of microvilli were highly variable.

The PC-3 Line

Isolation [15] and establishment of a culture of human prostatic adenocarcinoma cells has been reported [16]. This line, PC-3, was derived from a bone metastasis. Enzymatic dissociation was used. The morphology, ultrastructure, karyotype, and growth characteristics are those of an undifferentiated prostatic adenocarcinoma. Properties of this line are summarized in Table I.

PC-3 is now an established line. It grows in soft agar, in suspension culture [32], and forms tumors in nude mice. Cells identical to the original tumor-

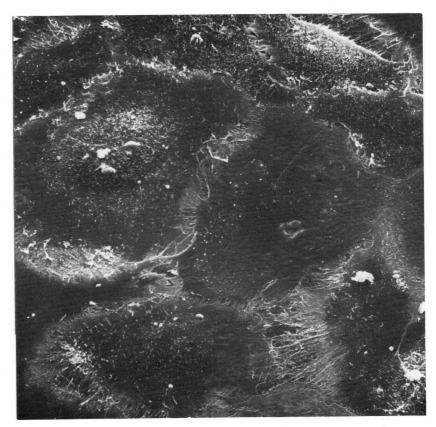

Fig. 1. Scanning electron micrograph of BPH (HP1-7) cells in vitro at seventeenth passage. The cells are typically epithelioid and show great variability in the number and length of microvilli per cell (magnification, × 650).

producing cells have been isolated and cultured from induced mouse tumors [16].

Both by phase-contrast and electron microscopy, PC-3 has epithelial characteristics [16]. A unique characteristic of PC-3 is its propensity to multilayer in loosely attached, grape-like aggregates (Figs. 2 and 3). These clusters consisted of viable but mostly nondividing cells. When examined by TEM, individual cells in these clusters (Fig. 4) appeared to be adhering to one another by junctional complexes. Such junctions were also seen between adjacent cells attached to the culture surface (Fig. 5) and between attached cells and cell clusters. Desmosomes with associated 10 nm filaments could be seen in PC-3 cells between the fourth

TABLE I. Properties of PC-3

Growth:
    1) Established line. Has undergone more than 300 population doublings.
    2) Grows in soft agar.
    3) Grows in suspension culture.
Heterotransplantation: Forms tumors in nude, athymic mice.
Chromosomes:
    1) Is 100% aneuploid with modes between 62 and 55.
    2) Has at least 11 marker chromosomes.
    3) Has unique karyotype.
Ultrastructure: Has characteristics of both epithelial and neoplastic cells.
Response to growth promoters:
    1) Has low serum dependence.
    2) Does not respond to EGF, FGF, HC.
    3) Does not respond to androgens.
Biochemical characteristics:
    1) Lacks acid phosphatase activity.
    2) Lacks 5 α-reductase activity.
    3) Has prostate-specific adenylate kinase isozyme pattern.
    4) Type B isozyme of glucose-6-phosphodehydrogenase.

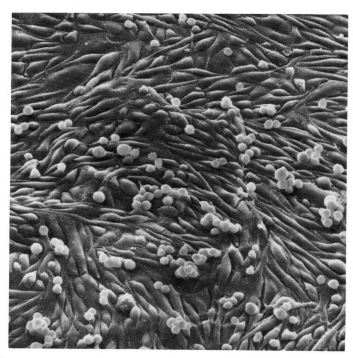

Fig. 2. Scanning electron micrograph survey of a dense culture of PC-3 cells showing the presence of spherical cells in grape-like clusters (magnification, × 200).

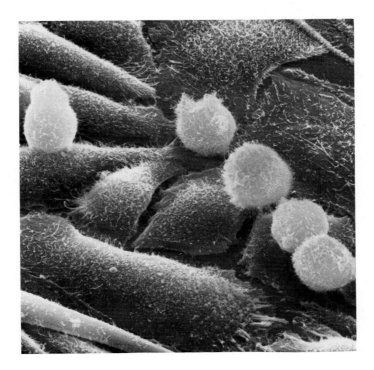

Fig. 3. Scanning electron micrograph of PC-3 cells showing the topography of rounded and attached cells at higher magnification. Note the close attachment of a rounded cell (singly at the left side of the micrograph) to a flattened cell (magnification, × 1,500).

and ninth passages (Fig. 6). Only the intermediate type of junctional complex was identified at later passages. Intercellular lumen-like spaces were often seen. No secretory granules could be identified.

Cells growing on the culture dish surface had a highly electron-dense cytoplasm. Their numerous tubular mitochondria often had structural abnormalities such as condensed matrices and aberrant cristae (Figs. 6 and 7). Free polyribosomes and lysosome-like structures were seen frequently (Figs. 5–7). Golgi structures and rough endoplasmic reticulum were rarely present. These cells also had annulate lamellae (Fig. 7). Their nuclei were often invaginated and contained homogeneously distributed euchromatin. Nucleoli were large, compact, and highly electron dense (Fig. 5).

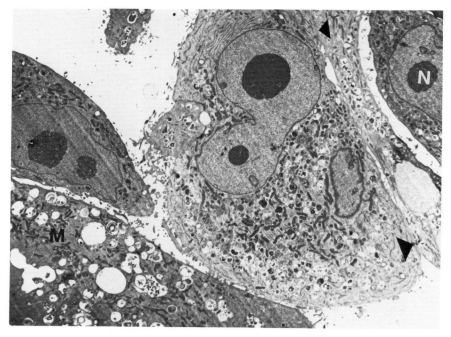

Fig. 4. Ultrastructure of spherical cells as seen by transmission electron microscopy of sections cut through the middle of an aggregate. Note the presence of large nucleoli (N), numerous dense mitochondria (M), and lysosomes (L). The electron micrograph also shows a few junctional complexes (arrows) (magnification, × 3,000).

Although ultrastructure of the cells in clusters was generally similar to that of cells attached to the surface, they differed in some respects. Their nuclear invaginations were more pronounced (Fig. 4). They also had increased numbers of abnormal mitochondria, abundant lysosomes, and dense bodies, many of which could be considered cytolysosomes or teleolysosomes (Fig. 4).

SEM studies showed that both attached and clustered cells had numerous microvilli of variable length (Fig. 3). Occasional cells showed blebs or other surface modifications.

PC-3 has a radically reduced dependence on serum for growth [26, 33]. It does not respond to growth factors (EGF, FGF), or to steroids (corticosteroids, androgens, and estrogens). Furthermore, clones have been isolated that are able to grow in serum-free medium (unpublished results).

The chromosomes of PC-3 are characteristic of advanced neoplasia. It is completely aneuploid with modes between 62 and 55 chromosomes [21]. It has

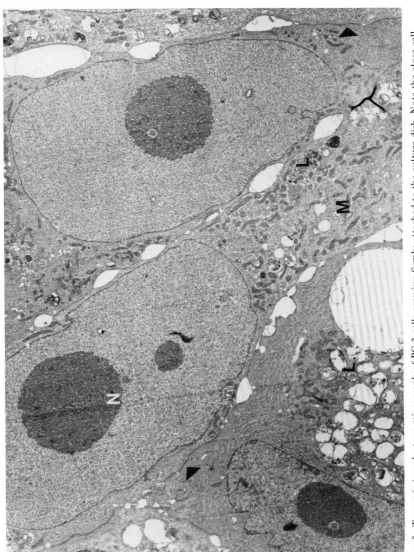

Fig. 5. Transmission electron micrograph of PC-3 cells growing firmly attached to the culture dish. Note the close cell–cell junctions (arrows), large compact nucleoli (N), numerous lysosomes (L), and mitochondria (M). The large membrane-bound granule in the lowermost cell in the micrograph is probably the remnant of an incompletely preserved lipid body (magnification, × 5,000).

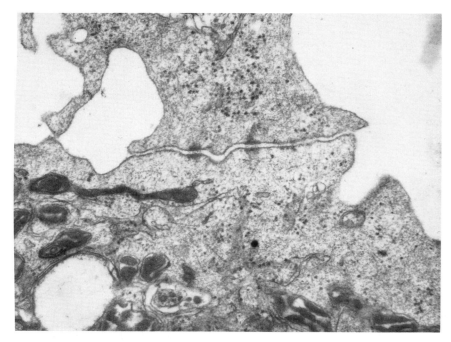

Fig. 6. Higher magnification of adherent PC-3 cells showing spot-desmosomes between two cells. Note the condensed dense matrices in the mitochondria (magnification, × 70,000).

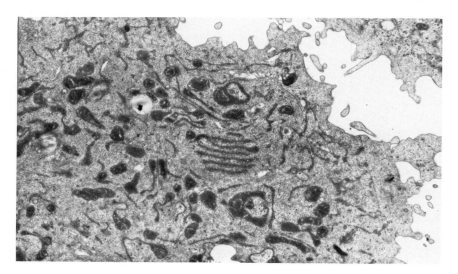

Fig. 7. Higher magnification of a spherical PC-3 cell showing the presence of annulate lamellae (arrow). Note also the presence of mitochondria with highly condensed matrices and aberrant cristae structure (magnification, × 14,000).

a characteristic karyotype with at least 11 distinct marker chromosomes. The overall karyotype and markers clearly distinguish PC-3 from HeLa or other established human lines (Fig. 8). Further, it has the fast-migrating, Type B glucose-6-phosphodehydrogenase isozyme found in Caucasians, as well as a prostate-specific adenylate kinase isozyme pattern [16]. Since PC-3 was derived from a metastasis nonresponsive to antiandrogen therapy, it is not surprising that it lacks testosterone 5 α-reductase and acid phosphatase activities [16].

Normal Cultures

Until recently, normal prostatic epithelial cells have not been successfully sub-cultured [17, 18]. Our experience has been that enzymes, especially trypsin, somehow destroy the division potential of these cells. For this reason we developed a two-step non-enzymatic method of subculture [19, 20]. Two cell types were observed in primary cultures. The smaller, cuboidal s-type, was found primarily in the supernatant of the tissue mince. The e-type was more commonly seen migrating from larger tissue fragments. No fibroblasts were seen. Both cell types were successfully subcultured with the "K-passing" procedure. After five such passages, both lines could be passed enzymatically. Both NP-2s and NP-2e were preserved in liquid N_2 at early passage levels [19].

Available criteria indicate that both lines have characteristics expected of normal glandular epithelium. Cytogenetic analysis by banding techniques demon-strated that both lines have the normal human male karyotype. At least until the ninth passage, equivalent to 25 population doublings, the karyotype remained unchanged (Fig. 9).

Scanning electron microscopy of subconfluent and confluent NP-2s cultures showed the surfaces of most cells to be smooth and devoid of major modifications (Fig. 10). The cells were typically polygonal in shape arranged in a closely opposed, nonoverlapping pattern. Closely adherent regions of adjacent cells had prominent ridges, which may represent the various types of junctional complexes distinguish-able by TEM.

The ultrastructure of NP-2s cells as seen in the TEM, showed the presence of spot desmosomes and 10 nm tonofilaments, thus establishing their epithelial nature. However, such complexes were less frequent than other types of junc-tional complexes. The intermediate type junctional complex, macula adherens, was clearly identified (Figs. 11 and 12). Although tight junctions or gap junctions were probably present, confirmation of their identity by freeze-fracture replica studies has not yet been done.

Groups of closely associated NP-2s cells often formed lumen-like regions reminiscent of glandular epithelia in vivo. Microvilli were often observed on the luminal surfaces (Fig. 11). The cytoplasm contained numerous mitochondria and clusters of free polyribosomes. The nuclei were ovoid with densely staining nucleoli, showing typical nucleolonemal structures (Figs. 11 and 12). The

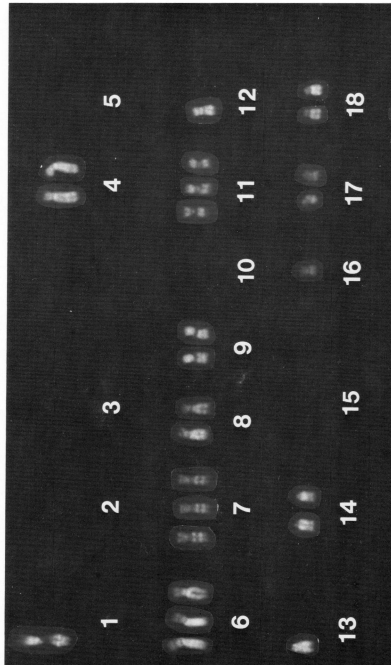

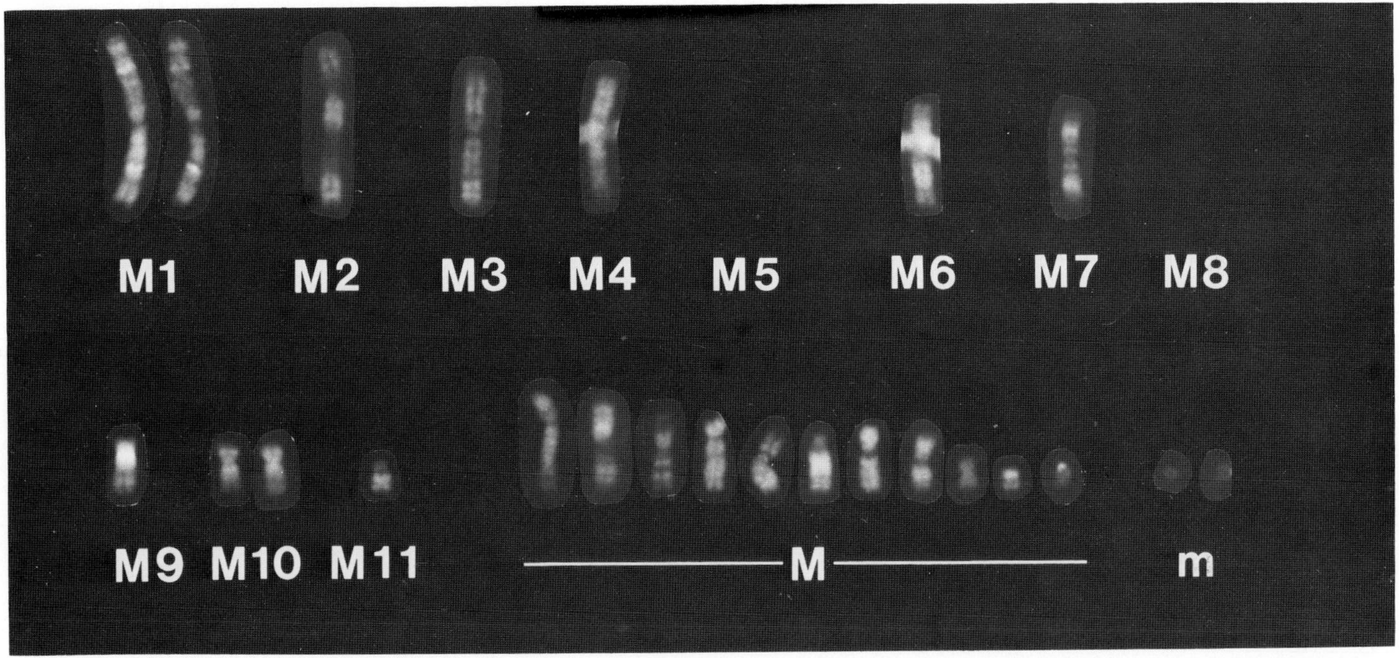

Fig. 8. Q-band karyotype of a PC-3 cell at the thirtieth passage with 59 chromosomes, including 22 markers (M1, M2, M3, M4, M6, M7, M9, M10, M11, and Ms). Besides these, two minute chromosomes (m) are observed.

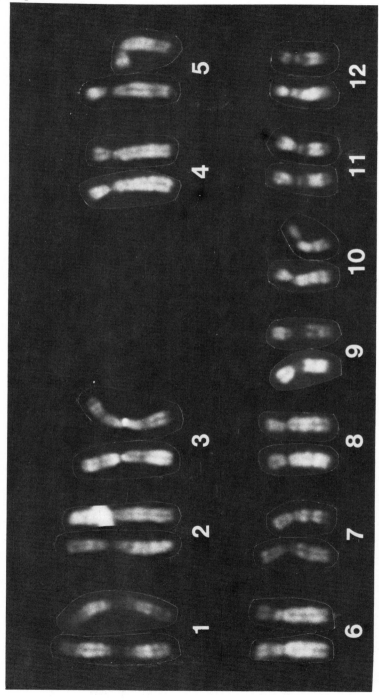

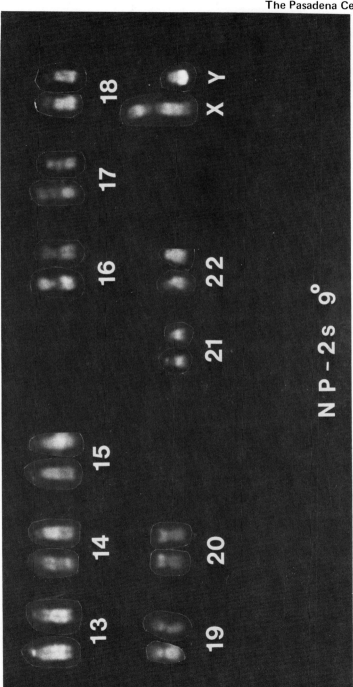

Fig. 9. Karyotype of a Q-banded metaphase of NP-2s cell line at the ninth passage. The gross morphology and banding patterns of individual chromosomes show normal human male karyotype.

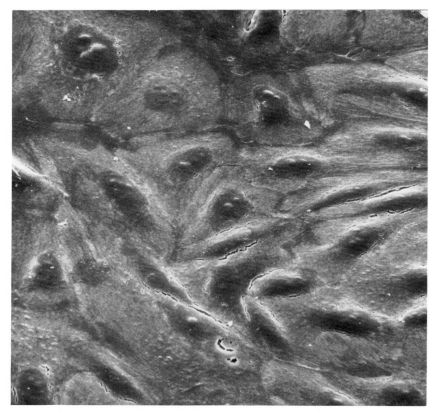

Fig. 10. Scanning electron micrograph of a group of normal prostate epithelial (NP-2s) cells in culture. The cells are epithelioid and are closely opposed to one another. Note the very smooth surface of the cells (magnification, × 680).

chromatin was predominantly homogeneous with moderate electron density. In addition to perinuclear Golgi, many small membrane-bound dense granules were usually found in close proximity to intercellular spaces (Fig. 12). They resembled secretory granules. The concomitant presence of Golgi, rough endoplasmic reticulum, and secretory-like granules provides evidence for the secretory nature of these cells.

The NP-2e line was larger and more flattened in monolayer culture than NP-2s cells [19]. TEM studies showed them to be composed largely of cells with oblong nuclei (Fig. 13). Cell—cell junctions were mostly of the intermediate type. The

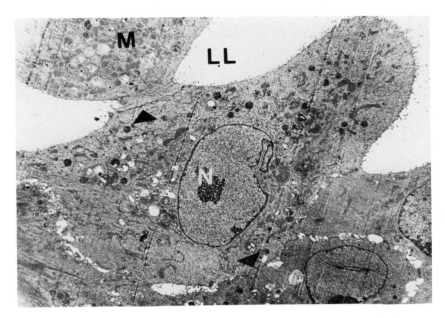

Fig. 11. Low magnification micrograph of a group of NP-2s cells showing overall ultrastruc-ture, cell–cell junctions (arrows), and tendency of the cells to form large intercellular lumen-like (LL) regions. Note the presence of microvilli on the free surfaces of the cells in the lumen-like regions. (N = nucleolus; M = mitochondria; magnification, × 2,100).

presence of 10 nm tonofilaments was easily recognized in these cells and served to establish their epithelial identity. Intercellular lumen-like areas were also observed. The mitochondria were more tubular than those of NP-2s cells. In contrast to the abundant free polyribosomes seen in the NP-2s cells, ribosomes were predominantly associated with the endoplasmic reticulum. Golgi and small, membrane-bound granules were seen less frequently than in NP-2s. Tonofilaments were more apparent in the perinuclear region than in NP-2s cells (Fig. 14).

A striking feature of the cytoplasm was the presence of many large lysosome-like structures containing closely packed membranous whorls, dense bodies that were sometimes identifiable as mitochondrial degradation products and multivesicu-lar bodies (Fig. 14). These, in all probability, were various stages of primary and secondary cytolysosomes.

Although there are some ultrastructural differences between the e and s lines, overall they are quite similar. The properties of NP-2s are summarized in Table II.

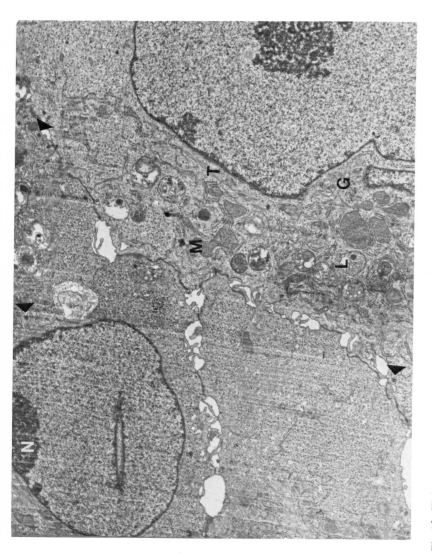

Fig. 12. Higher magnification of NP-2s cells showing some details of fine structure. Arrows point to small membrane-bound dense granules that could be secretory granules. Note the presence of both free and membrane-bound poly-ribosomes. (G = Golgi; L = lysosomes; M = mitochondria; N = nucleolus; T = tonofilaments; magnification, × 7,000).

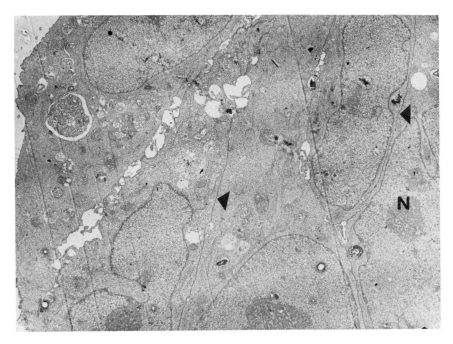

Fig. 13. Transmission electron micrograph of NP-2e cells showing oblong nuclei and long stretches of cell-cell junctional complexes (arrows). (N = nucleolus; magnification, × 3,000).

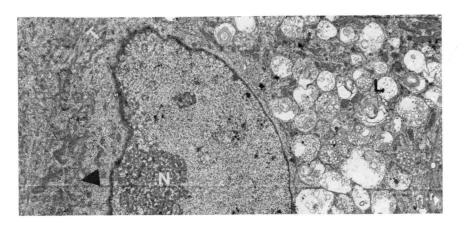

Fig. 14. Higher magnification of a portion of NP-2e cells. Note the presence of tonofilaments (T), many helical polyribosomes (arrow, for example), and many lysosomes (L). (N = nucleolus; magnification, × 11,700).

TABLE II. Properties of NP-2s

Growth:
1) Has finite life-span of 40–45 population doublings.
2) No growth in soft agar.
Heterotransplantation: Does not form tumors in nude mice.
Chromosomes: Euploid human male karyotype at all passage levels.
Ultrastructure: Has characteristics of normal glandular epithelium.
Response to growth promoters:
1) Serum requirement synergistically spared by HC with EGF or FGF.
2) Calcium requirement spared by EGF.
3) Growth rate increased by TPA.
Biochemical characteristics:
1) Converts testosterone to dihydrotestosterone indicative of 5 α-reductase activity.
2) Has low acid phosphatase activity.

The Effect of EGF on Culture Life-Span

Studies on the improvement and definition of media for prostatic cells are the subject of a companion paper [33]. These nutritional studies have shown that the growth rate of normal and benign prostatic epithelial cultures is enhanced by EGF and hydrocortisone [20, 26]. Since it had been shown that growth factors could extend the multiplication potential of some cell lines [20, 34], we determined the effectiveness of EGF to extend the division potential of these prostatic cell lines. The results were compared to studies using normal human fibroblasts (NF2). A modified clonal growth assay was used, since cells growing at clonal density do not alter medium composition [35]. Thus, the EGF concentration did not change appreciably during the experiment. The NP-2s cells had undergone 15 population doublings at the onset of the experiment, whereas HP1-7 and NF2 had doubled 39 and 24 times in culture, respectively. The cells had not been previously exposed to EGF.

The longevity data are summarized in Table III. A more detailed description of these experiments has been published [20]. The growth factors extended the division potential of NP-2s by 135%. Continuous exposure to EGF improved plating efficiency (400%) and decreased population doubling time (140%). It did not increase the division potential of HP1-7. However, compared with the normal epithelial cells, the culture life-span of HP1-7 was already significantly greater (180%). EGF also decreased the generation time of HP1-7, but did not influence its plating efficiency. The foreskin fibroblast line, NF2, which is genetically identical to NP-2s had a culture life-span 140% greater than that of NP-2s. EGF did not extend its life-span.

TABLE III. Effect of EGF on Multiplication Potential of Cultured Cells*

Cell line	CPD[a]		Enhancement %
	− EGF	+ EGF	
NP-2s	37.3	48.9	131
HP1-7	72.4	78.3	108
NF2	66.1	69.4	105

*A modified clonal growth assay was used to acquire these data. Initially, 16 replicate clonal plates were inoculated, each with 300 cells in 4 ml of growth medium. Eight of these plates received EGF (5 ng/ml), the other eight served as control. After 7–10 days of incubation, four plates each from both the control and experimental (EGF) groups were fixed and stained. The plating efficiency and the average population doublings/clone were determined (see Materials and Methods). A subsequent series of eight clonal plates was then established using the pooled cells dissociated from the four remaining unfixed replicate plates of each group. Cells that had been grown with EGF were replated in EGF-containing medium. Cells from control plates were replated without EGF. This procedure was continued until the cells no longer formed colonies. The CPD was the sum of the average population doublings per clonal passage series.
[a]Cumulative population doublings.

DISCUSSION

The basic objectives of our program have been to isolate replicative epithelial cell cultures from normal and neoplastic human prostatic tissue. Replicative cultures have been isolated from normal, benign prostatic adenoma and neoplastic human tissues by a combination of existing and newly developed methods. Previous methodologies used to culture differentiated cells were successfully applied both to BPH and metastatic carcinoma tissue [12, 15, 16]. However, for the isolation of normal prostatic epithelial cells from neonatal tissue, a new non-enzymatic procedure had to be developed [19, 20]. Careful selection of serum was essential in the early stages of this work and probably, in conjunction with the earlier developed techniques of cell dissociation, permitted isolation of the BPH and carcinoma lines. Although available methods are adequate, they are not routine. Much remains to be learned both about methods for dissociating epithelial cells and about their nutritional requirements.

Two types of cell have resisted our attempts to establish cultures. Although we have been successful in establishing cell lines from metastatic carcinoma, we have not had equivalent success in establishing cells from primary prostatic tumors. Of course, the problem of identifying tumor cells is much more difficult in a primary rather than a metastatic lesion. The second problem area is the culture of normal adult prostatic epithelium. Although, as in the case of other primary cultures, it is possible to obtain epithelial outgrowths in non-enzymatically treated cultures of this type of tissue, successful passage has not been achieved. Our second, probably more fundamental, problem involved with attempting to culture so-called normal adult tissue is that of identifying what is and what is not normal, since benign adenomas developed in an increasing percentage of adults with age [36]. The question could always be asked: "If the cell grows, has it arisen from normal epithelial cells or from an adenoma? "

What have we learned so far by use of these cell lines? Efforts to characterize the cells have revealed several important differences between normal and cancer-derived cultures. On the ultrastructural level, both surface and internal structures characteristic of normal and neoplastic prostatic tissue appear to persist in culture. Furthermore, chromosomal differences are noted early and are also perpetuated. However, as in the case of other cancer lines, karyotypic evolution occurs with continued culture. When PC-3 is passed through a nude mouse, its characteristic chromosomal constitution remains [16].

Major differences in response to nutrients and growth-controlling factors have been noted between normal and neoplastic cell types. Significant differences in such responses have also been observed between fibroblastic and epithelial cell types derived from the same individual [20, 26, 27]. In normal, but not in neoplastic cells, interesting interactions between growth-controlling factors have been observed. For example, synergistic reduction in serum requirements of normal cells have been observed when both hydrocortisone and EGF are added to the growth medium [20, 26].

Another observation that may be significant in the development of prostatic cancer is the possible interaction of growth-promoting agents with tumor promoters such as phorbol esters. TPA acts as a growth promoter in a dose-response fashion for the normal prostatic epithelial cell. On the other hand, if EGF is present in the medium the phorbol somehow inhibits the growth-promoting activity of EGF [33, 37].

In addition to the above findings, we have been able to transform a normal epithelial prostatic cell by the oncogenic virus, SV40 [38, 39]. The normal life-span of the NP-2s line is approximately 30–35 population doublings. If EGF is present in the medium, this is extended to 40–45 population doublings. Infection with SV40 virus extends this life-span manyfold. In fact, this extension in life-span, or escape from growth limitation, provides a simple means of isolating SV40-transformed cells. The transformed cells have altered responses to growth-promoting agents, ultrastructure similar to that of metastatic prostatic carcinoma cells, and variable, but significant, chromosomal changes [38, 39]. Thus, a system is now available for studying sequential changes in carcinogenesis of the human prostate in vitro.

It is obviously important to characterize the cell lines originating from different types of prostatic tissue. The question is what can and what cannot be identified? First, normal and frankly neoplastic cells are readily distinguished by several criteria. Most important of these are ultrastructural, chromosomal, and growth properties. Epithelial cells can generally be distinguished from their fibroblastic counterparts by virtue of their morphology in phase contrast and by ultrastructural differences. In particular, epithelial cells have extensive junctional complexes usually not found in fibroblasts. The presence of desmosomes, together with 10 nm tonofilaments, is characteristic of epithelial cells [40].

Another problem that must be considered is the possible adventitious contamination of prostatic cell cultures with other human cell lines. Two previously described presumptive prostatic carcinoma lines have been considered HeLa contaminants [10]. This type of problem can be essentially ruled out by karyotypic examination and determination of the glucose-6-phosphodehydrogenase isozyme pattern [10]. Thus, distinguishing normal from neoplastic and epithelial from other general cell types is quite straightforward in extreme instances.

When the differences between cell types are less dramatic, identification becomes more difficult. This overall problem can only be solved by a greater understanding of the characteristics of cultured cells derived from various tissues. It is important to stress that most of the reliable markers are genotypic or constitutive in nature. On the other hand, functional characteristics attributed to specific tissues are often under regulatory control. Such properties may not be expressed in dividing cells.

Obviously it would be desirable to be able to identify unequivocally the nature and origin of cell lines derived from prostatic tissue [42]. Unfortunately, established prostate-specific markers are not available. Those characteristics that have been suggested as specific markers (acid phosphatase, androgen responsiveness, androgen-metabolizing enzymes, and specific antigens) are based on studies of prostatic tissue in vivo [42]. The biologic nature of the prostate contributes to this problem of identification. In the adult organ the cells are probably terminally differentiated. In normal tissue cellular multiplication has not been observed. On the other hand, the neonatal cell population contains undifferentiated "stem" cells. These stem cells divide repeatedly to populate the organ, then differentiate and begin to express prostate-specific functions [43]. Thus, expression of prostate-specific characteristics would not be expected in cultures of neonatal prostatic stem cells. Understanding of the mechanism and conditions that promote prostatic differentiation poses a challenging problem for future research. Such understanding would furnish important clues to the mechanism of carcinogenesis of the prostate.

ACKNOWLEDGMENTS

Supported by Public Health Service (PHS) grant R26-CA19826-01 from the National Cancer Institute through the National Prostatic Cancer Project, and PHS contract N01-CP-75850 from the Division of Cancer Cause and Prevention,

National Cancer Institute (NCI). We thank B. Serar and T. Smith for technical assistance and Dr. D.D. Mickey, Duke University, for nude mice studies with the normal cells.

REFERENCES

1. Burrows MT, Burns JE, Suzuki Y: Studies on the growth of cells. The cultivation of bladder and prostatic tumors outside the body. J Urol 1:3–15, 1917.
2. Röhl L: Prostatic hyperplasia and carcinoma studied with tissue culture technique. Acta Chir Scand (Suppl)240:7–88, 1959.
3. Bergman RU, Bergman ET: Tissue culture of benign and malignant human genitourinary tumors. J Urol 86:642–649, 1961.
4. Fadei L, Nachtigal M: Primary cultivation of human tumors by trypsinization procedure. Archiv Geschwulst 21:201–207, 1963.
5. Schröeder FH, Sato G, Gittes RF: Human prostatic adenocarcinoma: Growth in monolayer tissue culture. J Urol 106:734–739, 1971.
6. Brehmer B, Riemann JF, Bloodworth JMB Jr, Madsen PO: Electron microscopic appearance of cells from carcinoma of the prostate in monolayer tissue culture. Urol Res 1:27–31, 1973.
7. Webber MM, Stonington OG, Poché PA: Epithelial outgrowth from suspension cultures of human prostatic tissue. In Vitro 10:196–205, 1974.
8. Franks LM: Research methods. Tissue culture in the investigation of prostatic cancer. Urol Res 5:159–162, 1977.
9. Fraley EE, Ecker S, Vincent MM: Spontaneous in vitro neoplastic transformation of adult human prostatic epithelium. Science 170:540–542, 1970.
10. Nelson-Rees WA, Flandermeyer RR: HeLa cultures defined. Science 191:96–98, 1976.
11. Okada K, Schröeder FH: Human prostatic carcinoma in cell culture: Preliminary report on the development and characterization of an epithelial cell line (EB 33). Urol Res 2:111–121, 1974.
12. Kaighn ME, Babcock MS: Monolayer cultures of human prostatic cells. Cancer Chemother Rep 59:59–63, 1975.
13. Mickey DD, Stone KR, Wunderli H, Mickey GH, Vollmer RT, Paulson DF: Heterotransplantation of a human prostatic adenocarcinoma cell line in nude mice. Cancer Res 37:4049–4058, 1977.
14. Stone KR, Mickey DD, Wunderli H, Mickey GH, Paulson DF: Isolation of a human prostate carcinoma cell line (DU 145). Int J Cancer 21:274–281, 1978.
15. Kaighn ME, Lechner JF, Narayan KS, Jones LW: Prostate carcinoma: Tissue culture cell lines. Natl Cancer Inst Monogr 49:17–21, 1978.
16. Kaighn ME, Narayan KS, Ohnuki Y, Lechner JF, Jones LW: Establishment and characterization of a human prostatic carcinoma cell line (PC-3). Invest Urol 17:16–23, 1979.
17. Webber MM: Effects of serum on the growth of prostatic cells in vitro. J Urol 112:798–801, 1974.
18. Mickey DD, Stone KR, Stone MP, Paulson DF: Morphologic and immunologic studies of human prostatic carcinoma. Cancer Treat Rep 61:133–138, 1977.
19. Lechner JF, Narayan KS, Ohnuki Y, Babcock MS, Jones LW, Kaighn ME: Replicative epithelial cell cultures from normal human prostate gland. J Natl Cancer Inst 60:797–801, 1978.
20. Lechner JF, Babcock MS, Marnell M, Narayan KS, Kaighn ME: Normal human prostate epithelial cell cultures. In Harris C, Trump BF, Stoner GD (eds): "Methods and Per-

spectives in Cell Biology; Cultured Human Cells and Tissues in Biomedical Research."
New York: Academic Press, Vol II, Ch 8 (in press).

21. Ohnuki Y, Marnell MM, Babcock MS, Lechner JF, Kaighn ME: Chromosomal analysis of human prostatic adenocarcinoma cell lines. Cancer Res (submitted).

22. Kaighn ME: Human liver cells. In Kruse PF Jr, Patterson MK Jr (eds): "Tissue Culture: Methods and Applications." New York: Academic Press, 1973, pp 54–58.

23. Kaighn ME: Characteristics of human prostatic cell cultures. Cancer Treat Rep 61:147–151, 1977.

24. Kaighn ME: Choice, treatment, and storage of sera for the growth of specialized cells. In Vitro Monogr 3:21, 1973.

25. Kaighn ME: "Birth of a Culture" – Source of postpartum anomalies. J Natl Cancer Inst 53:1437–1442, 1974.

26. Lechner JF, Kaighn ME: Application of the principles of enzyme kinetics to clonal growth rates: An approach for delineating interactions among growth promoting agents. J Cell Physiol 100:519–530, 1979.

27. Lechner JF, Kaighn ME: Reduction of the calcium requirement of normal human epithelial cells by EGF. Exp Cell Res 121:432–435, 1979.

28. Caspersson T, Zech L, Johansson C: Differential binding of alkylating fluorochromes in human chromosomes. Exp Cell Res 60:315–319, 1970.

29. Uchida IA, Lin CC: Quinacrine fluorescent patterns. In Yunis JJ (ed): "Human Chromosome Methodology," New York: Academic Press, 1974, p 47–58.

30. Arrighi FE, Hsu TC: Localization of heterochromatin in human chromosomes. Cytogenetics 10:81–86, 1971.

31. Kaighn ME: Measurement of acid phosphatase activity in various tissues and cultured cells. Natl Cancer Inst Monogr 49:59–60, 1978.

32. Russell P: Personal communication, 1978.

33. Lechner JF, Kaighn ME: Nutrition of prostate cells (this volume).

34. Rheinwald JF, Green H: Epidermal growth factor and the multiplication of cultured human epidermal keratinocytes. Nature 265:421–424, 1977.

35. McKeehan WL, Ham RG: Calcium and magnesium ions and the regulation of multiplication in normal and transformed cells. Nature 275:756–758, 1978.

36. Catalona WJ, Scott WW: Carcinoma of the prostate: A review. J Urol 119:1–8, 1978.

37. Lechner JF, Kaighn ME: Differential effect of phorbol esters on the growth rate of normal human epithelial and fibroblastic cells. In Vitro 15:225, 1979.

38. Lechner JF, Kaighn ME: Altered properties of human prostatic epithelial cells transformed by SV40 virus. In Vitro 15:227, 1979.

39. Narayan KS, Ohnuki Y, Babcock MS, Marnell M: Ultrastructural and karyologic changes in SV40 transformed human prostatic epithelial cell lines. In Vitro 15:207, 1979.

40. Franks LM, Wilson PD: Origin and ultrastructure of cells in vitro. Int Rev Cytol 48:55–139, 1977.

41. Bischoff R, Holtzer H: Mitosis and the process of differentiation of myogenic cells in vitro. J Cell Biol 41:188–200, 1969.

42. Merchant DJ: Prostatic tissue cell growth and assessment. Semin Oncol 3:131–140, 1976.

43. Franks LM: Primary culture of human prostate. In Harris C, Trump BF, Stoner GD (eds): "Methods and Perspectives in Cell Biology; Cultured Human Cells and Tissues in Biomedical Research." New York: Academic Press, Vol II, Ch 8 (in press).

The Miami Cell Line (UMS-1541)

Theodore I. Malinin and Alice J. Claflin

Tissues from consecutive human carcinomatous prostate glands were subjected to short-term in vitro cultivation in our laboratory during the past five years. In the course of these studies a culture initiated from pieces of tissue obtained at TUR for relief of obstruction behaved in an unusual manner. The growth of cells in this culture was more vigourous than in any other culture. Furthermore, no decline in cell growth occurred with ensuing passages, as was the case with all other cultures carried beyond a few initial passages. Additionally, the cells in culture maintained their epithelial appearance. Because of these characteristics of the culture, it was decided to allow it to continue instead of freezing the cells in early passages and terminating the experiment, as was our practice with all other cultures. After the culture exceeded 130 passages and the cells from frozen stock were passed over 60 passages a preliminary report was made at the 1978 meeting of the Tissue Culture Association describing this culture [1]. At the time the report was made it was stressed that the cells in the described cell line (UMS-1541) were not characterized and that a subsequent report on the culture would be made once such characterization was performed.

Initial chromosome karyotyping performed on cells in the twenty-ninth passage revealed 46 chromosomes of normocentric appearance. However, the predominant chromosome number was found to be 42 in virtually all subsequent cultures. Furthermore, the chromosomes in these cultures were acrocentric. These studies, the chromosome banding patterns, and the immunofluorescent studies with rat and human sera demonstrated the cells in the described culture to be of rat origin. Lactate dehydrogenase and the glucose-6-phosphate dehydrogenase isozyme mobilities of cells were comparable to rat cell control preparations.

The only cultures of rat tissue worked with in our laboratory were those of

Models for Prostate Cancer, pages 111–114

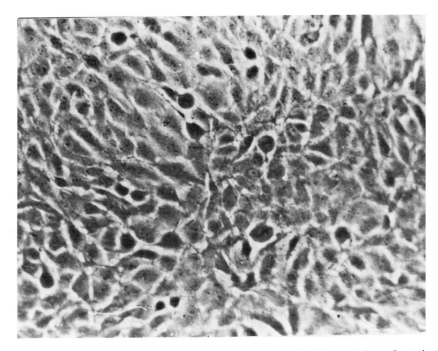

Fig. 1. Photograph of the cells in culture. The cells exhibit epithelial morphology. Several mitotic figures are present (unstained phase-contrast photomicrograph; magnification, × 120).

transplantable Dunning adenocarcinoma R-3327. The cells from these tumors were routinely dispersed for tansplantation as well as cultured in our laboratory. Thus, the presumptive evidence suggests that cell line UMS-1541 is a cell line of Dunning rat adenocarcinoma rather than human adenocarcinoma. The cell culture is still very interesting. It maintains its epithelial appearance even after 130 passages (Fig. 1) and is extremely fast growing. The doubling time of the cells calculated by the method of Hayflick [2] is approximately ten hours. In a further experiment 1.5×10^6 cells from this culture were injected subcutaneously into flanks of each of four aged Copenhagen male rats. Three weeks after the injection one rat had developed a hard nodule 4 mm in diameter. The animal was sacrificed and the nodule was examined histologically. This revealed islets of poorly differentiated neoplastic tissue and small islets of tissue with distinct glandular pattern (Fig. 2).

Interspecies contamination of cell cultures is a relatively frequent although unforunate occurrence [3] . It seems apparent that in this instance human cell

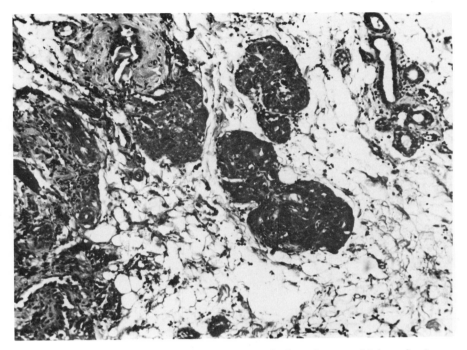

Fig. 2. Histologic section of a nodule from the flank of a Copnehagen rat 21 days after injection of the cultured cells into the site. The photograph shows solid tumor nodules and a glandular neoplastic structure (hematoxylin and eosin stain; magnification, × 120).

culture was cross-contaminated with rat cells and that rat cells eventually constituted the sole population of the culture. At which stage and how this contamination took place is impossible to determine. The resulting culture nevertheless may be of some biological interest. If our presumptions are correct, it is a culture derived from the Dunning rat adenocarcinoma.

The culture is no longer carried in our laboratory, but an adequate number of cells has been placed in the frozen repository.

ACKNOWLEDGMENTS

This investigation was supported in part by grant No 5R26CA15480-06 SRS, awarded by the National Cancer Institute, National Prostatic Cancer Project, DHEW.

We wish to thank Drs. E. Kaighn, S. Pathak, and W.D. Patterson, Jr., for their aid in identifying the cells.

REFERENCES

1. Malinin TI, Claflin AJ, Block NL, Garces MC: Isolation of human cell line (UMS-1541) from carcinoma of the prostate gland. In Vitro 14:367, 1978.
2. Hayflick L: Subculturing human diploid fibroblast cultures. In Kruse PF Jr, Patterson MK Jr (eds): "Tissue Culture, Methods and Applications." Academic Press, New York: 1973, pp 220–223.
3. Frogh J (ed): "Contamination in Tissue Culture." New York: Academic Press, 1973.

The LNCaP Cell Line—A New Model for Studies on Human Prostatic Carcinoma

Julius S. Horoszewicz, MD, DMSc, Susan S. Leong, PhD, T. Ming Chu, PhD, Zew L. Wajsman, MD, Moshe Friedman, MD, Lawrence Papsidero, PhD, Untae Kim, MD, Lee S. Chai, MS, Surabhi Kakati, PhD, Suresh K. Arya, PhD, and Avery A. Sandberg, MD

Human prostatic cancer each year claims over 18,000 lives in the United States. Clinical trials aimed at the development of the most effective methods of management of this disease are by their very nature and for obvious reasons necessarily limited in scope, because of long duration, high cost, and several constraints imposed by ethical considerations. Therefore the need for the most appropriate preclinical models of human prostatic neoplasia is apparent.

Experimental studies on the available models of rodent prostatic carcinoma reviewed by Coffrey et al [1] are highly useful in providing us with a better understanding of the biology of prostatic malignancy. These transplantable and easily grown in vitro tumors represent a collection of neoplasms originating in rat prostate. A wide spectrum of preserved biological and biochemical markers, hormonal responsiveness, malignancy, and drug sensitivity contributes significantly to their attractiveness as animal model systems. Their limitations are rooted in restrictions imposed by difficulties in direct translation of data obtained in an animal model system into the language of human disease.

Heterotransplantation of human prostatic tumors into nude mice has been attempted by several investigators, but the results, with few exceptions, were disappointing. Reid and co-workers [2, 3] reported that only one out of over 100 tumor specimens developed into a somewhat differentiated transplantable tumor

Models for Prostate Cancer, pages 115–132

in the nude mice. The properties of this tumor are modulated by androgens, and trace amounts of tartarate were observed to inhibit acid phosphatase. Similar and discouraging results are reported by Gittes (this volume).

None of the human cell lines described thus far derived from prostatic malignancies have gained wide acceptance as fully suitable human models, since they lack characteristic markers that could unequivocally identify their derivation from human prostatic malignant cells. The task of growing in vitro epithelial prostatic cells either from animals or from man is a difficult one, as evidenced by numerous publications focused on only short-term organ and cell cultures [4–12]. Prostatic cell lines MA 160 [13] and EB 33 [14] which were frequently used experimentally and widely quoted in literature, were found in fact to be HeLa cell contaminants [15]. New techniques for initiation of cultures from human prostates were described by Stonington and Hemmingsen [16]. Brehmer et al [17, 18] grew for approximately three months cells from protatic carcinoma and benign prostatic hyperplasia (BPH). Kaighn and Babcock [19] established a cell line from BPH which at three weeks showed intracellular tartarate-inhibited acid phosphatase. Webber et al [20, 21] were successful in propagating human prostatic epithelium as explant cultures over a period of a few weeks, and they were also able to make valuable observations on the morphology and properties of prepubertal prostate in vitro. Recently Mickey et al [22] and Stone et al [23] isolated an epithelial cell line, DU 145, from an individual with leukemia and prostatic adenocarcinoma metastasis to the brain. Similarly, Kaighn [24, 25] was able to grow epithelioid cells (line PC-3) from a CaP metastasis to a bone. Both cell lines are tumorigenic in nude mice. Neither line, however, appears to be responsive to sex hormones; no significant levels of acid phosphatase in cultures were observed, and organ-specific prostatic antigens were not reported.

In this chapter we summarize the results of our research directed toward isolation from metastatic lesions of human malignant cells that can be grown in vitro and are endowed with properties characteristic of prostatic epithelium.

CLINICAL HISTORY

The patient (S.I.) was a 50-year-old white male who one year prior to admission was diagnosed as having stage D_1 prostatic cancer. The diagnosis was based on needle biopsy of the prostate and retroperitoneal lymph node exploration. The review of pathology of primary biopsy had revealed moderately differentiated adenocarcinoma of the prostate (Fig. 1). He was treated initially with oral estrogen, but six months later disseminated bony metastases were found on bone scan. The patient has since undergone orchiectomy, with only mild subjective and temporary response.

One month before admission, pain in the right flank radiating to his right leg was observed, and the patient was referred to Roswell Park Memorial Institute. On physical examination, a hard enlarged prostate was palpated; no other

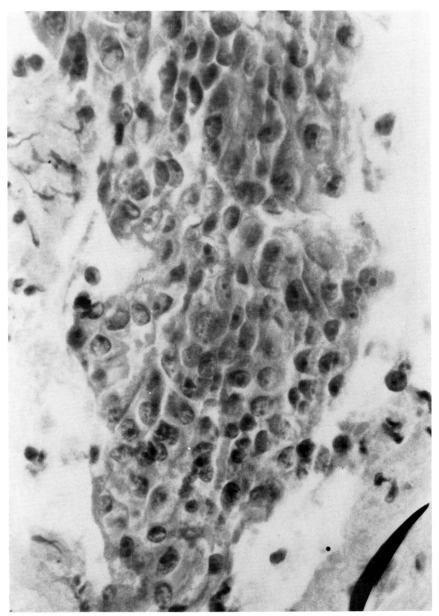

Fig. 1. Photomicrograph of histological section of prostatic needle biopsy from patient S.I. (hematoxylin and eosin stain; magnification, × 180).

abnormalities were found on physical examination. The serum acid phosphatase was 56 units (normal 0–3.7), and alkaline phosphatase was 235. The patient was randomized to be treated with methyl CCNU and Estracyt. One month later, in August 1977 a supraclavicular lymph node was palpated, and needle aspiration biopsy (Fig. 2) confirmed the diagnosis of metastatic carcinoma.

This material was used to initiate LNCaP cell culture in vitro. Transrectal biopsy of the prostate was consistent with carcinoma of the prostate. Further investigation revealed right hydronephrosis due to retroperitoneal lymph node pressure on the right ureter. The patient was treated at this time with cis-platinum. His disease continued to progress rapidly, with development of hoarseness, increased bone pain, and renal failure, which was temporarily improved by nephrostomy. He did show marked improvement with high dosage of Decadron, but this was also temporary, and the patient died at home six months after his admission to Roswell Park Memorial Institute, and one and one-half years after the diagnosis. In summary, this was a relatively young patient with rapidly progressing adenocarcinoma of the prostate, which showed only minimal and temporary response to hormonal therapy and no response to chemotherapy. Although not rare, this rapidly progressing course of the disease, unresponsive to conventional hormonal therapy and later to chemotherapy, was striking, and it was emphasized by a relatively short survival time of 18 months from the date of primary diagnosis.

THE LNCaP CELL LINE

Small fragments of tissue were obtained by needle aspiration biopsy of a metastatic lesion in the left supraclavicular lymph node. A single T-flask (15 cm^2) was inoculated, and the minute explants were fed twice a week with medium RPMI 1640 with added 1 millimolar glutamine, 15% fetal calf serum, and antibiotics (penicillin and streptomycin at $50\mu g/ml$). Seven such explants (0.5 mm) attached to the flask and grew very slowly as colonies with multilayered dense centers and a lucid periphery consisting of spreading epithelioid cells. Three months later (November 1977), the colonies reached a diameter of approximately 4 mm (Fig. 3). At that time the acid phosphatase was detected [26] in the cell culture medium ($7.9 \ \mu U/ml$ vs $0.1 \ \mu U/ml$ in the control medium). At no time were fibroblasts present in our primary culture or in subsequent passages. The first subcultures of LNCaP cells were carried out in December 1977. It was necessary to develop new "microtransplant" techniques for passaging these cells, since trypsinization or other methods of cell dissociation invariably resulted in the death of the cultures.

LNCaP cells have low anchoring potential, grow on plastic surfaces but not glass, usually do not produce smooth and uniform monolayers, rapidly acidify culture medium, and exhibit a much slower rate of growth in vitro than most of "typical" cell cultures (eg, the doubling of the area size of a transplanted LNCaP colony requires between five and seven days). The slow growth appears to be quite

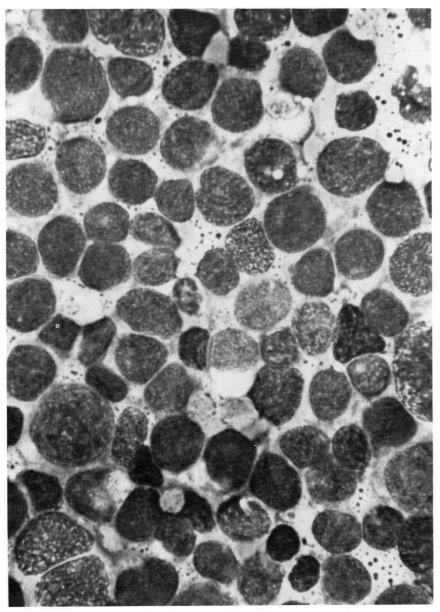

Fig. 2. Photomicrograph of a smear of needle aspiration biopsy from supraclavicular metastatic lymph node. This material was used to start LNCaP culture (Wright-Giemsa stain; magnification, × 600).

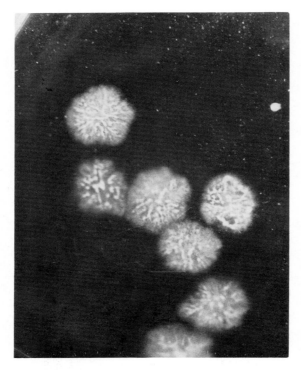

Fig. 3. Seventy-day old colonies formed by LNCaP cell in culture (dark field illumination; magnification, × 2.7).

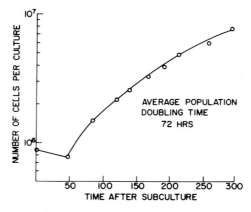

Fig. 4. Growth of LNCaP cells in monolayer culture. Medium changed at 72-hour intervals.

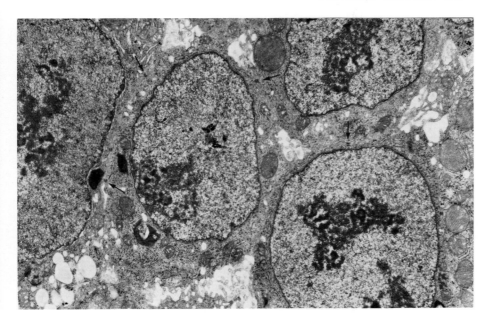

Fig. 5. Transmission electromicrograph of thin section of LNCaP cells in culture (magnification, × 5,840. Arrows point toward desmosomes.

consistent with the rate of multiplication of human malignant cells in vivo. Since June 1978 it has been possible to subculture LNCaP cells regularly every 30 days at a 1:8 split ratio.

Since January 1979 we have adapted one LNCaP subline to mild enzymatic dissociation procedures and obtained growth resembling conventional cell cultures. These cells are now propagated at 1:64 split every three weeks. This allowed is to determine that the average population doubling time is approximately 72 hours (Fig. 4). LNCaP cells are capable of growing to high saturation densities (over 2.5×10^5 cells/cm^2). LNCaP cells were cryopreserved at several different passage levels.

The morphology of cultured cells stained by the Wright-Giemsa method is similar to that of the original cells obtained at biopsy. Electron microscopic examination shows the presence of desmosomes, thus confirming the epithelioid nature of LNCaP cells (Figs. 5 and 6). A series of phase-contrast photomicrographs documents the stable epithelioid morphology over the period of the past 20 months (Fig. 7).

The malignant properties of LNCaP cells are maintained. Twenty out of 25 nude mice inoculated at different times with 1×10^7 of cultured cells developed rapidly growing, poorly differentiated adenocarcinomas at the injection site within

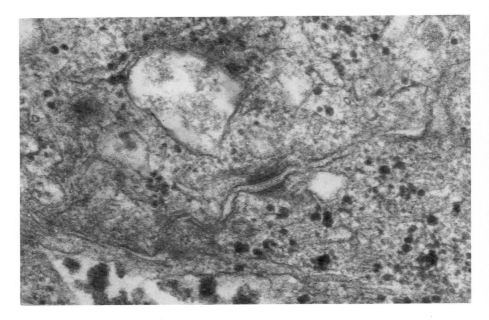

Fig. 6. Transmission electron micrograph of thin section of LNCaP cell in culture (magnification, × 91,840). Desmosome in the center.

eight weeks of inoculation (Figs. 8–11). No apparent distal metastases were observed; however, invasion of malignant cells into the muscle was noted. The tumors are highly vascular and usually kill mice within four months, by which time they are over 6 grams in size. This is in sharp contrast to our experience with other human tumors (eg, Burkitt lymphoma-Daudi line, which can grow for up to eight months, reaching a size in excess of 30 grams).

The unique property of the LNCaP cell line is the continuous production of acid phosphatase both in vitro and in vivo in the nude mice. The acid phosphatase was shown to be biochemically similar and immunologically identical to human prostatic acid phosphatase (PAP) by counter-immunoelectrophoresis and double-diffusion gel precipitation with monospecific antiserum. In cell culture fluids acid phosphatase was found to accumulate to a level in excess of 300 μU/ml/10^6 when measured by conventional spectrophotometric methods [28]. The kinetics of the acid phosphatase accumulation are shown in Figure 12. The acid phosphatase activity is also proportional to the cell density of tested cultures. We have examined cell culture fluids from six additional human tumor cell lines and one strain of diploid human fibroblasts for acid phosphatase activity. None of these fluids contained more than 1% of acid phosphatase activity observed in LNCaP cultures. In addition, by counter-immunoelectrophoresis [27–29] only fluids from LNCaP

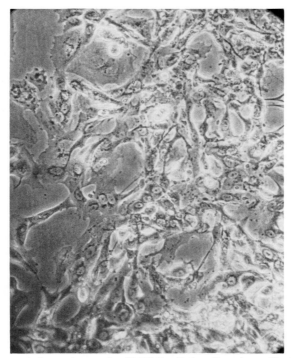

Fig. 7. Phase-contrast photomicrograph of LNCaP cells in culture (magnification, × 135).

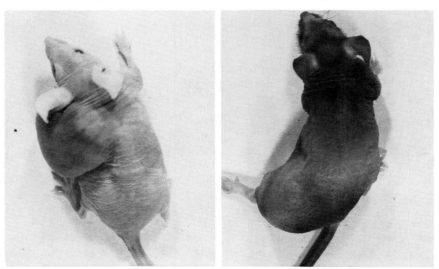

Figures 8 & 9. Tumors in nude mice 16 weeks after inoculation with LNCaP cells. Left: subcutaneous inoculation. Right intramuscular inoculation.

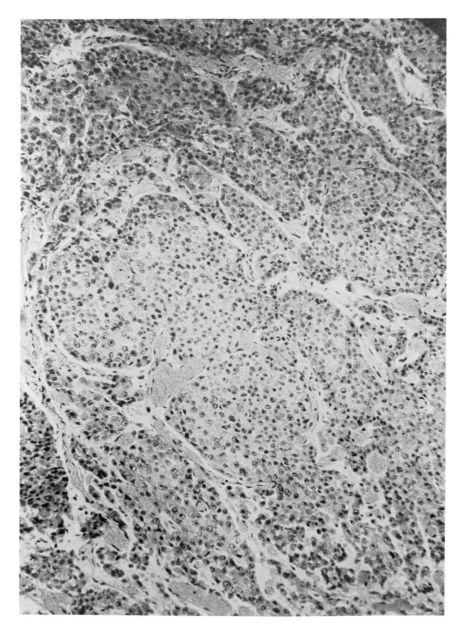

Fig. 10. Photomicrograph of histological section of LNCaP tumor growth in nude mouse (hematoxylin and eosin stain; magnification, X 100).

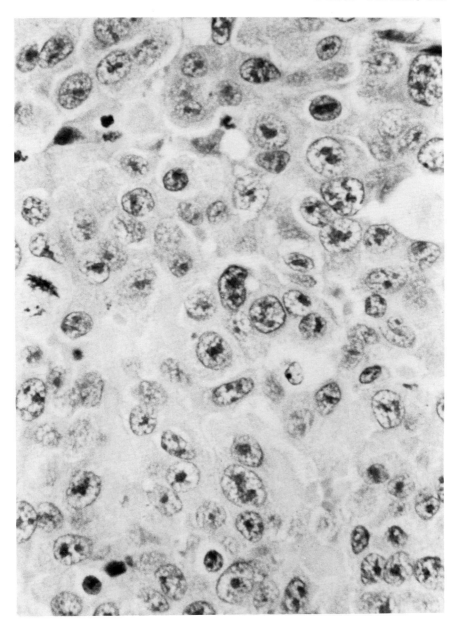

Fig. 11. Photomicrograph of histological section of LNCaP tumor grown in nude mouse (hematoxylin and eosin stain; magnification, × 350).

ACID PHOSPHATASE IN CULTURE
FLUIDS LNC$_a$P CELLS

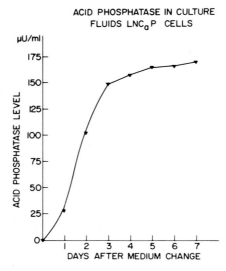

Fig. 12. Accumulation of acid phosphatase in culture medium from a confluent culture of LNCaP cells.

cells were reactive (Table I). It is noteworthy that we have not observed any significiant levels of acid phosphatase production in either of the two cell lines (DU 145 or EB 33) reported as being derived from human prostatic cancer.

By the indirect immunofluorescence method, using monospecific goat anti-PAP serum produced by Dr. Chu [27, 30], specific granular cytoplasmic staining of LNCaP cells was observed (Fig. 13). Its localization was similar to the histochemical localization of acid phosphatase within LNCaP cells using the Burstone method [31] (Fig. 14). The histochemical staining pattern was not changed following fixation of smears with formalin, which is also consistent with known properties of prostatic acid phosphatase.

Human prostatic acid phosphatase production by LNCaP cells is preserved in vivo following inoculation into nude mice. PAP is present in high concentrations in tumor homogenates and is readily detectable in the plasma of tumor-bearing animals (Table II). As controls, nude mice inoculated with human melanoma (ES-1) were used, since trace amounts of acid phosphatase are elaborated in vitro by these cells. This acid phosphatase, however, did not cross-react with antiserum specific against PAP.

In extracts of LNCaP cells an antigen specific to human prostate was detected by the rocket immunoelectrophoresis method.

Chromosomal analysis of LNCaP cells in culture, as well as of cells from tumors grown in nude mice, shows an aneuploid male human karyotype with several marker chromosomes (Figs. 15 and 16; Table III). A few cells with 46 chromosomes were

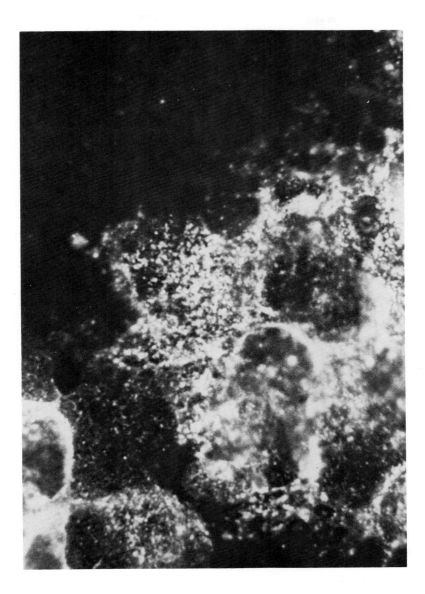

Fig. 13. Photomicrograph of LNCaP cells (from culture) stained by indirect immunofluorescence method with monospecific goat antiserum against human prostatic acid phosphatase and rabbit anti-goat IgG (fluorescein labeled).

TABLE I. Acid Phosphatase in Culture Fluids of Human Cells

Cell line	Origin	Acid phosphatase (μU/ml)
LNCaP	Prostatic cancer	343.0[a]
DU 145	Prostatic cancer	1.8
EB 33	Prostatic cancer	0.9
MDA-MB-231	Breast cancer	0.9
MCF7	Breast cancer	1.2
DAUDI	Burkitt lymphoma	1.0
ES-1	Melanoma	3.0
BG-9	Diploid fibroblasts	0.8
	Medium control	0.7

[a]Identified as human prostatic acid phosphatase by counter immunoelectrophoresis.

TABLE II. Acid Phosphatase in Tissue Homogenates and Plasma of Nude Mice

		Acid phosphatase (μU/ml)	
LNCaP	Tumor	21,488[a]	
	Plasma		57.0[a]
Melanoma (ES-1)	Tumor	720	
	Plasma		5.8
Normal mouse	Plasma		2.9

[a]Identified as human prostatic acid phosphatase by counter-immuno-electrophoresis.

TABLE III. LNCaP Cells Chromosome Number Distribution

	Number of chromosomes									
	26	40	45	46	47	48	54	57	64	80–94 and above
Cell culture Number of cells				3	2	1	1	1	1	15
Nude mouse tumor Number of cells	1	1	1	3		1			1	16

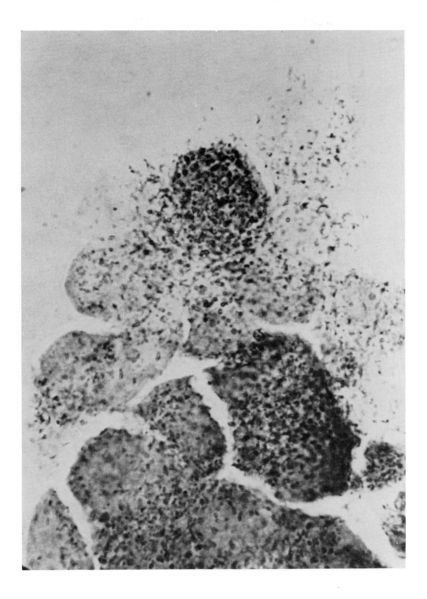

Fig. 14. Photomicrograph of LNCaP cells (from culture) stained by the Burstone-Sigma procedure for histochemical demonstration of acid phosphatase.

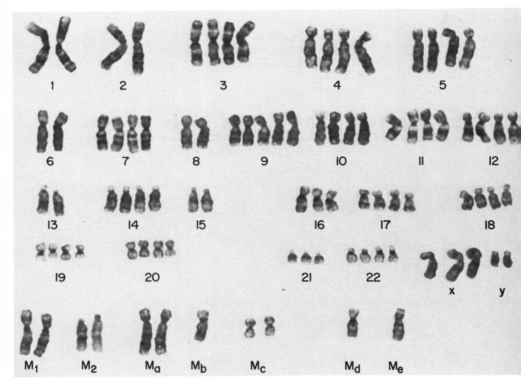

Fig. 15. A G-banded karyotype of a LNCaP cell from culture.

pseudodiploid, and they differ from each other karyotypically. Some marker chromosomes observed in cultured cells were not seen in material derived from tumors in mice, suggesting a possible selection process in vivo.

Cell culture fluids harvested from actively proliferating and stationary LNCaP cells were analyzed for the presence of reverse transciptase activity associated with particles of density characteristic for retroviruses (1.16 gm/cm^3). No such activity was found. This suggests that LNCaP cells in vitro do not spontaneoulsy release retrovirus like particles in quantities detectable by our assay procedure [32, 33].

In summary, the preservation of essential morphologic and functional properties by the LNCaP cell line suggest its utility as a new and relevant model for studies in the areas of etiology, biology, diagnosis as detection and treatment of human prostatic carcinoma [34].

REFERENCES

1. Coffey DS, Issacs JT, Weisman RM: Animal models for the study of prostatic cancer. In Murphy GP (ed): "Prostate Cancer." Littleton, Massachusetts: PSG Publishing Company, 1979.

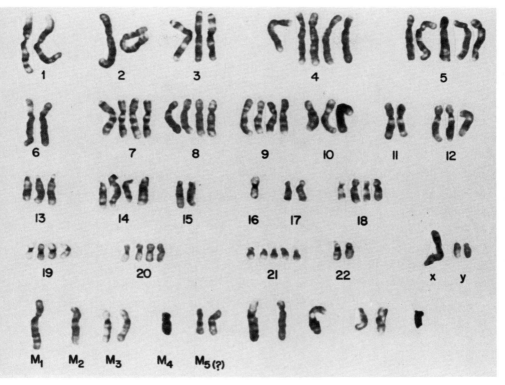

Fig. 16. A G-banded karyotype of a LNCaP cell from a tumor grown in a nude mouse.

2. Reid LC, Shin S: Transplantation of heterologous endoctrine tumor cells in nude mice. In Fogh J, Giovanella C (eds): "Experimental and Clinical Research." New York: Academic Press, 1978, pp 313–351.
3. Reid LC, Sato G: Development of transplantable tumors of human prostate gland implanted in nude mice. J Cell Biol 70:287a, 1976.
4. Lasnitski I: The effect of testosterone propionate on organ cultures of the mouse prostate. J Endocrinol 12:236–240, 1955.
5. Lasnitski I, Dingle JT, Adams S: The effect of steriod hormones on lysosomal activity of rat ventral prostate gland in culture. Exp Cell Res 43:120–130, 1966.
6. Richter KM, Akin RH: The cultivation of several genitourinary tract tumors. Trans South Central Section Am J Urol Assoc 67–91, 1957.
7. Rohl L: Prostatic and bladder tumors studied in vitro on the response to androsterone and on orthoaminophenol. Anio Inter Contra Cancrum Acta 20: 1316–1319, 1964.
8. Farnsworth WE: 10-Demethylation of testosterone by human prostate, in vitro. Steroids 6:519–530, 1965.
9. Heidelberger C, Iype PT: Malignant transformation in vitro by carcinogenic hydrocarbons. Science, 155:214–217, 1967.
10. Chen TT, Heidelberger C: Cultivation in vitro of cells derived from adult C3H mouse ventral prostate. J Natl Cancer Inst 42:903–914, 1969.

11. Mondal S, Embleton MJ, Marquardt H, et al: Production of variants of decreased malignancy and antigenicity from clones transformed in vitro methylcholanthrene. Int J Cancer 8:410–420, 1971.

12. Marquardt H, Kuroki T, Huberman E, et al: Malignant transformation of cells derived from mouse prostate by epoxides and other derivatives of polycyclic hydrocarbons. Cancer Res 32:716–720, 1972.

13. Fraley EE, Ecker S, Vincent MM: Spontaneous in vitro neoplastic transformation of adult human prostatic epithelium. Science 170:540–542, 1970.

14. Okada K, Schroeder FH: Human prostatic carcinoma in cell culture: Preliminary report on the development and characterization of an epithelial cell line (EB-33). Urol Res 2:111–121, 1974.

15. Nelson-Rees WA, Flandermeyer RR: HeLa cultures defined. Science 191:96–98, 1976.

16. Stonington OG, Hemmingson H: Culture of cells as a monolayer derived from the epithelium of of the human prostate: A new cell growth technique. J Urol 106:393–400, 1971.

17. Brehmer B, Marquardt H, Madsen PO: Growth and hormonal response of cells derived from carcinoma and hyperplasia of the prostate in monolayer cell culture. A possible in vitro model for clinical chemotherapy. J Urol 108:890–896, 1972.

18. Brehmer B, Riemann JF, Bloodworth JM, et al: Electron microscopic appearance of cells from carcinoma of the prostate in monolayer tissue culture. Urol Res 1:27–31, 1973.

19. Kaighn ME, Babcock MS: Monolayer cultures of human prostatic cells. Cancer Chemother Rep 59:59–63, 1975.

20. Webber MM, Stonington OG, Poché PA: Epithelial outgrowth from suspension cultures of human prostatic tissue. In Vitro 10:196–205, 1974.

21. Webber MM, Stonington OG: Ultrastructural changes in human prepubertal prostatic epithelium grown in vitro. Invest Urol 12:389–400, 1975.

22. Mickey DD, Stone KR, Wunderli H, Mickey GH, Vollmer RT, Paulson DF: Heterotransplantation of human prostatic adenocarcinoma cell line in nude mice. Cancer Res 37:4049–4058, 1977.

23. Stone KR, Mickey DD, Wunderli H, Mickey GH, Paulson D: Isolation of a human prostate carcinoma cell line (DU 145). Int J Cancer 21:274–281, 1978.

24. Kaighn ME, Narayan S, Ohnuki Y, Lechner JF: Establishment and characterization of a human prostatic carcinoma cell line (PC-3). Invest Urol (in press).

25. Kaighn ME, Lechner JF, Narayan KS, Jones LW: Prostate carcinoma: Tissue culture cell lines. Nat Cancer Inst Monogr 49:17–21, 1978.

26. Babson AL, Phillips GE: Improved acid phosphatase procedure. Clin Chim Acta 13:264–265, 1966.

27. Chu TM, Wang MC, Scott WW, Gibbons RR, Johnson DE, et al: Immunochemical detection of serum prostatic acid phosphatase: Methodology and clinical evaluation. Invest Urol 15:319–323, 1978.

28. Murphy GP, Karr J, Chu TM: Prostatic acid phosphatase: Where are we? CA 28:258–264, 1978.

29. Wajsman Z, Chu TM: Detection and diagnosis of prostate cancer. In Murphy GP (ed): "Prostate Cancer." Littleton, Massachusetts: PSG Publishing Co, 1979, pp 111–128.

30. Lee C, Wang MC, Murphy GP, Chu TM: A solid phase fluorescent immunoassay for human prostatic acid phosphatase. Cancer Res 38:2871–2878, 1978.

31. Burstone MS: Histochemical demonstration of acid phosphatases with naphthol AS-phosphates. J Natl Cancer Inst 21:523–532, 1958.

32. Arya SK, Zeigel RF, Horoszewicz JS, Carter WA: RNA tumor virus-like activities in human solid tissues: Endogenous RNA:DNA polymerase activities in the prostate. J Surg Oncol 8:321–332, 1976.

33. Arya SK, Zeigel RF, Horoszewicz JS, Carter WA: RNA tumor virus-like activities in human prostate: Possible novel pharmacologic approaches. Cancer Treat Rep 61:113–117, 1977.

34. Horoszewicz JS, Leong SL, Chu TM, Friedman M, Kim U, Chai LS, Kakati S, Arya SK, Sandberg AA: A new model for studies on human prostatic carcinoma. Proc Am Assoc Cancer Res 20:212, 1979.

In Vitro Models for Prostatic Cancer: Summary

Mukta M. Webber, PhD

Investigations on the etiology, the mechanism of carcinogenesis, and the modes of treatment for prostatic cancer can be made using in vitro and in vivo model systems.

As the many investigations reported in this volume show, considerable progress has been made in the last five years in developing in vitro cell models. Model systems using normal and malignant cells can be used for a variety of investigations. In this chapter I will primarily discuss the malignant cell models using human cells. I have described an in vitro cell model, derived from normal human prostatic epithelium, elsewhere in this volume.

The in vitro cell models derived from normal human cells are particularly well suited for studies on the etiology of cancer and on the mechanism of carcinogenesis. Normal cell systems further provide a basic understanding of the physiology of normal cells and of various growth-regulating mechanisms.

Models using malignant human cells are useful for testing different modes of treatment and for examining possible relationships between tumor resistance or sensitivity and related cell characteristics. Such a relationship, if established, can help in predicting the response of a tumor to a particular treatment.

Before I comment specifically on the normal and malignant cell lines discussed in the preceding chapters, I would like to begin with some simple terms in tissue culture and relate these to the cell systems that are available for studies on prostatic cancer. I do this for the benefit of those who are new to tissue culture and others who are considering cell or tissue culture for their investigations. These terms were proposed by the Committee on Nomenclature, Tissue Culture Association, Inc., in June 1966.

PRIMARY CULTURES

"This term implies a culture started from cells, tissues or organs taken directly from organisms." Such cultures (eg, Dr. Lewis' [1] cultures of monkey prostate and mine of normal human prostate [2]) are particularly important because cells are not kept in culture for a long time, hence the in vitro changes do not have the time to occur. Cells in primary cultures closely resemble the cells from which they originated.

Models for Prostate Cancer, pages 133–147

CELL LINES

"A 'cell line' arises from a primary culture at the time of the first subculture. The term 'cell line' implies that cultures from it consist of numerous lineages of the cells originally present in the primary culture." Although these cultures have a finite life, their importance and usefulness must be recognized in that they generally maintain properties of primary cultures (eg, our cultures of normal human prostatic epithelium [2] and NP-2 cells of Dr. Kaighn [3, 4]). These cells go through a limited number of passages.

ESTABLISHED CELL LINE

"A cell line may be said to have become established, when it demonstrates the potential to be subcultured indefinitely in vitro." These cells have the ability to propagate indefinitely. PC-3 [4] and DU 145 [5, 6] prostatic cancer cell lines are good examples of this.

CELL STRAIN

"A 'cell strain' can be derived either from a primary culture or a cell line by the selection or cloning of cells having specific properties or markers. The properties or markers must persist during subsequent cultivation." Dunning tumor cell strains showing specific properties of hormone resistance or sensitivity could be used as examples of cell strains [7].

CLONE

"This term denotes a population of cells derived from a single cell by mitoses. A clone is not necessarily homogeneous and therefore the term 'clone' or 'cloned' should not be used to indicate homogeneity in a cell population." Usually cloning is done to select specific mutants. This may be done when we select cells with a specific chromosome pattern, which eg, may be associated with sensitivity or resistance to a specific drug.

The important features of primary cultures and cell lines discussed in the preceding chapters are summarized in the paragraphs that follow.

NONHUMAN PRIMATE PROSTATE

Dr. Lewis [1] described a system using nonhuman prostate (Table I). I am concerned about the use of terms like "nonhuman" or "canine" prostate, because these terms encompass a large number of species. I recommend that species be clearly identified, because it might become important in the future to know the

TABLE I. Nonhuman Primate Prostate (Normal)

Origin	Cranial and caudal prostate
In vitro	Primary explant cultures in monolayer
Characterization	Positive for acid phosphatase
Needed research	Growth and nutrient requirements to be established
	Defined medium to be developed
	Methods for subculturing to be developed
	Further characterization

From Lewis and Kaack (this volume).

species from which a certain cell line arose, in case species differences are observed at a later date. This system is likely to be a useful model. However, a tremendous amount of work needs to be done before this system can be used.

NP-2 CELL LINE

This cell line is derived from neonatal human prostatic epithelium [3]. My major concern about this cell line is its neonatal origin. These cells do not respond to insulin or testosterone. Adult prostatic epithelium, from which carcinoma cells arise, is responsive to both of these hormones [2]. Prostatic epithelium does not become fully functional until puberty. Therefore, I suggest to Dr. Kaighn that some studies on hormone responsiveness, characterization and differentiation be done on these cells to establish their prostatic epithelial origin and to determine their usefulness as a model system for studies on prostate physiology and carcinogenesis.

The questions to be asked are:

Do these cells show characteristics of prostatic epithelium?
Can these cells differentiate into secretory epithelium?
Are these cells hormone responsive?

I would now like to spend a little time on the malignant cell models discussed in the previous chapters and others developed in the past.

MA-160 CELL LINE

In 1970 MA-160 cell line was reported by Fraley et al [8] (Table II). The cells for primary culture were derived from benign prostatic hyperplasia. These cells were thought to have undergone malignant transformation in vitro. This cell line shows some HeLa cell markers and may be a HeLa cell contaminant [9, 10].

EB-33 CELL LINE

In 1974 EB-33 [11] cell line came into existence (Table III). The cells, thought to be malignant, were derived from the primary site — ie, the prostate. The origin of these cells is doubtful, and their identity has not been firmly established.

TABLE II. MA-160 Cell Line

Site	Prostate, BPH[a]
Response	Inhibited by androgens and estrogens in vitro
In vitro	Grows in monolayer
Environment	Eagle's MEM[b] + 10% FBS[c]
Characterization	Considered a HeLa cell contaminant
	HeLa markers

[a]BPH = benign prostatic hyperplasia.
[b]MEM = minimum essential medium.
[c]FBS = fetal bovine serum.

TABLE III. EB-33 Cell Line

Site	Prostate, primary tumor
Response	Hormones ± in selected clones
In vitro	Grows in monolayer
Environment	Ham's F_{10} + 12.5% HS[a] + 2.5% FBS
Characterization	Considered a HeLa all contaminant, HeLa markers

[a]HS = horse serum.

HPC-36 CELL LINE

Lubaroff [12] in 1977 reported HPC-36 cell line (Table IV), originating from a prostatic carcinoma. However, cells for culture were derived from the primary site. This leads to some doubts about the malignant origin of HPC-36 cells because normal, benign, and malignant cells are present in the prostate and the possibility of in vitro transformation of normal or benign cells has to be considered. Further work needs to be done to establish characteristics of these cells.

The two cell lines that seem to be the most promising at present are DU 145 and PC-3.

DU 145 CELL LINE

The DU 145 cell line [6] arose from a metastatic lesion of prostatic adenocarcinoma in the central nervous system (CNS). These cells are unresponsive to hormone therapy and possess a Y chromosome. Their other characteristics are listed in Table V. This cell line is considered to be of prostatic carcinoma origin.

TABLE IV. HPC-36 Cell Line

Site	Prostate, primary tumor
In vitro	Grows in: monolayer
	: suspension
Environment	Dulbecco's MEM + 10% HS
Characterization	Positive for acid phosphatase
	Further characterization needed

TABLE V. DU·145 Cell Line

Site	Metastatic CNS lesion, prostatic adenocarcinoma
Response	Unresponsive to hormone therapy
In vitro	Grows in: monolayer
	: soft agar
Environment	Medium 199 + 20% bull serum
Characterization	Weakly positive for acid phosphatase
	Modal chromosome 64 (p 57)
	Y chromosome present
	Considered of prostatic origin
Heterotransplantation	In nude mice

PC-3 CELL LINE

The PC-3 cell line [4] was derived from a metastatic lesion of prostatic adeno-carcinoma in a lumbar vertebra (Table VI). These cells are unresponsive to hormones and lack a Y chromosome. This cell line is considered to be of prostatic carcinoma origin.

The positive features of DU 145 and PC-3, which make them useful cell lines for studies on chemotherapy, are listed in Table VII. Both DU 145 and PC-3 are unresponsive to hormones. This feature is of significance because although a majority of prostatic carcinomas are initially responsive to hormone therapy, they eventually become unresponsive. It is these unresponsive cells that are responsible for death of the cancer patient. Therefore, a study of these cells is of utmost importance. In order to bring about an effective control of these cells, it is particularly important to find the drugs to which they are sensitive. Therefore, the fact that these cells are unresponsive to hormones does not distract from the usefulness of these cell models.

Another point worth noting is that cell lines PC-3 and DU 145 have been derived from metastatic tumors from sites other than the prostate. This essentially makes them pure cultures of malignant prostatic epithelial cells, since there is no possi-

TABLE VI. PC-3 Cell Line

Site	Metastatic, lumbar vertebra, prostatic adenocarcinoma
Response	Unresponsive to hormone therapy
In vitro	Grows in: monolayer
	: soft agar
Environment	PFMR-1[a] + 1% FBS
Characterization	Negative for acid phosphatase
	Modal chromosome 58 (p 30)
	Y chromosome absent
	Considered of prostatic origini
Heterotransplantation	In nude mice

[a]PFMR-1 — Pasadena Foundation for Medical Research-1 medium.

TABLE VII. Positive Features of PC-3 and DU 145 Cell Lines

1. For culture, origin from a metastatic tumor is preferred.
2. Unresponsiveness to hormones is not a drawback.
3. Useful models for 20% of the tumors that are unresponsive at the outset and for the remaining 80% which eventually become unresponsive to hormones.

bility of contaminating them with normal or benign cells, which could occur if the tissue specimen for culture was taken from the primary site.

LNCaP CELL LINE

This cell line (Table VIII) was developed by Julius Horoszewicz and collaborators in 1977 and was derived from a metastatic lesion [13, 14]. Cells were collected by needle biopsy of a supraclavical lymph node of a 50-year-old patient with disseminated prostatic carcinoma. The tumor was unresponsive to hormone therapy. These cells are positive for prostatic acid phosphatase, whereas other cell lines described earlier, are not. With further characterization, this cell line may also become a useful model for studies on the treatment of prostatic cancer.

The malignant cell lines described above have not so far been used for evaluating the effectiveness of different modes of treatment, for testing synergism between drugs, or for testing new drugs. This work remains to be done, and it is hoped that these model systems will make significant contributions in the area of the treatment of prostatic cancer.

There are often doubts raised about the malignant nature of cell lines. Heterotransplantation into nude mice and the resulting tumors has been considered a good test to prove the malignant nature of cells. However, Dr. Gittes [15] has

TABLE VIII. LnCaP Cell Line

Site	Metastatic, supraclavical lymph node, prostatic adeno-carcinoma
Response	Unresponsive to hormone therapy
In vitro	Grows in monolayer
Environment	RPMI 1640 + 15% FBS
Characterization	Positive for acid phosphatase
	Modal chromosome number between 80 and 95
	Y chromosome present
	Further characterization needed
Heterotransplantation	In nude mice

TABLE IX. Characteristics of Malignant Cells

1. Escape from normal growth regulation
2. Loss of contact inhibition
3. Reduced serum requirement
4. Growth in soft agar
5. Fibrinolytic activity
6. Karotypic changes
7. Agglutination with plant lectins
8. Antigenic changes
9. Greater cloning efficiency
10. Changes in cyclic nucleotide system
11. Changes in surface architecture
12. Ability to metastasize

raised some doubts about the reliability of this test. Also, facilities to use nude mice are not widely available. In view of this, even if a nude mouse system is used, it is important to use some other in vitro tests to prove the malignant nature of cells. I would like to review briefly some of these tests (Table IX).

CHARACTERISTICS OF MALIGNANT CELLS

In order to be able to use the normal and tumor cell systems, it is important to know how tumor cells differ from normal cells, so that one may try to reverse or block these changes. Certain characteristics of malignant cells that can be used to establish their malignant nature are described in the following sections. These characteristics may not all be shown by all malignant cell lines. However, the presence of several of these in a cell line would substantiate its malignant nature.

Escape From Normal Growth Regulation

Once a cell has undergone malignant transformation, it no longer responds to the normal growth regulation of the body [16]. In essence it shows an altered response to

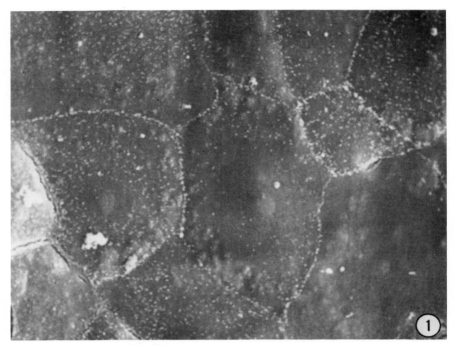

Fig. 1. Scanning electron micrograph of cells from a hamster embryo cell line transformed by Herpes simplex virus Type 1. Cells show contact inhibition, have relatively smooth surface architecture, and are nontumorigenic (magnification, × 1,518).

growth-controlling factors, so that it can multiply at a rate quite independent of other cells in the tissue from which it originated.

Loss of Contact Inhibition

When cancer cells are grown in culture, they show decreased sensitivity to contact inhibition of movement and to density-dependent growth inhibition [16]. In a culture of normal cells, as soon as a cell comes into contact with another cell, its further movement in that direction stops and it does not grow over or under the other cell. Thus, once the available space is occupied (as in a confluent culture) and a monolayer is formed, the culture does not grow any further if the medium is not replenished. Virus-transformed but nontumorigenic cells may also show these properties exhibited by normal cells. Malignant cells, however, do not respond to contact-inhibition signals. They continue to grow, underlapping each other, thus forming several layers, even under depleted nutrient conditions. This difference is demonstrated in Figures 1 and 2.

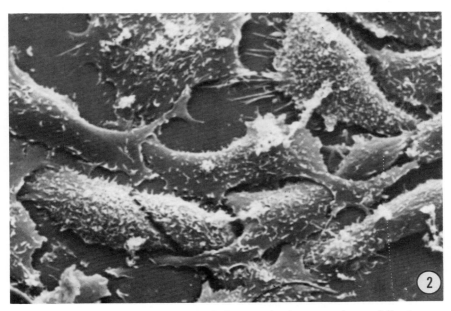

Fig. 2. Scanning electron micrograph of cells from another hamster embryo cell line transformed by Herpes simplex virus Type 1. These cells are not contact inhibited, show underlapping, have a more active cell surface, and are tumorigenic (magnification, × 1,650).

Reduced Serum Requirements

Cells in culture require serum or serum factors for growth in vitro [17]. Up to a certain limit, the higher the serum concentration, the better the growth. In low serum levels, the growth of normal cells is poor. Malignant cells, however, continue to grow rapidly even in low serum levels in the culture medium; eg, PC-3 cells grow well in 1% serum, whereas normal cells may require 5% to 20% serum.

Growth in Soft Agar

Cancer cells have the ability to grow and form colonies in soft agar, whereas normal cells do not [18]. This property results from a loss of anchorage dependence in malignant cells. This property is now being used by many investigators as a test for detecting cancer cells and for separating cancer cells from normal cells, from a mixture of the two. This test could be used for separating cells — eg, when the cancer cells for culture are obtained from the primary site, as was the case with HPC-36.

Fibrinolytic Activity

Malignant cells have the ability to lyse fibrin, whereas normal cells do not [19]. Tumor cells produce a plasminogen activator. Serum in culture media contains plasminogen, and in the presence of the activator it is converted to an active, fibrinolytic enzyme, plasmin. When tumor cell cultures are overlaid with agarose containing fibrin, lysis of fibrin occurs at sites where there are tumor cells, and this can be detected by several different methods. The reaction takes place as follows:

$$\text{Serum plasminogen} \xrightarrow[\substack{\text{from cancer} \\ \text{cells}}]{\substack{\text{Plasminogen} \\ \text{activator}}} \text{Plasmin (the fibrinolytic enzyme)}$$

$$\text{Fibrin} \xrightarrow{\text{Plasmin}} \text{Fibrinolysis}$$

This property is also frequently being used as a test for transformation.

Karyotypic Changes

A large number of animal and human tumors show chromosomal changes. Generally, there is an increase in the number of chromosomes from the normal diploid, or there are morphological changes in the chromosomes without a change in number. Virus-induced tumors generally do not show a change in number. These changes in chromosomal structure and number lead to a general instability in the cancer cell karyotype. This feature must be given important consideration in chemotherapy.

Agglutination With Plant Lectins

Tumor cells have the ability to agglutinate when mixed with plant lectins — eg, concanavalin A or wheat germ agglutinin — but normal cells do not [20].

Antigenic Changes

As a result of malignant transformation, cells acquire new surface antigens [21].

Greater Cloning Efficiency

Cancer cells have a greater ability to form clones in culture than do normal cells; eg, if 1,000 normal cells are plated in a culture dish and 1,000 cancer cells are plated in another dish, after a period of about 14 days, normal cultures may only have 100 to 200 clones, whereas the cancer cell cultures may have as many as 600–700 clones.

Changes in Cyclic Nucleotide Systems

Cyclic AMP (cyclic adenosine monophosphate) is considered to be an important cell growth regulator. Changes in the cyclic nucleotide system have been associated with growth rate, malignancy and differentiation of mammalian cells in culture. Also, changes in cyclic nucleotide phosphodiesterase are important events associated with neoplasms [22].

TABLE X. Malignant, Human Cell Models

Useful for studies on

1. Effectiveness of different modes of treatment (radiation, hormone, and chemotherapy)
2. Testing new drugs for chemotherapy
3. Potentiation and synergism in therapy
4. Prediction of response to therapy
5. Association of chromosomal and other characteristics with resistance or sensitivity to specific treatment
6. Tumor progression

Changes in Surface Architecture

The cell surface architecture changes as a result of transformation [23]. This is shown in the scanning electron micrographs of nontumorigenic and tumorigenic cells (Figs. 1 and 2).

Ability to Metastasize

An important characteristic of cancer cells, which has implications directly in the cancer patient, is their ability to metastasize [24]. The cells lose their natural affinity to remain in contact with other cells of their own kind. They separate and move to other parts of the body, where they form new tumors.

With this background, we can now move on to examining the usefulness of malignant cell models. Studies for which such cell models can be used are listed in Table X. When these models are used to study toxicity of drugs to malignant cells, it is also important to know their effects on normal cells. Therefore, both normal and malignant cell systems should be used simultaneously for testing drugs (Fig. 3). The most important uses of normal human cell models are listed in Table XI. In vitro systems for activation of suspected carcinogens or drugs can be designed; therefore, meaningful studies on carcinogenesis and target-cell specificity can be performed. A summary of in vitro cell models available for studies on the etiology and treatment of prostatic cancer is presented in Table XII.

Finally, I would like to make some comments about the cellular aspects of tumor progression and the development of resistance to therapy. Such studies can be made in in vitro systems. Tumors generally consist of a very heterogeneous cell population with cells containing many different chromosome combinations [25]. When a tumor is treated with a drug, a certain population sensitive to the drug is killed. However, a smaller, resistant cell population remains and contributes to regrowth of the tumor (Fig. 4). In essence, the drug acts as a selection factor and selects for resistant cells. Therefore, therapy involving a combination of drugs or a combination of different

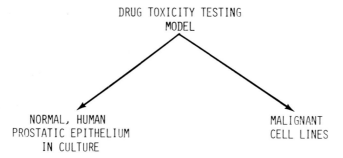

DRUG TOXICITY TESTING
MODEL

NORMAL, HUMAN
PROSTATIC EPITHELIUM
IN CULTURE

MALIGNANT
CELL LINES

Fig. 3. A diagram showing the two major components of a model for in vitro testing of the effectiveness of chemotherapeutic agents against malignant cells. The model consists of a normal cell system and one or more malignant cell lines.

TABLE XI. Normal, Human Cell Models

Useful for studies on

1. Etiology
2. Early steps in prostatic carcinogenesis
3. Metabolic activation of carcinogens and their cell specificity
4. Mechanism of transformation with viral, chemical, and physical agents
5. Cell nutrition and metabolism of hormone-dependent cells
6. Growth factors and regulation
7. Aging
8. Screening of suspected carcinogens and toxic environmental agents

TABLE XII. In Vitro Human Cell Models Available

1. Normal, postpubertal prostatic epithelium
2. Normal, neonatal prostatic epithelium
3. Malignant, prostatic adenocarcinoma, PC-3, DU 145 cell lines
4. Potential malignant cell models, prostatic adenocarcinoma, HPC-36, LnCaP cell lines

modes of treatment is more effective, because this results in killing more than one type of cell.

Selection at the cellular level is very similar to what happens in nature among insect or animal populations and can be described as evolution at the cellular level in a tumor cell population. As a result of selection by changes in environmental factors, new species of animals or insects arise. These new species are well adapted to the changed environment. Similarly, resistant tumor cells are better adapted to the environment in the presence of a chemotherapeutic drug than was the original tumor cell population, thus allowing tumor recurrence and continued growth.

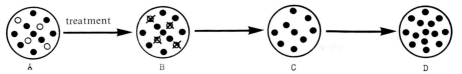

Fig. 4. A diagram illustrating selection of resistant cells from a heterogeneous tumor cell population exposed to a therapeutic agent. For convenience, only two cell types are shown. ○, Sensitive cells; ●, resistant cells. A, original cell population; B, action of selective environment resulting in the death of the sensitive cell population; C, the remaining resistant cell population; D,
regrowth of tumor from the resistant cell types (after Webber et al [25]).

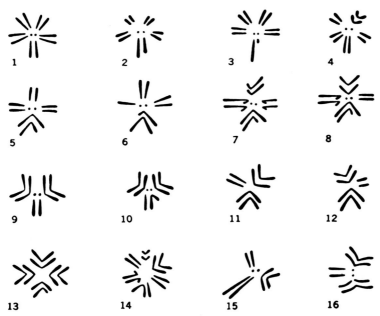

Fig. 5. Evolution and selection of Drosophila species resulting from rearrangements in the ancestral chromosomal complement. This evolution of species is compared with tumor progression, selection of resistant cells, and development of resistance in a tumor cell population exposed to chemotherapeutic agents or hormones (from Sinnot et al [25], used with permission
of McGraw-Hill Book Company).

I would like to demonstrate evolution and selection of species and chromosomal changes that go along with this selection by using the example of Drosophila
species [26] (Fig. 5). The simplest and perhaps the ancestral chromosome complement present in species of the genus Drosophila, consists of five pairs of rod-shaped
and one pair of dot-like chromosomes, as shown in Figure 5(1). Variations shown
in Figure 5(2–16) have resulted from chromosomal rearrangements, primarily trans-
locations. In a natural population of Drosophila, these variations may have been

present. Certain variations may have had specific advantages over others in the changing environment or in new niches. These environmental changes acted as selection factors and selected those flies which were better adapted to the new situation. These flies eventually developed into new species (Fig. 5, 2–16).

I have used this example to emphasize the importance of chromosomal changes. Chromosomal changes may be significant in the development of resistance, metastases, and progression of tumors; resistant cells can be considered new species, equivalent to new species at the organism level.

In conclusion, I would like to list areas in which further work is needed in the development of in vitro models (Table XIII). As emphasized by Dr. Merchant [16], there is need for multiple model systems for studies on the normal and malignant prostate. I believe that many questions on the etiology and treatment of prostatic tumors will be answered by using in vitro models of normal, benign, and malignant cells.

TABLE XIII. In Vitro Models

What is needed?

1. Additional in vitro systems using normal and malignant human cells
2. Chemically defined media
3. Enhancement of growth and maintenance
4. Growth controlling factors and growth regulation
5. Specific markers for prostatic epithelium
6. The use of several tests to establish malignant transformation

REFERENCES

1. Lewis RW, Kaack B: Non-human primate prostate culture (this volume).
2. Webber MM: Growth and maintenance of normal prostatic epithelium in vitro. A human cell model (this volume).
3. Lechner JF, Narayan KS, Ohnuki Y, Babcock MS, Jones LW, Kaighn ME: Replicative epithelial cell cultures from normal human prostate gland: Brief communication. J Natl Cancer Inst 60:797–801, 1978.
4. Kaighn ME, Lechner JF, Babcock MS, Marnell M, Ohnuki Y, Narayan KS: The Pasadena cell lines (this volume).
5. Stone KR, Mickey DD, Wunderli H, Mickey GH, Paulson DF: Isolation of a human prostate carcinoma cell line (DU-145). Int J Cancer 21:274–281, 1978.
6. Mickey DD, Stone KR, Wunderli H, Mickey GH, Paulson DF: Characterization of a human prostate adenocarcinoma cell line (DU-145) as a monolayer culture and as a solid tumor in athymic mice (this volume).
7. Smolev JK, Coffey DS, Scott WW: Experimental models for the study of prostatic adenocarcinoma. J Urol 118:216–220, 1977.
8. Fraley EE, Ecker S, Vincent MM: Spontaneous in vitro neoplastic transformation of adult human prostatic epithelium. Science 170:540–542, 1970.

9. Webber MM, Horan PK, Bouldin TR: Present status of MA-160 cell line. Prostatic epithelium or HeLa cells? Invest Urol 14:335–343, 1977.
10. Nelson-Rees W, Flandenmeyer R: HeLa cultures defined. Science 191:96–98, 1976.
11. Okada K, Schröder FH: Human prostatic carcinoma in cell culture: Preliminary report on the development and characterization of an epithelial cell line (EB-33). Urol Res 2:111–121, 1974.
12. Lubaroff DM: Development of an epithelial tissue culture line from human prostatic adenocarcinoma. J Urol 118:612–615, 1977.
13. Horoszewicz JS, Leong SS, Chu TM, Friedman M, Kin U, Chai LS, Kakati S, Arya SK, Sandberg AA: A new model for studies on human prostatic carcinoma. Proc Am Assoc Cancer Res 20:212, 1979.
14. Horoszewicz JS: A new model for studies on human prostatic carcinoma (this volume).
15. Gittes RF: The nude mouse – Its use as a tumor-bearing model of the prostate (this volume).
16. Poste G, Weiss L: Some considerations on cell surface alterations in malignancy. In Weiss L (ed): "Fundamental Aspects of Metastasis." New York: American Elsvier Publ Co, 1976, pp 25–47.
17. Dulbecco R: Topoinhibition and serum requirements of transformed and untransformed cells. Nature 227:802–806, 1970.
18. Macpherson I, Montagnier L: Agar suspension culture for the selective assay of cells transformed by polyoma virus. In Pollack R (ed): "Readings in Mammalian Cell Culture." New York: Cold Spring Harbor Laboratory, 1973, pp 288–291.
19. Unkeless J, Dano K, Kellerman GM, Reich E: Fibrinolysis associated with oncogenic transformation. J Biol Chem 249:4295–4305, 1974.
20. Burger MM: Surface changes in transformed cells detected by lectins. Fed Proc 32: 91–101, 1973.
21. Coggin JH Jr, Anderson NG: Cancer, differentiation and embryonic antigens: Some central problems. Adv Cancer Res 19:105–165, 1974.
22. Ryan WL, Curtis GL: Chemical carcinogenesis and cyclic AMP. In Schultz J, Gratzner HG (eds): "The Role of Cyclic Nucleotides in Carcinogenesis." New York: Academic Press, 1973, pp 1–18.
23. Porter KR, Todaro GJ, Fonte V: A scanning electron microscope study of surface features of viral and spontaneous transformants of mouse Balb 3T3 cells. J Cell Biol 59:633–642, 1973.
24. Weiss L (ed): "Fundamental Aspects of Metastasis." New York: American Elsvier Publ Co, 1976, pp 443.
25. Webber MM, Joneja MG, Connolly JG: Observations on Fortner tumor – A transplantable carcinoma of the hamster prostate. Invest Urol 5:348–357, 1968.
26. Sinnot EW, Dunn LC, Dobzhansky T: Genetics of species formation. In "Principles of Genetics." Ed 5. New York: McGraw-Hill, 1958, pp 286–302.
27. Merchant DJ: Requirements of in vitro model systems (this volume).

The Anatomic Heterogeneity of the Prostate

John E. McNeal, MD

The prostate gland is not a homogeneous organ. Within its capsule resides a diversity of tissues, both glandular and nonglandular. Aging further alters the composition of these different regions in ways that vary from person to person. Even as early as the fifth decade of life the same anatomic area may be quite different in appearance between different prostates. The results of tissue culture and other analyses must be profoundly affected by sampling problems resulting from this heterogeneity. However, the variables fall into a limited number of specific patterns, and these are discussed here in order to define the role of regional anatomic factors in tissue sampling.

REGIONAL ANATOMY OF THE PROSTATE

There are within the capsule of the normal adult prostate four different anatomic regions of substantially different composition [1, 2]. In precisely defining and locating these regions the prostatic urethra forms a valuable anatomic reference point. Its course through the gland brings it into contact with each region in a unique way (Fig. 1). The major ducts of the two main glandular regions of the prostate enter the urethra exclusively in its distal or prostatic segment, extending from the upper end of the verumontanum to the apex of the gland. A nonglandular. fibromuscular region lies anterior to the glandular prostate and contacts the urethra only at the bladder neck proximally and again distally at the prostate apex. Another region surrounds the proximal or preprostatic half of the prostatic urethra above the verumontanum. This is a complex region of mixed glandular and nonglandular tissue, which in the normal prostate is very small. These four regions of the prostate will be defined in detail in the sections that follow.

Models for Prostate Cancer, pages 149–160

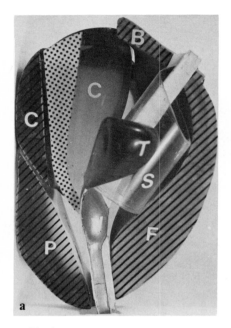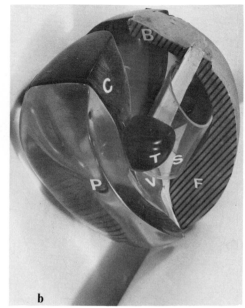

Fig. 1a. Three-dimensional model of prostate anatomy, side view. Sagittal cuts (lined areas) have been removed near side of fibromuscular stroma (F), bladder neck (B), central zone (C), and peripheral zone (P). Transition zone (T), sphincter (S), and urethra with verumontanum (V) are seen in full. Periurethral ducts hidden behind transition zone. Ejaculatory ducts (stippled) traverse center of central zone.

Fig. 1b. Three-dimensional model of prostate anatomy, ¾ view. Near side of fibromuscular stroma and bladder neck only removed by sagittal cut. Same symbols as Figure 1a.

The Anterior Fibromuscular Stroma

The anterior fibromuscular stroma is about one-third the total bulk of the normal adult prostate [3]. It is entirely lacking in glandular elements and is not of interest for tissue analysis except for its large size and the fact that its location totally conceals the anterior aspect of the glandular prostate and makes accurate dissection difficult. It consists of a thick sheath of tissue that takes origin from the detrusor muscle. Surrounding and blending with the internal urethral sphincter at the bladder neck, it sweeps distally as an apron over the anterior prostate surface, contacting the urethra again at the prostate apex. In its course it fans out laterally to merge with the capsule covering the anterior border of the glandular prostate. As it passes in front of the distal or prostatic segment of the urethra, it incorporates on its inner surface circular bands of sphincteric striated muscle which encircle the anterior aspect of the distal urethra and are continuous with the striated external sphincter distal to the prostate apex [4, 5]. At mid-urethra, just anterior to the verumontanum and proximal to most of the striated muscle fibers, the inner aspect of the sheath has a large fibrous component into which many of the smooth muscle fibers extending downward from the detrusor are anchored.

Peripheral Zone

The peripheral zone is the larger of the two major glandular regions of the prostate and represents roughly 75% of the total glandular tissue. This is the region where almost all carcinomas arise [6], and because of its accessible location and large size, most random biopsies of the prostate consist of tissue from this region. It is a flat disc of secretory tissue whose ducts branch out laterally from the distal segment of the prostatic urethra. It arises from ducts that exit as a double row of orifices along the posterolateral recesses of the urethra extending from the proximal end of the verumontanum to the prostate apex. Though extending mainly laterally, the more proximal ones also spread proximally but fail to complete the proximal quadrant of the glandular disc, which lies directly behind and above the verumontanum. Laterally, some of the terminal duct branches of the peripheral zone curve anteriorly to form a shallow cup around the striated sphincter and then anchor into the lateral extent of the fibromuscular stroma.

Central Zone

The central zone is the second component of the functioning glandular prostate and makes up about 25% of its mass. It completes the proximal quadrant of the glandular tissue above and behind the verumontanum. Its lateral margins are therefore apposed to the most proximal of the peripheral zone ducts, forming a smooth-surfaced complete disc whose two compartments are not evident from external inspection. The central zone ducts contact the urethra only in a single small area immediately surrounding the orifices of the ejaculatory ducts on the convexity of the verumontanum. They are remote from the peripheral zone duct orifices, which lie in the recesses lateral to the verumontanum. The central zone ducts course proximally, surrounding closely the course of the ejaculatory ducts. They branch mainly laterally to form a flat wedge of glandular tissue with its apex at the verumontanum and its base at the base of the prostate posterior to the bladder neck.

The definition of central zone versus peripheral zone depends on differences in gland architecture and cytologic detail in addition to clear-cut anatomic boundaries between these zones [4, 7]. The peripheral zone ducts are long, narrow, and straight, with short terminal branches ending in small, simple, round acini (Fig. 2). The central zone ducts are larger with more complex arborization. They produce large acini of irregular contour, partially compartmentalized by septa (Fig. 3). The peripheral

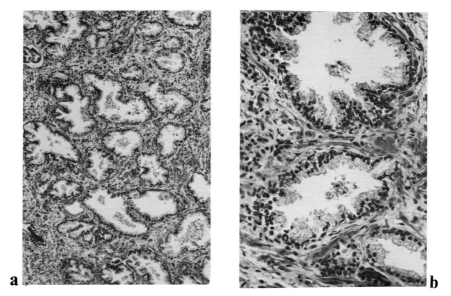

Fig. 2. Normal peripheral zone: a) at 35×; b) at 140×.

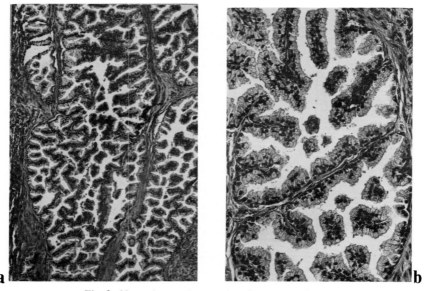

Fig. 3. Normal central zone: a) at 35×; b) at 140×.

zone epithelium consists of pale cells in simple columnar arrangement with basal, small, dark nuclei and distinct cell borders. The central zone cells have granular, opaque cytoplasm. They are irregularly crowded so that nuclei lie at different levels. The nuclei tend to be larger than those of the peripheral zone and more variable in size.

The distinction between these two zones is important for tissue sampling because carcinomas arise frequently in the peripheral zone but are quite uncommon in the central zone. Furthermore, the striking morphologic differences suggest a major difference in basic biologic function, though there is no evidence to confirm this possibility. The architectural and histologic features of the central zone closely resemble those of the seminal vesicle [7]. This has led to the suggestion that the central zone may be of Wolffian duct origin, while the remainder of the glandular prostate arises from the urogenital sinus. This possibility might correlate with the observation that both central zone and seminal vesicle are resistant to the development of carcinoma.

The variation between prostates of different species is considerable. In several animals used for experimental purposes, the existence of regions homologous to the human central and peripheral zones is not obvious [7]. In the dog and cat, the glandular prostate appears homogeneous, having some resemblance to human peripheral zone but with significant morphologic differences. Central zone appears not to be represented, and perhaps significantly, the seminal vesicle is absent in both species. Rhesus monkeys, on the other hand, have prominent seminal vesicles and possess a region called the cranial lobe, which is histologically similar to their seminal vesicle and has the same anatomic location as the human central zone [8]. A recent electron microscopic study [9] indicates that the rhesus cranial lobe is homologous with the human central zone. If this homology can be confirmed, it might be of great value in prostate research.

Preprostatic Tissue

The preprostatic tissue, which surrounds the urethra proximal to the upper end of the verumontanum, is the smallest of the four regions but the most complex in its arrangement of both glandular and nonglandular elements. Its main component is a cylindrical smooth muscle sphincter surrounding the entire preprostatic urethra. Closely related to this sphincter are two tiny areas of glandular tissue, one of these inside the sleeve of sphincteric tissue and the other immediately outside it [1]. Of these two the smaller component, the periurethral glands, consist of simple straight ducts of near microscopic size arising from the urethral wall inside the sphincter and coursing for a few millimeters proximally parallel to the urethra. Their levels of origin and their numbers are inconstant. They have few branches, few or no acini, and no periductal smooth muscle, since their only stroma is that of the nonglandular urethral submucosa. Hence, they are unlikely to play any role in adult prostatic function.

At the distal border of the cylindrical preprostatic sphincter, in a very short segment hear the upper end of the verumontanum, the lateral urethral wall receives the orifices of the transition zone ducts. These small ducts pass around the distal end of the sphincter and branch proximally toward the bladder neck immediately outside the sphincter. They have a fairly elaborate system of duct branching which fills the shallow cleft between the peripheral zone and the sphincter but extends for only a short distance proximally toward the bladder neck. The acini in part have their own smooth muscle slings, but there is much intermingling of sphincteric stroma with transition zone glandular tissue. Thus, the duct systems originating in the lateral recesses of the urethral wall have three components. The peripheral zone ducts are located in the distal or prostatic urethral segment, the tiny periurethral ducts are limited to the preprostatic segment, and the transition zone system arises at the junction of the two segments. These three duct systems form a continuous double row of duct orifices extending from the prostate apex to the bladder neck. The three duct systems are histologically similar, probably reflecting a common embryologic derivation. Their major difference is their striking dissimilarity in degree of duct development and in the character of the stroma with which each is associated. The peripheral zone is at least twenty times larger than the other two components. It shows elaborate acinar development with extensive periacinar muscle slings. At the other extreme, the entire bulk of the periurethral glandular tissue can be measured in cubic millimeters. It has no stroma of its own and only imperfectly developed acini. The transition zone is a miniature model of the peripheral zone, but its acinar tissue is often less well developed, and its stroma shows a mixture of appropriate periacinar slings with a foreign element of circular smooth muscle fibers from the preprostatic cylindrical sphincter.

Though these three ductal systems are probably of common embryologic origin, their adult fate is dramatically different, as demonstrated by the unique propensity of transition zone and periurethral glandular tissue to give rise to benign nodular hyperplasia (BPH) [1]. Thus, in many glands from which tissue samples are taken for tissue culture and other analyses these two tiny regions may be markedly expanded. The normal peripheral zone may weigh 15–20 grams. The abnormal overgrowth of BPH may cause the tiny periurethral and transition zone to outweigh the peripheral zone by 100 grams or more. The peripheral zone becomes flattened into a thin shell encapsulating the nodular masses — the "surgical capsule" of urologic surgery. The peripheral zone then undergoes compression atrophy and becomes very difficult to sample because of its thinness. Biopsies taken from the usual peripheral zone areas may consist mainly of BPH tissue when the disease process is advanced. Microscopic examination may not always reveal the true tissue origin because of the close histologic resemblance between the acinar tissue in these three regions.

DIVERGENT VIEWS OF PROSTATE ANATOMY

The above morphologic description does not reflect uniformity of opinion on the anatomy of the prostate. Not only differing concepts of morphology but also a proliferation of conflicting terminologies have made this historically a very confusing subject. Such inconsistencies become a critical hindrance to the proper selection of tissue samples for culture. It is important therefore to explain the differences between these opposing views and also to outline their points of similarity, which are often obscured by differences in terminology. Lowsley [10] in 1912 divided the prostate into lobes, and his lobe concept has determined much of the thinking about prostate anatomy even into recent years. It should be remembered, however, that Lowsley worked entirely with prostates from embryos and newborn infants. He regarded the prostate as histologically homogeneous, but he would not have been able to appreciate histologic differences between the central and peripheral zones since these are not obvious in the prepubertal gland. He declared that prostate carcinoma arose only in the posterior lobe, but this was anecdotal information and was obviously not a conclusion from any of his own data. During the half century since his investigation, the existence of the posterior lobe as an entity in the postnatal prostate has been frequently contested [11, 12]. Most investigators have found that the distribution of carcinoma in the prostate does not correspond at all to the boundaries that Lowsley set for his posterior lobe. Therefore, it must be questioned whether Lowsley's conclusions contribute in any significant degree to the understanding of adult prostatic anatomy or disease.

The periurethral ducts above the verumontanum were identified and described by Lowsley. He was unaware of their relationship to BPH and he specifically stated that they did not belong to any of the prostate lobes he had described. He did not even consider them to be part of the prostate. It remained for Franks in 1954 [12] to establish that these ducts, and perhaps other ducts very close to the urethra, were responsible for BPH. He referred to these glandular structures as the "inner prostate," whereas the duct systems belonging to Lowsley's lobes were called the "outer prostate." Franks supported the conclusions of previous studies that the lobe distinctions proposed by Lowsley for the outer prostate do not exist in the adult gland and do not have significance for the distribution of cancer in the prostate. Franks supported the conclusions of previous studies that the lobe distinctions proposed by Lowsley for the outer prostate do not exist in the adult gland and do not have significance for the distribution of cancer in the prostate. Franks stated that carcinoma occurred diffusely throughout the outer gland. Unfortunately, much of these data appears to have been collected from single transverse sections through the middle of the prostate. Hence, it went unrecognized that the periurethral ducts are present only above the verumontanum and represent a proximal extension of the peripheral zone ducts. The existence of the transition zone and the association of both these regions with a preprostatic cylindrical sphincter must also have been overlooked in the absence of efforts to examine the third (vertical) dimension of this organ. For the same reason, Franks would not have been able to visualize the superior segment of the glandular prostatic disc — that which represents the central zone. Hence, in these two major studies of prostate anatomy, the central zone could not be recognized in one because of the exclusive use of prepubertal material and in the other probably because of inadequate sections taken from the area of interest. Therefore, the prostate was regarded until recently as being histologically homogeneous, and investigators with confidence took sections at random from any part of the gland, even including BPH tissue.

CHANGES IN THE PROSTATE WITH AGE

In many men at a relatively early age the characteristic anatomic features described above undergo a variety of alterations, both focal and diffuse. The commonest early change is focal atrophy, first described by Moore [13] as beginning in the fifth decade, and subsequently studied by other investigators. The commonest form of atrophy is focal and is characterized by marked gland shrinkage, frequent chronic inflammation, and stromal fibrosis (Fig. 4). Moore did not distinguish this as a separate pattern. Franks [14] thought that this special variety of "sclerotic atrophy" was premalignant. The nearly constant inflammatory reaction and the damage done to both glands and stroma suggest that this is a basically inflammatory process. It is quite common, but there is no evidence at present that it has any clinical symptomatology. Its significance for tissue collection for culture and analysis is that it may be quite severe in relatively young men and produce a large area of gland atrophy in an otherwise normal prostate [4]. It is possible that such atrophic epithelium might behave normally when removed from its natural environment into tissue culture conditions, but there is no evidence available on this possibility.

Observation of prostates at autopsy suggests that the atrophy associated with aging and presumably due to androgen withdrawal has a different histologic pattern [4]. The gland spaces remain large, stromal fibrosis is less conspicuous, inflammation is absent, and the atrophy tends to be diffuse (Fig. 5). Although this type of atrophy is not normally seen in younger men, it can be produced by chronic debilitating diseases such as malignancy. Without such disease, its age of onset in many men is delayed until the eighth decade. However, it often occurs earlier for no apparent reason. Because of the occurrence of these two types of atrophy, plus the pressure atrophy produced by BPH, the histologic features and presumably the biologic characteristics of prostates from men over the age of 40 cannot be presumed to be similar between different glands, or even between different areas of the same gland. Thus, the accurate study of tissue for culture

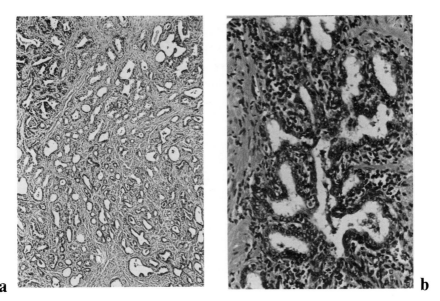

Fig. 4. Sclerotic atrophy: a) at 35×; b) at 140×.

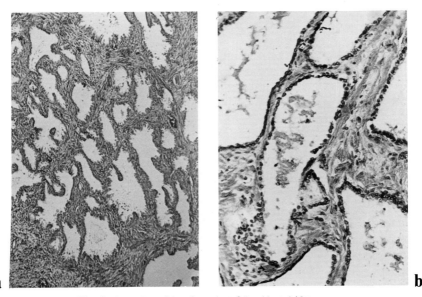

Fig. 5. Atrophy with aging: a) at 35×; b) at 140×.

or other analysis requires histologic confirmation of the nature of the tissue sampled.

In addition, a variety of hyperplastic changes of premalignant nature occur focally in the peripheral zone [6, 15]. These appear inconstantly, most often affect glands with a high degree of epithelial activity, and become progressively more common over the age of 40. Their focal nature and the bizarre changes of architecture or cytology seen with them suggest that these represent spontaneous focal emergence of autonomous growth potential. In one variety of alteration, the dominant change is the appearance of marked nuclear pleomorphism and hyper-chromatism within the epithelial cells of preexisting ducts (Fig. 6). There also appears prominent cellular crowding, suggesting a degree of uncontrolled cellular growth. In its fully developed state, this change deserves the designation of "carci-noma in situ," and in selected cases, invasive cancer can be seen developing in such areas.

Another type of premalignant hyperplasia results from the budding of new small acini out of preexisting acini with preservation of entirely normal nuclear characteristics (Fig. 7). This creation of new architecture suggests the reemergence of embryonic capacities. It can be seen on favorable sections to blend into areas of very well differentiated carcinoma. Both these atypicalities are usually seen in small foci, but occasionally they may cover very large areas of the prostate and certainly represent marked changes in the biologic characteristics of any epithelial tissue sampled from these areas.

SUMMARY

In selecting tissue samples for culture or other analysis, it must be recognized that the prostate gland is an organ of heterogeneous composition. Fortunately, that component showing great susceptibility to carcinoma is also the largest and the most easily accessible to biopsy. However, this area is often susceptible to secondary changes with aging. These include several types of atrophy and several varieties of hyperplasia which are probably premalignant. These changes may begin focally in the fifth decade and produce in time a regional heterogeneity within the previously homogeneous peripheral zone. Furthermore, the increasing mass of the transition zone and periurethral glands as BPH develops often compresses the pe-ripheral zone and increases the possibility of erroneously sampling the abnormal tissue.

These problems can be partly circumvented by careful attention to the anatomy and using material from men under the age of 40. Over this age, material can still be useful and representative of normal tissue, providing histologic study of the sam-ple shows it to be the area desired for study and of normal morphology.

The central zone has never been adequately studied with sophisticated tech-niques and might be of interest because of its relative immunity to carcinoma.

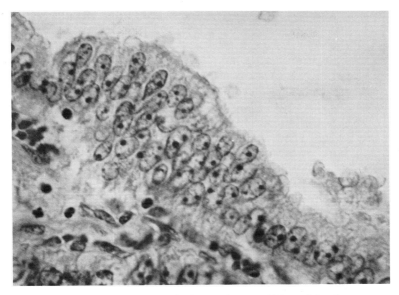

Fig. 6. Severe epithelial dysplasia and in situ carcinoma within peripheral zone prostatic duct, 560×.

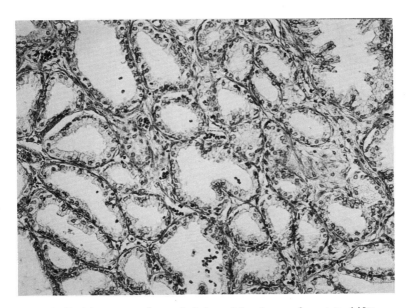

Fig. 7. Adenomatous hyperplasia in peripheral zone of prostate, 140×.

Within the peripheral zone, the premalignant hyperplasias deserve further study but will invariably be difficult to sample properly because they are usually of small size and inconstant in occurrence and location. Tissue from nonhuman sources may also be of value. However, it should be kept in mind that at present there is insufficient evidence of valid homologies between species. There is no reason to believe that the dog prostate is any more like the human prostate than the human central zone is like the peripheral zone. Conclusions from one species may not then be generalized with confidence.

REFERENCES

1. McNeal JE: Origin and evolution of benign prostatic enlargement. Invest Urol 15:340–345, 1978.
2. McNeal JE: New morphologic findings relevant to the origin and evolution of cancer of the prostate and BPH. UICC Monograph – Cancer of the Prostate (In press).
3. McNeal JE: The prostate and prostatic urethra: A morphologic synthesis. J Urol 107:1008–1016, 1972.
4. McNeal JE: Regional morphology and pathology of the prostate. Am J Clin Pathol 49:347–357, 1968.
5. Blacklock NJ: Surgical anatomy of the prostate. In Williams DI, Chisholm, GD (eds) "Scientific Foundations of Urology." Chicago: Yearbook Medical Publishers, 1977, pp 113–125.
6. McNeal JE: Origin and development of carcinoma in the prostate. Cancer 23:24–34, 1969.
7. McNeal JE: Developmental and comparative anatomy of the prostate. In Benign Prostatic Hyperplasia, 1–10, DHEW (NIH) 76–113, 1976.
8. Blacklock NJ, Bouskill K: The zonal anatomy of the prostate in man and in the rhesus monkey. Urol Res 5:163–167, 1977.
9. Battersby S, Chandler JA, Harper ME, Blacklock NJ: The ultrastructure of rhesus monkey prostate. Urol Res 5:175–183, 1977.
10. Lowsley OS: The development of the human prostate gland with reference to the development of other structures at the neck of the urinary bladder. Am J Anat 13:299–349, 1912.
11. LeDuc IE: The anatomy of the prostate and the pathology of early benign hypertrophy. J Urol 42:1217–1241, 1939.
12. Franks LM: Benign nodular hyperplasia of the prostate: A review. Ann Roy Coll Surg 14:92–106, 1954.
13. Moore RA: The evolution and involution of the prostate gland. Am J Pathol 12:599–624, 1936.
14. Franks LM: Atrophy and hyperplasia in the prostate proper. J Pathol Bacteriol 68:617–621, 1954.
15. McNeal JE: Age related changes in prostatic epithelium associated with carcinoma. In "Some Aspects of the Aetiology and Biochemistry of Prostatic Cancer." Cardiff: Tenovus Workshop Publications, pp 23–32, 1970.

Establishment of Primary Cell Cultures From Normal and Neoplastic Human Prostate Gland Tissue

Theodore I. Malinin, MD, Alice J. Claflin, PhD, Norman L. Block, MD, and Arnold L. Brown, MD

Several reports on the in vitro cultivation of human prostate gland cells have appeared in the literature [1—4] during the last decade. Most of these deal either with the attempts to propagate pure "epithelial" cell cultures or to use such cultures for testing hormonal sensitivity of same. The outcome of these endeavors was not always clear, mainly because of the difficulties encountered with characterizing the morphologic nature of cell populations in cultures or quantitating the biological response of cells in cultures [3]. The early experience gained by the authors of this report indicated that when explants of either embryonic or normal adult prostate tissues began to grow in culture, the initial cell sheet thus produced was usually composed of cells having an "epithelial" morphologic appearance [5]. Similar observations have been reported by Webber et al [1]. Histologic sections of the explants showed the cells growing out of alveoli and ducts of the prostate gland. Whether such cells from normal glands can produce a continuous growth in tissue culture if isolated from supporting connective tissue and vascular elements is open to question. Carefully conducted experiments of Franks and co-workers [4] suggested such may not be the case.

Subsequent experiments conducted on larger numbers and on greater varieties of the prostate gland tissue explants indicated that in many instances epithelial cells, once they migrated away from the explant, soon either elongated or became mixed with fibroblast-like cells [6]. These studies suggested that the biology of the in vitro growth of normal and neoplastic cells from human prostate glands would perhaps lend itself to the study in primary cell cultures. Having developed an explant technique that produced consistent results in our laboratory [7], tissues from 168 prostate glands with and without tumors were subjected to in vitro cultivation under identical standard conditions.

The cultivation of the prostate gland by the explant technique is not new. All-

Models for Prostate Cancer, pages 161—180

göwer placed pieces of prostatic adenoma in plasma clots in 1949 and noted that outgrowing cells lysed the clots [8]. Roehl [9] reported hormone dependency of prostatic cancer cells in culture. Lasnitzky, in a review article [10], states that hormonal response of human prostate adenoma cells in culture is still controversial, but the same author demonstrated cellular changes in "organ cultures" of adenomatous prostate glands suggestive of androgen sensitivity of these cells. In a widely quoted paper, Wojewski and Przeworska-Kaniewicz reported the results of explant cultivation of 2,429 specimens of human adenoma and 1,085 specimens of human prostatic cancer [11]. However, this large number of explants was obtained from the prostate glands of but 18 patients. The majority of the above-cited studies employed the plasma-clot explant technique. This technique is somewhat cumbersome inasmuch as the clot lysis occurs in many cultures. For that reason, an alternate technique was employed in the present studies. It was selected by a trial-and-error method from several existing explant techniques [12].

The subject of this report is the initial behavior of cells in the explant cultures obtained consecutively from a relatively large number of normal and abnormal human prostate glands. In addition, an attempt was made to determine whether the initial cell outgrowth from the explants can be stimulated by the addition of testosterone to culture media. Since several thousand explants were used in these experiments, the results are presented in an overall summary fashion. The volume of data obtained from each experiment and the scope of the report preclude a detailed description of individual results obtained in these studies.

MATERIALS AND METHODS

The prostate glands studied were obtained at surgery or were excised under sterile conditions from cadavers [5]. Of 168 prostate glands, 94 were surgical specimens obtained either by perineal, suprapubic, or retropubic prostatectomies; 52 were autopsy specimens, and 22 were pieces of the prostate gland removed by cold transurethral resection. Seven lymph node biopsies with histologically confirmed metastatic carcinoma from the prostate gland were also subjected to study, but these were not included in the total number of 168 prostate glands. In addition, six specimens, one from autopsy and five from TURs, were received contaminated with microorganisms. These were also not included in 168 prostate glands which are the subject of this report.

Surgical specimens were examined and step-sectioned transversely at 2—4 mm intervals from within a few minutes to one-half hour after resection. The slices of tissue removed from the prostate glands thus sectioned were placed into sterile containers with tissue culture medium CMRL 1415 ATM and brought to the laboratory. At autopsy, the prostate glands were removed retropubically in toto. Resected prostate glands were then handled in the same manner as the surgical specimens. However, all pieces of tissue obtained by TURs were collected at the Mayo

Clinic, Rochester, Minnesota, and shipped to Miami in tissue culture medium. These specimens did not reach the tissue culture laboratory for about 48 hours after excision.

Of the total number of prostate glands subjected to tissue culture studies, 21 were from fetuses, 34 were normal, 22 were with adenomas, and 98 including metastatic lymph nodes were carcinomatous.

Upon receipt in the tissue culture laboratory, appropriate prostate gland tissue samples were selected for culturing. The tissue used for explants was that distant from the connective tissue capsule of the prostate gland. The explants consisted of blocks of tissue approximately 1 mm^3. The preparation of the explants was carried out on a Teflon board covered with tissue culture medium. The explants were transferred into plastic tissue (250 ml) culture flasks, the bottoms of which were barely covered with medium consisting of CMRL 1415 with sodium bicarbonate buffer and 30% fetal calf serum with 100 units/ml penicillin, 100 mcg/ml streptomycin, and 2 mcg/ml of fungizone. From five to 12 explants were placed into each culture vessel. Usually five culture flasks were prepared for each experiment, but this obviously varied with the amount of tissue available. Only one or two flasks could be set up with fetal tissues. The culture flasks were gassed with 10% CO_2 in 90% air before they were stoppered and placed into an incubator at 37°C.

Individual explants became attached to the bottoms of the culture vessels usually within 24 hours, but a small percentage of explants never attached at all.

The medium was not changed for the first seven days, and then only after cellular outgrowth was noticed or when there was a perceptible drop in the pH of the fluid. Once cell growth took place, the serum concentration in the medium was reduced to 10%. In the cultures in which the cellular outgrowth did not take place the medium was changed either when there was a noticeable shift in its pH or every two weeks.

The flasks were observed under a phase-contrast microscope initially every day, and after the onset of cell growth every two to three days. Observations on each flask were continued until the cultures became confluent. If cell growth did not occur, the flasks were discarded in about two months.

For morphologic observations, cells were fixed in 10% formalin in Earle's balanced salt solution and stained with Wright-Giemsa stain, hematoxylin and eosin, or iron hematoxylin. For ultrastructural studies cells were fixed in flasks with 3% glutaraldehyde in phosphate buffer for one hour, post-fixed in Dalton's fixative for 45 minutes, dehydrated in graded alcohols, and embedded in Epon. After polymerization the plastic flasks were cracked by immersion in boiling water. Cells remained embedded in Epon. These were sectioned with a diamond knife on a Sorvall MT-2 ultramicrotome, double stained with uranyl and lead salts, and examined in a Philips EM-500 microscope.

To determine the possible effect of testosterone on the growth of cells from prostatic tissue explants, 1 mcg/ml of testosterone was added to randomly selected tissue culture flasks from 60 experiments with sufficient tissue to set up duplicate

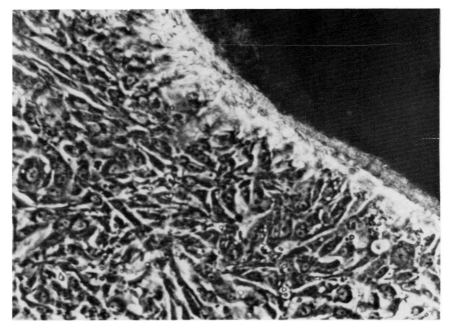

Fig. 1. Cells from human fetal prostate gland at the edge of the explant. The cells are densely packed and epithelial in appearance (unstained phase-contrast photograph; magnification, × 100).

experiments. The growth of cells from explants in these flasks was compared to that in cultures to which testosterone was not added. The explant cell cultures grown in medium with testosterone were observed and fluid was changed in an identical manner to all other cultures.

RESULTS

Cell growth was obtained from all 21 fetal prostate glands. Cellular outgrowth from these explants was noted from one to eight days of cultivation, with the average time of occurrence of cell growth being 4.1 days. The cells which surrounded and migrated away from fetal explants had an epithelial-like appearance (Fig. 1). Serial histologic sections of explants showed that the cells which produced the cell sheet and encapsulated the relatively acellular explants originated from the tubules or the alveoli of the prostate gland (Fig. 2). The rate with which the fetal cells proliferated in cultures varied, but these cells grew faster than any other cells from prostate glands studied. Cellular confluence was achieved between 12 and 34 days, despite the fact that, because of the small size of the glands, only a few explants

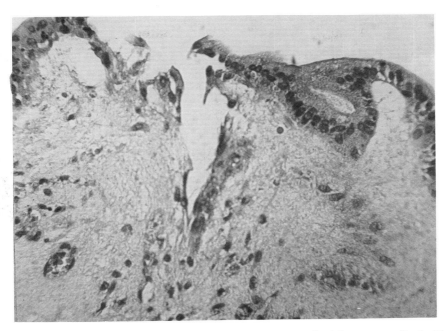

Fig. 2. Section of the explant of the fetal prostate gland. Note aglandular structure lined with columnar epithelial cells. These cells appear to be the main contributors to the initial cell outgrowth emanating from the explant (hematoxylin and eosin stain; magnification, × 250).

could be placed in a flask. The average time for reaching cellular confluence was 23.4 days from the time explants were placed in culture. However, if the time of confluence was estimated from the onset of cellular outgrowth rather than from placing the explants in cultures, the average time to confluence was reduced to 20.6 days, but the range was still wide — from nine to 31 days.

Of 34 normal adult prostate glands studied, explants from 18 produced cellular outgrowth. The explants from the other 16 glands failed to grow altogether. However, in five of 18 experiments in which the explants produced cellular outgrowth, the cells failed to form confluent cell sheets and the cultures degenerated and died. The first cellular outgrowth was noted, on the average, in 10.2 days, with the range from two to 21 days. The average time to confluence in 13 cultures was 51.4 days, with the range from 22 to 113 days from the time of the initiation of culture. The time to confluence calculated from the onset of cellular outgrowth was 49.3 days with a range of 24 to 96 days. Initially, cells near the explants from normal prostate glands had an epithelial-like appearance (Fig. 3). However, as the cells migrated away from the explants, elongated cells made their appearance (Fig. 4).

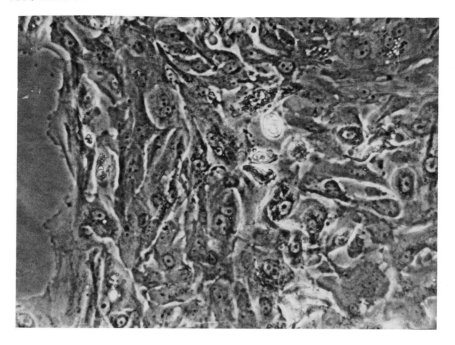

Fig. 3. The sheet of large epithelial cells in the primary, but not yet confluent culture of the normal adult prostate gland (unstained phase-contrast photograph; magnification, × 250).

In some but not all cultures, these became predominant by the time confluence was reached. No clear-cut relation between the cell growth or lack thereof from the explants of the normal adult prostate glands and the postmortem period of four to 24 hours, or the patient's age, could be established. However, all three prostate glands from the kidney donors grew. The summary of the growth of the normal prostate glands, donor's age, and the postmortem interval is given in Table I.

Of 22 prostates with adenomas, five of which were obtained at autopsy, 19 produced cellular growth in culture, while three did not. The cultures from three donors did not reach confluence. Of five autopsy specimens, one failed to grow and cells from another one failed to reach confluence. The average time for the first cell outgrowth was 9.2 days, with a range of three to 45 days. The time to confluence was 43.8 days, with a range of 23 to 57 days. The time to confluence from the appearance of the initial cellular outgrowth was 41.7 days, with a range of 14 to 54 days. The cells in these cultures were large and maintained an epithelial character, as is shown in Figure 5.

Explants from 98 prostate glands including seven lymph nodes with carcinomas (four autopsies, 72 prostatectomies, 22 TURs) produced cellular outgrowth in 85

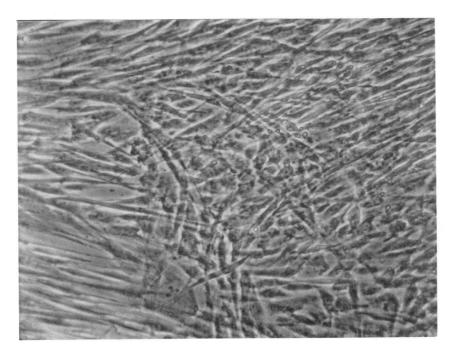

Fig. 4. Confluent primary culture of normal adult prostatic cells. The epithelial cells visible in the center of the cluster of cells are overgrown by elongated fibroblast-like cells (unstained phase-contrast photograph; magnification, × 100).

experiments. However, cells from cultures from seven donors failed to become confluent. Of these, one was from a prostate gland tumor obtained at autopsy. The average time for cellular outgrowth was 9.75 days, with a range of three to 34 days. The average time needed for the cultures to reach confluence was 44.9 days, with a range of 19 to 103 days. If calculated from the time of cellular outgrowth rather than initiation of the cultures, the average time to confluence was 32.5 days, with a range from 14 to 102 days. These cells were rounded or polyhedral and usually had large nuclei (Fig. 6). However, many cultures produced cell clusters with cells piling up on one another.

The explant cultures from all seven lymph nodes with metastases produced cellular growth that became confluent. In the cultures the average time to cellular outgrowth was 11.5 days, with a range of six to 18 days. Confluence was reached on the average in 44.5 days, with a range of 26 to 60 days. Calculated from the time of cellular outgrowth, confluence was reached on the average in 34.7 days, with a range of 11 to 49 days. The summary of the growth patterns of all tissues studied is given in Table II.

TABLE I. Summary of Results Obtained With Adult Normal Prostate Glands Obtained at Autopsy

Number	Age	Postmortem interval (hours)	Cell growth	Confluence
1	60	8	yes	yes
2	65	14	yes	yes
3	76	16	yes	no
4	23	22	yes	no
5	53	12	yes	no
6	49	11	no	
7	61	24	no	
8	54	12	yes	no
9	62	17	yes	yes
10	55	10	no	
11	32	8	yes	no
12	66	6	no	
13	60	15	yes	yes
14	13	14	yes	yes
15	50	6	no	
16	31	4	yes	yes
17	16	6	yes	yes
18	36	8	yes	no
19	48	8	yes	no
20	68	8	yes	yes
21	53	7	no	
22	47	17	yes	no
23	57	9	yes	yes
24	54	9	no	
25	77	19	no	
26	51	1	yes	yes
27	64	10	no	
28	50	19	no	
29	76	8	no	
30	16	3	yes	no
31	11	0.5	yes	yes
32	37	0.2	yes	yes
33	18	0.2	yes	yes
34	49	5	yes	yes

There was no perceptible difference in the cell growth in 50 out of 60 experiments between the cultures treated with testosterone and the control cultures. In the remaining ten experiments (six carcinomas, three BPHs, and one normal) differences in the cell growth were noted. In these experiments the average time of cellular outgrowth was 9.0 days for testosterone-treated cultures and 7.1 days for paired untreated cultures.

Electron microscopic study of the cells derived from normal human prostate

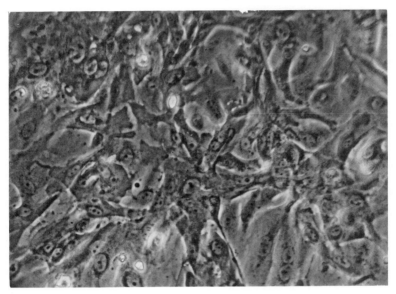

Fig. 5. Primary cell culture from an adenocarcinoma of the prostate gland. The epithelial cells are round with large nuclei and relatively scant cytoplasm (unstained phase-contrast photograph; magnification, × 100).

glands showed many cells examined to be of similar appearance. The nuclei were either oval or slightly elongated. Most contained indentations. Nucleoli, when included in the section planes, were eccentric and prominent. The cytoplasm contained large numbers of organelles, including aggregates of rough endoplasmic reticulum, free ribosomes, polysomes, Golgi complexes, and mitochondria. However, the well-defined regional polarization and differentiation of cell organelles was lost. The rough endoplasmic reticulum was distended and filled with finely granular material. The periphery of the cells contained filamentous bundles, presumably myofilaments. Desmosomes and desmosomal junctions were present. Scattered throughout the cytoplasm were numerous secretory vacuoles containing granular material, polymorphic material, and darkly staining lamellar structures, possibly derived from phospholipids (Fig. 7).

The ultrastructural appearance of cells derived from adenomatous prostate gland explants differed from that of cells derived from normal prostate glands. These cultures were composed of two predominant cell types. The cytoplasm of some cells was packed with organelles, the predominant ones being dense, relatively amorphous structures reminiscent of residual bodies (Fig. 8). Although these bodies were present throughout the cytoplasm, they appeared to be more numerous in the supranuclear regions. On higher magnification, the residual bodies contained

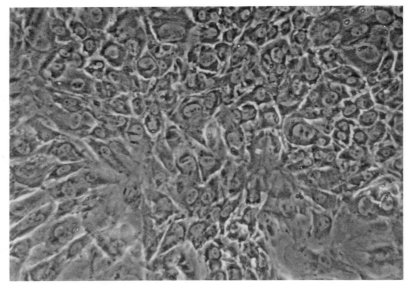

Fig. 6. Primary cell culture from an adenocarcinoma of the prostate gland. The epithelial cells are round with large nuclei and relatively scant cytoplasm (unstained phase-contrast photograph; magnification, × 100).

TABLE II. Summary of Results With Growth of Explant Cultures of Human Prostate Gland

	Fetal	Normal adult	BPH	Carcinoma	Lymph node metastases
Number of prostates studied	21	34	22	91	7
Percent of prostates failing to produce cell growth	0	47	3	6	0
Time of the appearance of first cellular outgrowth	4.1	10.2	9.2	9.7	11.5
Total average time to confluence	24	51.4	43.8	44.9	44.5
Average time to confluence from the appearance of cell growth	20.6	49.3	41.7	35.2	34.2

some ill-defined lamellar-like arrangements of granular material (Fig. 9). The mitochondria were generally large, with a dense granular matrix and widely separated cristae. Free ribosomes were found between the structures. The other type of cells contained numerous secretory vacuoles, some of which contained clusters of dense particles and lamellar bodies and secretory granules with a rim of electron-dense material in the periphery. The lamellar bodies, the myelin nature of which becomes apparent on higher magnification, were apparently extruded by the cell with finger-, like cytoplasmic extensions (Fig. 10).

Cultures of cells from explants of carcinomatous prostate glands presented a variegated appearance. Cells growing at the edges of the explant among abundant collagen fibers were either compact with well-organized cytoplasm or had their cytoplasm grossly distorted by many large vacuoles filled with amorphous material and dense residual bodies (Fig. 11). The nuclei of many cells were lobulated and contained prominent nucleoli composed of dense, presumably ribonucleic acid particles. However, in many other cells nuclei showed atypical alterations, including pleomorphism, extensive invaginations, and accumulation of dense chromatin. In the cells the loss of the usual cytoplasmic organellar arrangement was complete (Fig. 12). The cells away from the explant also showed changes compatible with those described for poorly differentiated prostate adenocarcinoma cells [16] (Fig. 13).

DISCUSSION

The tissue culture studies conducted on the cells derived from explants of fetal, normal adult, adenomatous, and cancerous prostate glands reaffirmed the reliability of the explant technique for assessing growth potential of the tissue. The observations on the growth patterns of the prostate cells in vitro demonstrate a high proliferative capacity of fetal cells, as compared to adult cells, including those derived from neoplastic glands. The growth of these cells was more consistent and rapid than the growth of cells of carcinoma of the prostate. Since the slow growth of prostatic carcinoma is a well-documented phenomenon, this finding does not appear surprising. The same held true for the explants obtained from the lymph node metastases, which, in their cell growth pattern, did not differ appreciably from the explants of the carcinoma of the prostate gland itself. The growth pattern of the adenomatous glands did not differ markedly from that of the carcinomatous glands, but the behavior of the explants from the adult normal prostate glands did. The percentage of the prostate glands failing to produce cell growth from explants was considerably higher in the normal glands (47.0%) than in BPH (13.6%) and carcinomas (6.5%). The average time of first cellular outgrowth and the time needed to reach confluence of the cell sheet was also greater for the normal than for the tumorous prostate.

However, it may be said that a comparison between normal prostate glands ob-

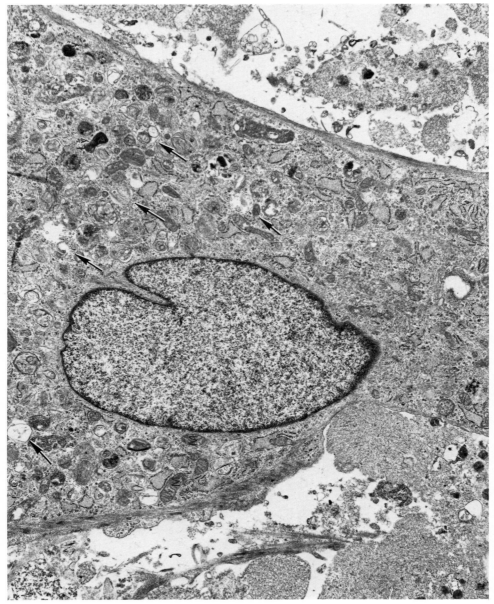

7

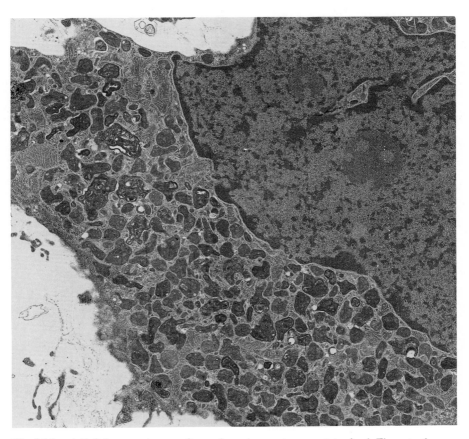

Fig. 8 (above) Cell from a primary culture of an adenomatous prostate gland. The cytoplasm is packed with residual bodies (original magnification, × 4,000).

Fig. 7 (facing page). Cell from a culture from normal adult prostate gland. The secretory vacuoles (arrows) are found predominantly in one portion of the cytoplasm, possibly the original apical pole. Many of these are filled with polymorphous material and lamellar structures. Mitochondria (M) are not numerous. The spherical electron-dense structures, possibly lysosomes (ly), represent areas of focal cytoplasmic degradation (original magnification, × 12,540).

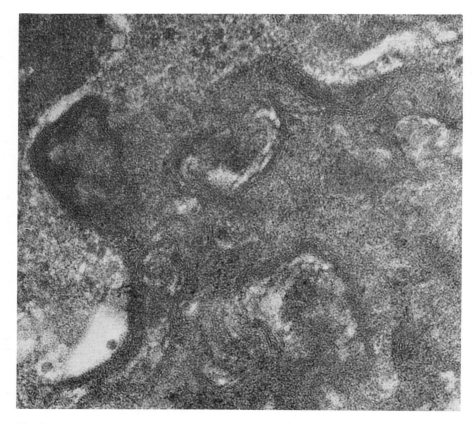

Fig. 9. The residual bodies are composed of irregular granular material arranged in parallel arrays near the margin of the bodies (original magnification, × 60,420).

tained primarily at autopsy and diseased glands obtained primarily at surgical operations may not be valid. True, the comparison between postmortem and surgical material would be difficult to make were it not for the prostate gland from the cadaver kidney donors and the diseased glands obtained at autopsy. Although a clear-cut correlation between the postmortem interval and the growth of the explants was difficult to make, it must be noted that the explants from prostate glands collected after 17 hours postmortem did not grow at all, whereas the ex-

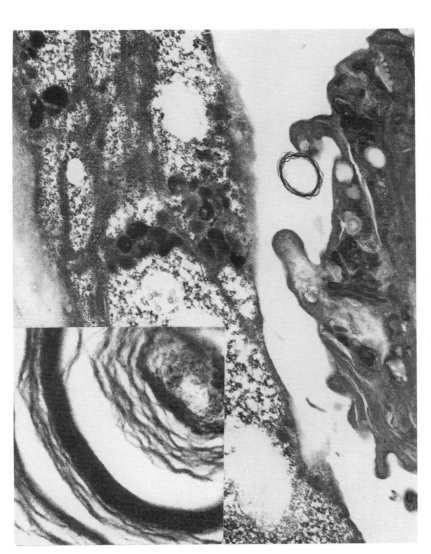

Fig. 10. Two cells from a culture from an adenomatous prostate gland. Both cells exhibit considerable degradative changes. The cell on the bottom is extruding a lamellar structure from a cytoplasmic pseudopol (original magnification, × 8,094). The myelin nature of the lamellar structure becomes apparent in the insert (original magnification, × 60,420).

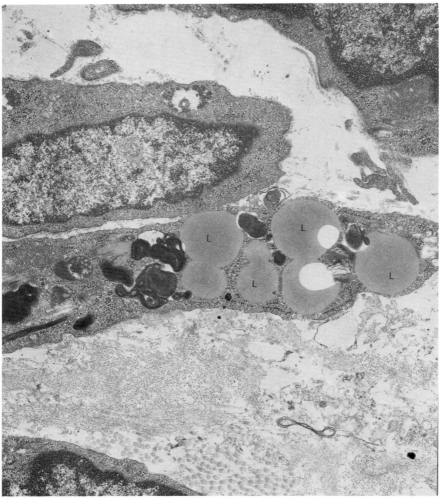

Fig. 11. Carcinomatous cells at the periphery of an explant after ten days of cultivation. Large lipid vacuoles (L), residual bodies, and myelin bodies are present in the cell in the center. The cytoplasm of other cells is compact. Collagen and the amorphous material are part of the supportive tissue framework of the explant (original magnification, × 4,560).

plants from all glands collected less than four hours postmortem produced cell growth.

The mode of the cellular outgrowth of cells from alveolar structures of the explants reported in this study appears to be the same as described by Webber et al [1]. In most cultures, the initial cell outgrowth was epithelial in character. How-

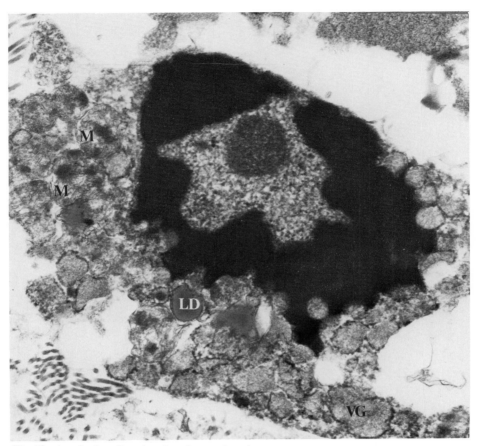

Fig. 12. Anaplastic cell at the edge of an explant from a carcinoma of the prostate. Atypical nucleus shows multilobulation. Irregular cytoplasm contain lipid droplets (LD), disarranged mitochondria (M), and vacuoles with granular material (VG), which probably represent distended channels of the endoplasmic reticulum. The large clear area may represent the intracytoplasmic lumen (original magnification, × 12,000).

ever, cell populations in some cultures exhibited mixtures of fibroblast-like cells with epithelial-like cells. Each of these cell types seemed to form individual cell islets. The initial presence of predominant "epithelial" cells in primary cultures suggests that in the early stages of culture development the epithelial cells may possess preferential growth characteristics over stromal elements.

The ultrastructural studies of the cells in primary cultures show that characteristics of these cells are similar to those described for solid tissues [13]. The presence of lammelar myelin bodies in the cytoplasm may be due to autophagy or heterophagy [14]. The cytoplasmic changes observed in cells from adenomatous

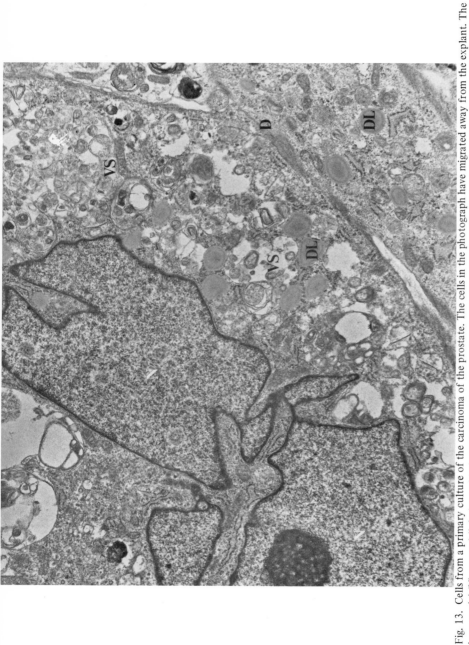

Fig. 13. Cells from a primary culture of the carcinoma of the prostate. The cells in the photograph have migrated away from the explant. The large nuclei (N) are multilobular and indented. Normal cytoplasmic organelles have been pushed aside by large secretory vacuoles (SV) with myelin lamellar structures and lipid droplets (DL), Desmosomes (D) are present, and the cells are connected to one another (original magnification, × 6,840).

prostates are similar to those described by Brandes for aging [15]. The presence of bundles of myofilaments in some cells spoke for their myoepithelial nature.

The loss of cytoplasmic organelle organization, which was evident in most cultures, may be a reflection of the disruption of the normal secretory activity of the cells [16]. The abundant vacuoles with their degenerative content may be distorted secretory vacuoles. The mitochondrial changes and the large number of dense residual bodies, which were particularly prominent in the cells from adenomatous prostate glands, may be related to biochemical abnormalities described in tumor cell mitochondria.

The nuclear changes in the cells from carcinomatous prostate glands, although easily discernible, were not as severe as those described in anaplastic prostatic carcinomas [16]. The experience with the addition of testosterone, in rather low doses, to the culture media proved interesting. In the majority of cases it had no noticeable effect on the cultures, but in some 10% of experiments a difference was noted, mainly in cancer cells, between testosterone-treated cultures and untreated cultures. However, the testosterone effect observed in these experiments was uniformly inhibitory rather than stimulating. Thus a categorical statement to the effect that determination of hormonal sensitivity in prostatic cancer is impossible in vitro [11] may not be warranted. Not all prostate cancers respond uniformly and in a predictable way to hormonal manipulation in vivo. If such were not the case the biologic control of the disease would be an easy matter. Therefore, it seems that further study of the in vitro response of various cells from the prostate gland to various agents may provide us with some measure of understanding the basic biologic properties of these cells. The results of such studies would be difficult to interpret if these are derived from studies on tissue samples obtained from a few patients as, in general, are the results from a small sample of patient population.

The technique of the preparation of a large number of primary cultures of prostate cells described herein was developed in order to overcome these difficulties. If correctly applied, it will produce for the investigators a large number of primary human cell cultures suitable for a large variety of individual studies. As can be judged from the ultrastructural studies, the alterations in the cells cultured under the conditions described resemble those found in the cells of the parent tissues. The cells in these cultures were not uniform, as are the cells in serially propagated cultures, but neither are the prostate glands from different individuals or the cancers they so frequently contain. Thus, the lack of uniformity in the primary cultures of the prostate cells may constitute their main advantage, for it may mimic biological phenomena encountered in vivo.

SUMMARY

Explants of embryonic, normal adult, and tumor-containing prostate gland tissue in culture produced outgrowths of cells having an "epithelial" appearance. The fetal cells exhibited by far the highest potential for growth in vitro. Growth of prostate gland adult cells did not appear to depend on the age of the donor. Ultrastructural characteristics of cells from normal human prostates differed from cells derived from adenomatous prostate glands, which had many cytoplasmic characteristics similar to those described in solid tissues. These studies suggest that the characteristics of prostate gland cells in explant primary culture are similar to those in the parent tissues.

ACKNOWLEDGMENTS

This investigation was supported by grant CA 15480-06SRC awarded by the National Cancer Institute, National Prostatic Cancer Project, DHEW.

REFERENCES

1. Webber MN, Stonington OG, Poche P: Epithelial outgrowth from suspension cultures of human prostate tissue. In Vitro 10:196–205, 1974.
2. Schroeder FH, Sato G, Gittes RF: Human prostatic adenocarcinoma. Growth in monolayer tissue culture. J Urol 106:734–739, 1971.
3. Kaighn ME, Babcock MS: Monolayer cultures of human prostatic cells. Cancer Chemother Rep 59:59–64, 1975.
4. Franks LM, Ridde PN, Carbonell AW, Gey CO: A comparative study of the ultrastructure and lack of growth capacity of adult human prostate epithelium mechanically separated from stroma. J Pathol 100:113–119, 1970.
5. Malinin TI: Collection of postmortem prostate tissue under sterile conditions. Cancer Chemother Rep 59:91–95, 1976.
6. Malinin TI: Explant cultivation of normal and neoplastic human prostatic gland tissue. Fed Proc 36:1066, 1977.
7. Claflin AJ, Malinin TI, Block NL: Explant culture of normal and tumor bearing human prostate glands. In Vitro 13:179, 1977.
8. Allgöwer M: The cultivation of human prostate adenoma in vitro. Exp Cell Res Suppl 1: 456–459, 1949.
9. Roehl L: Hormone dependency of prostatic cancer studied by cell culture technique. Br J Urol 30:450–454, 1958.
10. Lasnitzki I: Growth and hormonal response of prostatic tumors. In Tannenbaum M (ed): "Urologic Pathology: The Prostate." Philadelphia, Lea & Febiger, 1977, pp 215–222.
11. Wojewski A, Przeworska-Kaniewicz A: The influence of stilbesterol and testosterone on the growth of prostatic adenoma and carcinoma in tissue culture. J Urol 93:721–724, 1965.
12. Malinin TI, Claflin AJ, Block NL: Technique of cultivation of the prostate gland tissue. In Vitro (in press).
13. Brandes D, Kirchheim D, Scott WW: Ultrastructure of the human prostate. Normal and neoplastic. Lab Invest 13:1541–1560, 1964.
14. Trump BP, Valigorsky JM, Jones RT, Mergner WJ, Garcia JH, Cowley RS: The application of electron microscopy and cellular biochemistry to the autopsy. Hum Pathol 6:499–516, 1975.
15. Brandes D: The fine structure and histochemistry of prostatic glands in relation to sex hormones. Int Rev Cytol 20:207–276, 1966.
16. Brandes D, Kirchheim D: Histochemistry of the prostate. In Tannenbaum M (ed): "Urologic Pathology: The Prostate." Philadelphia: Lea & Febiger, 1977, pp 99–128.

Growth and Maintenance of Normal Prostatic Epithelium In Vitro—A Human Cell Model

Mukta M. Webber, PhD

Investigations into the etiology, mechanism of carcinogenesis, and the modes of treatment for prostatic cancer can be made using in vivo and in vitro model systems. Considerable progress has been made in the last five years in developing such models. Three animal models that can be used to study modes of treatment and tumor progression have recently become available and are discussed elsewhere in this volume (see chapters by Lubaroff; Pollard).

Studies on the etiology of prostatic cancer and on the mechanism of carcinogenesis have been hampered primarily by the rarity of spontaneous prostatic cancer in common laboratory animals and by difficulties in inducing the same. In view of this, the importance of in vitro cell models for the prostate has recently been recognized [1], and great emphasis is being placed on the development of in vitro systems using normal prostatic epithelial cells. In order to understand the malignant prostatic epithelial cell, it is important first to have a thorough understanding of the physiology — ie, of growth controls, cell interactions, and hormone responses — of the normal prostatic epithelial cell.

The major objective of studies being conducted by this investigator is to develop an in vitro cell model using postpubertal, normal human prostatic epithelium, which could be used 1) to study early steps in prostatic carcinogenesis; 2) to identify specific carcinogens for these target cells; 3) to elucidate the metabolic activation of carcinogens and their organ specificity; and 4) to examine the mechanism of transformation.

Models for Prostate Cancer, pages 181—216

The value of establishing an in vitro model using normal human cells is based on the following facts: 1) First and most important of all is that in an isolated cell system, one is more likely to be able to pinpoint the specific changes involved in carcinogenesis. 2) Until recently, long-term experiments with animals provided the only means for detecting the potential of various agents as carcinogens. The bioassay of compounds by in vivo testing seems to be an insurmountable task. Therefore, in vitro models have proved to be very useful for screening potential carcinogens for man. Also, such in vitro procedures can provide results in a shorter time, are less costly, and are reliable, sensitive, and practical. 3) Concern and doubts have been expressed time and time again on the usefulness and applicability of animal model systems for studying problems of human disease. Although it is difficult to obtain and culture normal human epithelial cells, it is believed that the ultimate answer to the question of cancer etiology can be provided only by testing various agents on human cells. Therefore the use of cells derived from man is naturally appropriate for studies on human cancer.

Further, current information suggests that 80% of all human cancers may be caused by environmental carcinogens. Considerable emphasis is therefore being placed on the identification of these carcinogens and on the methods of interfering with the process of malignant transformation. It is also known that nearly 85% of all human tumors arise from epithelial cells. It is therefore important to identify and determine the mechanism of carcinogen—target cell interaction in organs that show a high incidence of cancer. The incidence of benign tumors of the prostate may be as high as 80% in men over the age of 40 [2]. Also, at least 30% of all men over 50 years may have histologic carcinoma, and this figure increases to 50% after the age of 70 [3]. In view of this, it is important to understand the mechanism of carcinogenesis in the prostate. For these reasons, it is necessary to develop an in vitro model using human prostatic epithelium. In order to develop such a model, it is necessary to meet certain basic requirements, which are to isolate normal epithelium, to establish its growth and maintenance requirements in vitro, and to characterize it to establish its prostatic epithelial origin (Fig. 1).

Very few studies have been made on the isolation and growth and maintenance of normal human prostatic epithelium in vitro. One of the major problems has been the acquisition of normal viable tissue. The major source of tissue has been cadaver organ transplant donors and autopsies. Lechner et al [4] have reported successful cultivation of neonatal human prostatic epithelium. These cultures were initiated from cells spilled after mincing the tissue. No work, other than that done in my laboratory and which is the subject of this and other forthcoming papers [5–9], has been reported on the successful isolation, cultivation, and maintenance of normal, postpubertal, human prostatic epithelium. The significance of using postpubertal prostate must be emphasized. Since prostatic carcinomas arise from adult, androgen-responsive epithelium, it is important to use such epithelium for developing an in vitro model. All other studies on in vitro cultivation of human prostatic epithelium have used benign or malignant prostate.

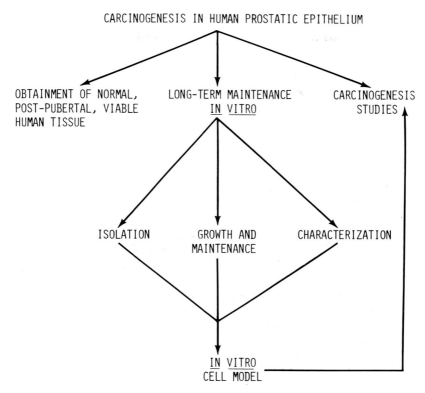

Fig. 1. A diagram showing the basic requirements for developing an in vitro cell model using normal human prostatic epithelium for studies on prostatic carcinogenesis.

It has generally been difficult to grow and maintain normal human epithelial cells in vitro. This is paradoxical when one realizes that the majority of human cancers are of epithelial origin. One of the reasons for this failure has been the general dependence on standard commercially available media and the failure to recognize that prostatic epithelial cells are specialized secretory cells whose growth, maintenance, and differentiation in vivo are controlled by several hormones, vitamins, and other growth-controlling factors. It is, therefore, logical to assume that these cells would have certain specific requirements of the above substances for their growth and maintenance in vitro. My investigations were therefore based on the premise that, since prostatic cells did not grow well under the environmental tissue culture conditions provided so far, the first logical step would be to modify the environment for their optimum growth and survival — ie, to design a special medium to satisfy growth requirements of normal prostatic epithelium in vitro.

One of the basic requirements for establishing this in vitro model is to establish pure cultures of prostatic epithelium, and for this, one must first isolate the cells.

ISOLATION OF NORMAL PROSTATIC EPITHELIUM FOR IN VITRO CULTIVATION

Introduction

Various methods for epithelial cell isolation and culture have been used — eg, nonenzymatic isolation by scraping of bovine pancreatic duct [10]; explant cultures [11—14]; enzymatic digestion (eg, minced pancreatic tissue [15] and human endometrium [16]); and collection of normal epithelial cells from human milk [17]. Waymouth [18] has recently reviewed various methods for tissue digestion and subculturing.

Cultures of animal prostatic epithelium to date have primarily been established from explant cultures [19—24]. Human prostatic epithelium has also primarily been grown in vitro using explant cultures [11—14, 25—33]. Enzymatic digestion of prostatic tissue using trypsin and pronase has been tried [26, 29, 34]. Stone et al [35] used collagenase for dispersal of benign prostatic tissue.

One of the major problems in culturing human epithelial cells has been the contamination with fibroblasts. When ordinary tissue culture methods are used, prostatic epithelial cultures are generally contaminated with stromal fibroblasts [28, 30, 36, 37]. The investigations reported here, which examine the usefulness of collagenase in establishing pure monolayer cultures of prostatic epithelium, began in 1974. There were two major reasons for conducting these investigations: 1) To isolate prostatic acini from prostatic tissue, which could then be used to initiate pure cultures of prostatic epithelium (also, it was felt that by this method a large number of cultures could be set up in a fraction of the time — two to three days — spent on cutting explants for 200—300 cultures); and 2) to inhibit the growth of fibroblasts in mixed cultures initiated from explants. In order to eliminate these fibroblasts, collagenase was tested for its cytotoxicity to fibroblasts, especially with the knowledge that it did not have deleterious effects on epithelial cells and did not damage their cell membranes. Work was begun on both normal and benign human prostatic tissue [38].

Physiological breakdown of collagen in many mammals and amphibians is accomplished by the action of specific collagenases, produced in very small amounts as needed. These are apparently not stored in vivo [39, 40]. Collagenase activity has been detected in normal and diseased human skin, in the edges of healing wounds, in growing bone, in involuting uterus, in inflamed human tissues (eg, rheumatoid arthritis), and in regenerating newt limbs [39]. On the basis of these observations it is logical to conclude that the same enzyme might be used for isolation of cells from tissues after digestion with collagenase.

Collagenases by definition are enzymes capable of dissolving fibrous collagen by peptide bond cleavage under physiological conditions of pH and temperature. The specific substrate, collagen, represents 33% of the total protein in mammalian organisms [40].

Lasfargues [41] pioneered the use of collagenase for digestion of tissue for cell dispersal in the preparation of primary cultures of mouse mammary epithelium. Since prostate has a histologic composition similar to that of the mammary glands, I have used collagenase for the isolation of prostatic epithelium.

Collagenase has been used in recent years for dissociation of animal tissues and for isolation of epithelial cells of various types — eg, aortic endothelium [42]; liver [43]; endocrine pancrease [44]; and mammary epithelium [41, 45]. In the majority of these cultures some fibroblasts did get carried over into the cultures.

Stromal elements form a major part of prostatic tissue. Separation of epithelial cells from the stroma using collagenase is an interesting phenomenon. Electron microscopy was used to pinpoint the site of action of collagenase, which facilitated isolation of acini [5].

Collagenase is nontoxic at a neutral pH, is active within a pH range of 6.5—7.8, and requires Ca^{++} ions for its activity and stability. It can therefore be dissolved in complete tissue culture medium. Since it has its specific action on collagen, it is active even in medium containing 5—10% serum. Thus, minced tissue can be placed in a complete culture medium enriched with serum and still be exposed to the dissociating activity of collagenase. This results in improved cell viability as compared to serum-free dissociating medium containing proteolytic enzymes.

Methods

Collagenases of bacterial origin (Clostridium histolyticum and Clostridium perfringens) have been found to be the most efficient agents for cell dispersal. The impure enzyme preparations are more effective for tissue digestion, and their stability is excellent even at room temperature [40]. Stock solutions should, however, be kept frozen, and media containing collagenase should be refrigerated (4°C). Temperatures above 56°C inactivate the enzyme rapidly and completely [46]. All antibiotics are compatible with collagenase. Gibco* collagenase (Clostridiopeptidase A from Cl histolyticum) was found to be the best for digestion of prostatic tissue [5].

Specimens of normal prostatic tissue were collected from cadaver organ transplant donors and autopsies. Tissue was collected aseptically in cold transport medium [5] consisting of Puck's Saline G containing 500 units/ml penicillin, 500 μg/ml streptomycin, and 50 μg/ml gentamicin. The tissue was brought to the laboratory, washed twice with fresh cold transport medium, and then processed further. In earlier experiments explant cultures were used. Explants measuring 0.5 to 1 mm were cut and plated according to the method described earlier [14]. Later experiments employed collagenase digestion of tissue. Superficial connective tissue was removed from the specimen and discarded, and the remaining tissue was dissected into 3—4 mm cubes and processed as shown in the protocol in Figure 2. The volume of the cut tissue was measured, and the tissue was divided into 100 mm Petri

*Grand Island Biological Company, Grand Island, NY 14072.

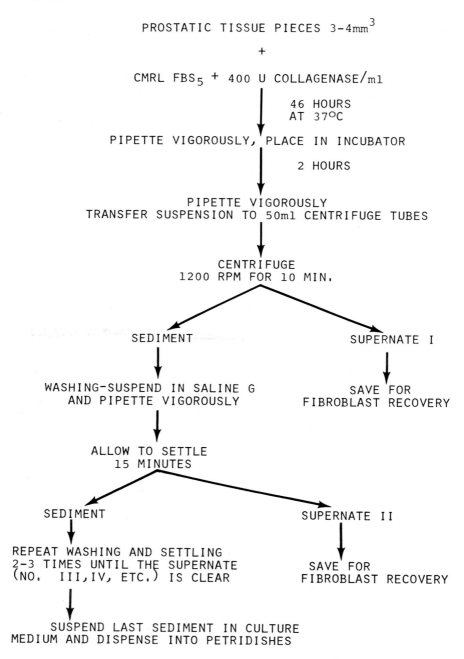

Fig. 2. Protocol for collagenase dispersal of human prostatic tissue and isolation of prostatic acini (from Webber [5]).

dishes, with each dish containing approximately 2 ml of tissue. To each dish 12 ml of medium containing collagenase was added.

The medium used for dissociating the tissue consisted of CMRL 1066 with 5% fetal bovine serum (FBS) and 100 units/ml penicillin, 100 μg/ml streptomycin, and 10 μg/ml gentamicin. To this medium collagenase was added at a level of 200 units/ml or 400 units/ml. Collagenase is freely soluble in tissue culture media. It should be pointed out that the concentration of collagenase must be expressed in units/ml rather than μg/ml because the activity of collagenase (ie, units/μg) varies from lot to lot. Tissue can be incubated at 37°C, in 400 units/ml collagenase medium for 24 to 48 hours and in 200 units/ml collagenase for up to 60 hours without loss of epithelial cell viability. After this time the tissue was pipetted vigorously to break it up and placed in the incubator for further digestion for one to two hours. The digested tissue was again pipetted vigorously, centrifuged, and resuspended in Puck's Saline G. This was followed by repeated washing of the sediment with Saline G and settling by gravity in 50 ml conical centrifuge tubes. All supernates were saved, and fibroblasts were recovered from these by centrifugation. Although these cells have low viability, sufficient cells can be collected and are being used for studies on stromal–epithelial interaction. The last sediment consisted of acini of various sizes. The volume of these was measured, which, for tissue with normal histology, was 1/20th the original volume of the tissue digested. Various plating dilutions of the acini were tested.

In earlier experiments CMRL 1066 medium containing 10% fetal bovine serum (FBS), 10% horse serum (HS), 100 units/ml penicillin, 100 μg/ml streptomycin, 10 μg/ml gentamicin, and 2 mM L-glutamine was used. Recent experiments were conducted using RPMI 1640 plus the supplements listed above. The reasons for this change in culture medium will be described in a forthcoming paper [8]. The cultures were maintained at 37°C with 5% CO_2 in air in a humidified atmosphere.

For transmission electron microscopy, cells were prepared according to the method described earlier [47]. Briefly, cells were grown in a monolayer on 60 mm plastic tissue culture Petri dishes (Falcon), rinsed quickly with warm (37°C) Puck's Saline G, and fixed in situ in 4% gluteraldehyde in 0.1 M Sorenson's phosphate buffer (pH 7.4) for two hours. Cells were postfixed in 2% osmium tetroxide in 0.1 M phosphate buffer (pH 7.4) for one hour. Cells were then washed three times in triple-distilled water, dehydrated through an ethyl alcohol series, and embedded in Epon. Sections were stained with a saturated aqueous solution of uranyl acetate and then in Reynold's lead citrate solution. Sections were examined with a Philips EM-300 transmission electron microscope.

For scanning electron microscopy cells were prepared according to the method described by Porter et al [48]. Cells were grown on glass coverslips and were fixed at 37°C for 20 minutes with 3% gluteraldehyde buffered with 0.05 M cacodylate at pH 7.2 and 0.5X Puck's Saline G. After a brief wash in Saline G (37°C) they were postfixed for 15 minutes at room temperature with 1% osmium tetroxide buffered with 0.2 M cacodylate buffer at pH 7.2 and dehydrated rapidly in acetone. Cells were critical-point dried with liquid CO_2. Cells were then coated with carbon followed by a thin film of gold. The cells were examined with a Cambridge S-4 stereoscan electron microscope operated at 20 kV. For light microscopy, cells were fixed and stained by a Giemsa method [49].

Results

Figure 3 shows results of experiments that demonstrate that collagenase, when incorporated into the culture medium, does have cytotoxic and growth-inhibitory effects on fibroblasts. Cultures containing 50 units/ml collagenase show vigorously growing epithelium with no fibroblasts or only minute colonies of fibroblasts. It can be concluded that fibroblasts can be eliminated to some extent from mixed cultures by the use of collagenase as a component of the tissue culture medium.

Prostatic acini were isolated according to the protocol shown in Figure 2. Using this procedure, intact acini (Fig. 4a) could be isolated. These acini maintained normal arrangement of the epithelium in two layers around the lumen (Fig. 4b). When these acini were plated, pure cultures of vigorously growing epithelium resulted (Fig. 4c, sediment). Occasional colonies of fibroblasts did appear in some cultures. Cells isolated from the supernate and washings were predominantly fibroblasts (Fig. 4c, supernate). Figure 4d shows the typical morphology of epithelial cells grown from acini isolated after collagenase digestion.

Normal prostatic epithelium rests on a basal lamina that separates it from the underlying stromal elements (Fig. 5). When prostatic tissue is exposed to collagenase, the basal lamina is one of the sites of action, in addition to the collagen in the stroma. As a result, the epithelial cells separate from the underlying stromal elements. Figure 6 shows stromal cells (primarily fibroblasts) separating from the epithelium. These cells are partly digested and degenerating, thus losing cell viability, whereas epithelial cells remain viable and have a clean outer epithelial surface. As a result of collagenase action, the collagen of the lamina propria and of the remaining stroma is digested. Cells are held together by desmosomes, as they are in vivo, and the outer surface of the acinus is free of stromal elements. This is also clearly demonstrated in the scanning electron micrograph of the surface of an acinus (Fig. 7).

It has generally been difficult to initiate cultures from explants prepared from autopsy tissue specimens or samples obtained from transurethral resection of the prostate (TURP). However, good epithelial cell growth has been initiated from acini isolated from these tissues after collagenase digestion [5]. Cultures from TURP specimens may contain some fibroblast colonies due to incomplete separation of acini from the stroma. This results from incomplete digestion with collagenase of denatured tissue, which is caused by electrocauterization during surgery.

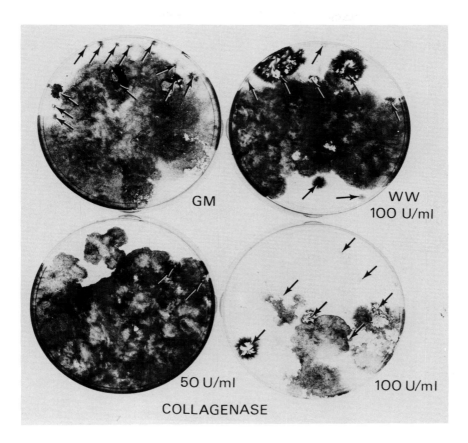

Fig. 3. Cytotoxicity and inhibition of fibroblast growth with collagenase incorporated into the culture medium. Mixed cultures of prostatic epithelium and fibroblasts were exposed to culture medium containing collagenase. Cultures were initiated from explants. Arrows indicate fibroblast colonies. GM: control culture maintained on growth medium consisting of CMRL 1066 + 10% FBS + 10% HS shows numerous fibroblast colonies. The remainder of the dish was covered with epithelial cells. WW: this culture was treated once a week with growth medium containing 100 units/ml collagenase for 48 hours. The fibroblast colonies persisted. There is no inhibition of fibroblasts in this culture. In fact, the colonies are larger than in the control. 50 units/ml: cultures maintained on 50 units/ml collagenase show good epithelial growth. These cultures showed a dramatic loss of fibroblasts, while the epithelium grew vigorously. 100 units/ml: collagenase at a level of 100 units/ml in the culture medium was toxic to monolayers of both epithelial cells and fibroblasts (Giemsa stain; from Webber [5]).

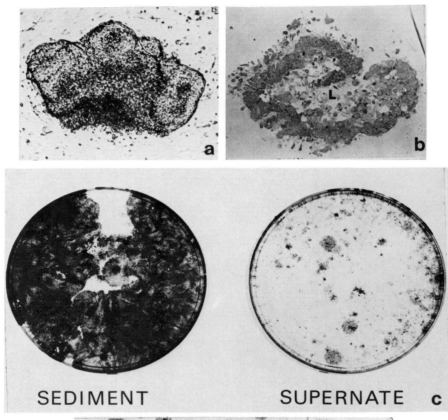

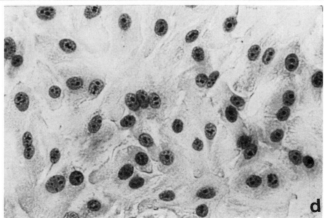

4

Discussion

Results presented here clearly demonstrate that the growth of epithelial cells is enhanced when 50 units/ml collagenase is incorporated into the culture medium, whereas growth of fibroblasts is inhibited. Collagenase was first used by Lasfargues and Moore [50] as a component of the culture medium to remove collagen secreted by fibroblasts and deposited on epithelial cells. Lasfargues [41] believed that this deposit of collagen prevented epithelial cells from multiplying and spreading. Various other methods have also been used to inhibit growth of fibroblasts in mixed culture — eg, D-valine media [51] and 5-bromodeoxyuridine [37].

Crude collagenase is a mixture of hydrolytic enzymes containing some peptidase and trypsin-like proteinase in addition to collagenase. Crude collagenase is most effective in prostatic tissue digestion. Pure collagenase is not as effective. High levels of collagenase in the culture medium are toxic because the other enzyme impurities have deleterious effects on the cell membranes. At lower levels, which are nontoxic to epithelial cells, collagenase inhibits fibroblastic growth and shows cytotoxicity for fibroblasts.

The effectiveness of digestion of tissue with collagenase depends in part upon the age of the donor, which may be related to the amount of collagen present. Soukupova et al [52] found that tissue from young rats could be digested more easily than that from older rats, using the same concentration of collagenase. Our observations on human prostate show the same effect.

Collagen in organs is considered to form a three-dimensional matrix, and collagen molecules closely coat epithelial cells. The intercellular matrix consists of mucopolysaccharides and soluble collagen fibers. At the basal surface of epithelia is found a continuous mucopolysaccharide layer, the basal lamina, which at higher magnifications under the electron microscope has a texture. The fine filamentous component of the basal lamina is collagen in the form of soluble tropocollagen molecules. This collagen and that forming the fibrous network in the intercellular matrix is attacked and digested by collagenase, resulting in the separation of acini from the stroma.

Since collagenase is not toxic to epithelial cells, its use is not as limited with respect to time and concentration as trypsin. Organs with heavy collagen matrices like the prostate, can therefore be incubated for as long as 60 hours without loss of cell viability. Trypsin does not act on collagen of the intercellular matrix, therefore it

Fig. 4. 4a) A group of prostatic acini isolated from prostatic tissue after collagenase digestion (magnification, × 144). 4b) Histologic section of an isolated acinus showing the arrangement of epithelial cells. The stroma attached to the surface is lost after collagenase digestion and by repeated washing of the preparation. L = lumen (toluidine blue, 1 μ thick section; magnification, × 276). 4c) Cultures derived from collagenase dispersed tissue. The culture arising from the isolated acini, which constitute the sediment, is epithelial, whereas that arising from the supernate primarily contains fibroblast colonies and some epithelial cells (Giemsa stain). 4d) Morphology of prostatic epithelium in a culture derived from collagenase isolated acini (magnification, × 360; from Webber [5]).

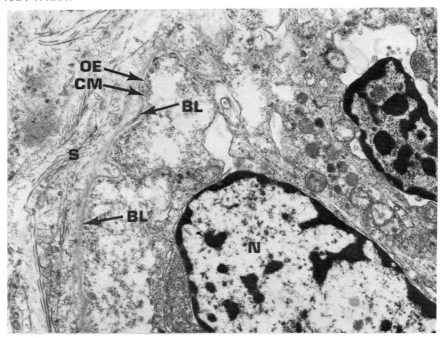

Fig. 5. Electron micrograph of prostatic epithelium in a tissue specimen showing basal lamina (BL) and underlying stromal matrix (S). The cell membrane (CM) adjacent to basal lamina is shown. OE = outer epithelial surface. (Age of tissue donor, 19 years; magnification, × 7,300; from Webber [5]).

Fig. 6. Composite electron micrograph showing the process of separation of acini from the stroma after collagenase digestion of the tissue. The bottom of the picture shows the outer epithelial layer (OE) of cells in the acinus, with their outer surface clear of stromal elements. Two stromal cells (SC) are shown separating from the glandular epithelium. Collagen (C) is shown in a partly digested state. (N = nucleus; magnification, × 4,658; from Webber [5]).

is not effective in dissociating tissues rich in connective tissue. It is also harsh on cells, digests cells, and causes considerable cell membrane damage. The great selectivity of collagenase and lack of damage to cell membranes makes it highly desirable for tissue dissociation. One should bear in mind that some proteolytic enzymes inactivate collagenase by digesting it like any other protein. Therefore, the use of collagenase in combination with trypsin or pancreatin is incompatible. Similarly, chelating agents like EDTA are also incompatible with collagenase, because calcium is essential for its activity and stability.

On the basis of results presented above, it can be stated that viable, postpubertal prostatic epithelium of normal human origin has been successfully isolated for in vitro cultivation. Isolated acini give rise to vigorously growing epithelial cultures. A certain minimum number of acini is required per culture in order to obtain a vigorously growing culture and increase the life-span of the cells [5] . This behavior

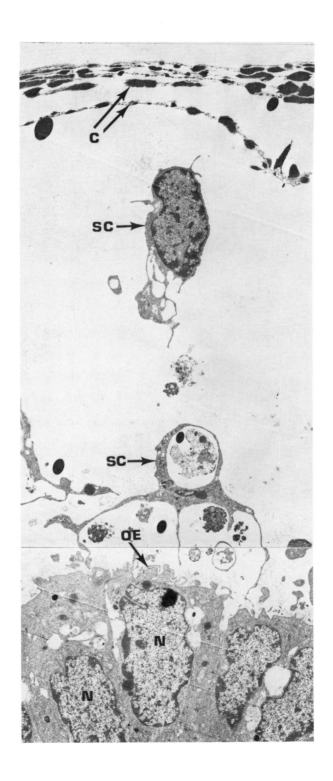

6

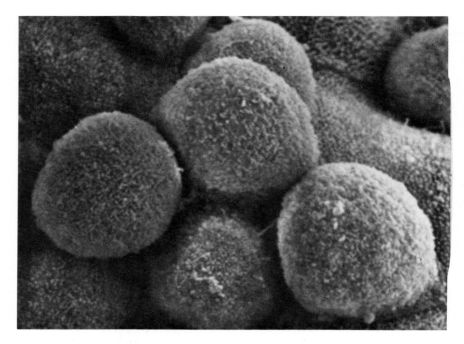

Fig. 7. Scanning electron micrograph of the surface of an isolated prostatic acinus. The surface is free of stromal elements and has numerous microvilli (magnification, × 6,720; from Webber [5]).

may be related to the ability of cells to condition media. Also, cells in primary cultures tend to grow better when plated in large numbers. Epithelial cultures derived from autopsy specimens have been similarly established.

GROWTH AND MAINTENANCE OF NORMAL PROSTATIC EPITHELIUM IN VITRO

Introduction

After isolation, the next objective is to grow and maintain prostatic epithelial cells in culture for long periods. Only limited studies have been made [26, 28, 30, 37] on the maintenance of human prostatic organ cultures, derived from benign and malignant prostate. However, no concerted effort had been made to define nutrient and growth requirement of normal prostatic cells in vitro. This has been one of the major objectives of our studies, and to date several growth requirements of normal prostatic epithelium have been established. These factors enhance the growth and life-span of the cells and maintain a normal cell morphology at the ultrastructural level.

Lasnitzki [23] has been a pioneer in the studies on the maintenance of mouse prostatic tissue organ cultures. She has examined the effects of sex hormones, chemical carcinogens, and vitamins on cell viability, and on the maintenance of normal

cell morphology, and function. However, when the present studies began, successful cultivation and maintenance of normal human prostatic epithelium had never
been accomplished.

Criteria for adequacy of growth and nutrition for prostatic cells in vitro are
only now being established. Culture media commonly used for established cell
lines have been used in the past for prostatic cell cultures with disappointing results. Since prostatic epithelial cells are specialized secretory cells and since their
growth is affected directly by certain hormones and vitamins in vivo, a tissue culture medium must be designed to satisfy their growth requirements. In order to
achieve this, a number of different serum types and media were first tested for
their growth-supporting properties for these cells. In vivo, testosterone, insulin,
and vitamin A control growth, secretory activity, differentiation, and cell morphology of prostatic epithelium. On this bases, these three agents were selected
for an intensive study of their effects on the growth and maintenance of prostatic
epithelium in monolayer cultures.

Methods

Primary cultures derived from explants or from collagenase-isolated acini were
used for testing the effects of serum, media, and other test agents on the growth
and maintenance of prostatic epithelium. For explant cultures, tissue was cut into
0.5–1 mm pieces under a dissecting microscope, and a specific number of explants
(eg, 15 explants per 60 mm Petri dish) was plated into each Petri dish. In order to
allow the explants to settle and attach, only 1.5 ml of medium was initially added
per dish. The growth medium consisted of RPMI 1640 supplemented with 10%
HS, 10% FBS (mycoplasma and virus screened), 100 units/ml penicillin, 100 μg/ml
streptomycin, 10 μg/ml gentamicin, and 2 mM L-glutamine. Cultures were maintained at 37°C in a humidified atmosphere containing 5% CO_2 in air. After an
initial two-to-three-day lag phase, during which the majority of explants attached
to the substrate, the cells began to spread on the dish surface. Growth was extensive
by the sixth day. Cells were placed on medium containing the test substances on
day 3, the day of plating being day 0.

Insulin (Schwartz/Mann*, bovine pancreas, activity 27.17 international units
(IU)/mg) was dissolved in 0.1 N hydrochloric acid in the basal medium without the
supplements. Stocks containing different levels of insulin were prepared so that although, the level of insulin was different in each test medium, the percentage of
0.1 N hydrochloric acid, used as the vehicle, was always the same (ie, 1 ml/100 ml
medium). A wide range of insulin levels, varying from 0.01 IU/ml to 100 IU/ml of
the culture medium, were tested.

Retinol acetate (Sigma†, all trans, Type 1, crystallin, activity 2,747,000 USP
units/gm) was used to examine the effects of vitamin A on the growth and maintenance of prostatic epithelium. Stock solutions were prepared in absolute ethyl

*Schwartz/Mann, Division of Becton, Dickinson & Company, Orangeburg, NY 10962.
†Sigma Chemical Company, St. Louis, MO 63178

alcohol and were kept in the dark in liquid nitrogen. Vitamin A levels varying from 0.01 units/ml to 200 units/ml of medium were tested, and stocks were prepared so that, although the level of vitamin A was different in each test medium, the percentage of ethyl alcohol was always constant.

Testosterone (Sigma*, Δ^4-Androsten-17β-ol-3-one) and 5α-dihydrotestosterone (Sigma*, 5α-Androstan-17β-ol-3-one) were also dissolved in absolute ethyl alcohol. Levels of these hormones varying from 0.01 μg/ml to 100 μg/ml in the culture medium were tested. The level of alcohol, added to the culture medium as the vehicle, remained constant at 0.05%.

Cultures were fed at two-day intervals and were maintained for ten to 21 days. At the end of an experiment, cells were fixed and stained by a Giemsa method described earlier [49].

Quantitation of cell growth in vitro is necessary to establish the growth enhancing effects or toxicity of the test substances. When using fibroblasts or other cells that can be easily dissociated and dispersed into single cell suspensions, it is easy to determine the extent of growth on the basis of cell number. However, many epithelial cells in primary culture − eg, prostatic epithelium − do not dissociate easily into single cells but remain as sheets or clumps after enzymatic treatment. Assessment of growth on the basis of cell counts is, therefore, not reliable. A Datacolor scanning densitometer [53] was used for quantitation of growth in cell cultures. Growth measurements are based on the measurement of the dish area covered with cells.

Selection of Serum and Medium

Serum is an important component of tissue culture media. Studies by this investigator [12] and by Puck et al [54] suggest that serum in the culture medium may act as a selection factor and favor the multiplication of one cell type over another. Results show that horse serum favors the growth of epithelial cells in culture [12]. Similar observations have recently been made by other investigators [55]. We have examined the effects of horse serum (HS), fetal bovine serum (FBS), and calf serum (CS) on the growth of prostatic epithelium. These sera were incorporated into the culture medium individually at 5%, 10%, and 20% levels and also in various combinations. The basic medium consisted of CMRL 1066 with 50 μg/ml gentamicin and 2 mM L-glutamine. Cultures were maintained for 14 days on these media. Results (Fig. 8) show that the best growth of prostatic epithelium occurred in cultures maintained on medium containing 10% FBS + 10% HS, and these cultures were also purely epithelial. Details of this work are reported elsewhere [7].

Having established the serum requirements, we proceeded to examine the effects of six different media on the growth of prostatic epithelium.

Effects of CMRL 1066, RPMI 1640, medium 199, Earle's minimum essential medium (EMEM), medium F12, and Earle's basal medium (BME), containing 10%

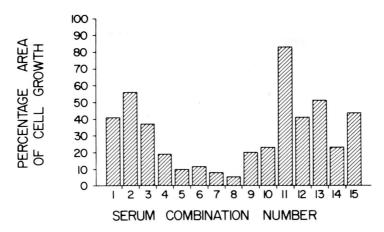

Fig. 8. Effects of different serum types and serum combinations on the growth of normal human prostatic epithelium in vitro. HS = horse serum; FBS = fetal bovine serum; CS = calf serum. The numbers on the histogram refer to the following serum combination numbers: 1) 5% FBS; 2) 10% FBS; 3) 20% FBS; 4) 5% HS; 5) 10% HS; 6) 20% HS; 7) 5% CS; 8) 10% CS; 9) 20% CS; 10) 5% FBS + 5% HS; 11) 10% FBS + 10% HS; 12) 5% FBS + 5% CS; 13) 10% FBS + 10% CS; 14) 5% HS + 5% CS; 15) 10% HS + 10% CS. Maximum growth occurred in combination #11, consisting of 10% FBS + 10% HS (age of cell donor, 20 years; from Webber et al [7]).

FBS and 10% HS, were examined on the growth and maintenance of prostatic epithelium [8]. Results show (Fig. 9) that both CMRL 1066 and RPMI 1640 stimulate good growth of epithelial cells, whereas F12 showed the poorest growth. Cell growth in RPMI was, however, the best, and cells could also be maintained in this medium longer than in CMRL. Hence RPMI 1640 has been selected for growing normal and benign prostatic epithelium in vitro.

Effects of Insulin

Introduction. Insulin has been added every now and then to tissue culture media for many years because it was thought to stimulate the uptake of glucose and increase cell growth [56–58]. There are, however, very few commercially available media — eg, Trowell's T-8 and Waymouth's MAB 87/3 — that contain insulin.

Insulin was first found to have a stimulatory effect on tissue cultures by Gey and Thalmier (see [56]). It has been shown to stimulate in vitro cell growth of a variety of cells, including certain human cells; eg, Blaker et al [59], using HeLa cells, showed that the serum supplement in a defined medium could be replaced by insulin. Flaxman and Lasfargues [60] showed that insulin increased the number of DNA-synthesizing cells in cultures of human mammary epithelium.

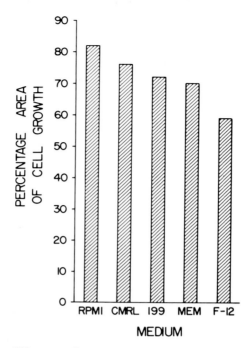

Fig. 9. Effects of five different media on the growth of normal human prostatic epithelium in vitro. All media contained 10% FBS + 10% HS. Results show that RPMI supported the best growth. Media used were RPMI 1640, CMRL 1066, 199, MEM (Earle's minimum essential medium) and Ham's F-12 (age of cell donor, 19 years; from Webber and Jankowsky [8]).

Very few studies on the in vitro cultivation of prostatic epithelium have used insulin in the culture medium [61–67]. Insulin stimulated growth of mouse prostatic epithelium in vitro [62]. It also stimulated protein synthesis in explants of the ventral prostate from orchiectomized mice, whereas testosterone had no effect [66]. Insulin prevented cell atrophy and regression in rat ventral prostate in organ culture [63] and stimulated protein, RNA and DNA synthesis in rat ventral prostate, and human benign hyperplasia tissue explants [61, 64]. Injections of insulin in castrated rats induced growth and secretory activity in the prostate [67].

From the above information, it is quite clear that very little work has been done on the role of insulin in prostatic growth control in animal and human systems in vivo or in vitro, and nothing has been done especially on its effects on normal human prostate.

Insulin not only stimulates carbohydrate metabolism but also protein, RNA, and DNA synthesis, and cell multiplication [68, 69]. Insulin potentiates the effect of fibroblast growth factor [70] and increases pinocytosis and uptake of glucose by increasing the cell membrane permeability [58, 71, 72]. Changes in cell membrane ultrastructure have been described in adipose tissue after insulin treatment [73].

In addition to the usefulness of insulin for the growth of cells in vitro, insulin is particularly important because of its specific effects on prostatic epithelium and on the accessory sex organs. Hunt and Bailey [74] observed that severe diabetes in rats resulted in failure of descent of testes, failure in the development of germinal epithelium, and in castrate-type accessory glands. Treatment with insulin corrected all the deleterious effects of diabetes on the reproductive system. With regard to prostate, Hunt and Bailey [74] found that at 23 days of age, the prostate gland of the rat is in an active secretory state. However, prostate from diabete rats from 37 to 72 days of age showed little evidence of secretory activity. The secretory state could be restored by insulin administration. Whether this effect of insulin on the prostate is direct or involves feedback mechanisms involving other hormones is not clear. Diabetic condition does result in a reduction of pituitary gonadotrophins, which in turn affect the production of androgens. This may be considered one explanation for the above observations.

However, other results point to a more direct effect of insulin on male accessory sex organs. Diabetic, castrated male rats show a decreased response to exogenous testosterone [75]. However, administration of insulin restored their ability to respond to testosterone. Although partial testosterone action is possible in the case of insulin deficiency, the presence of insulin is required for the full restorative effect. Insulin, therefore, must be considered to be a hormone that modifies the action of testosterone on the accessory sex organs. The importance of insulin in growth regulation of prostatic epithelium is clearly demonstrated by this investigator [9].

Results. The increased pinocytotic activity induced in cells exposed to insulin in vitro is well demonstrated in Figure 10. The number of pinocytotic vesicles and microvilli increases dramatically in exposed cells. Formation of these vesicles and their movement to the interior of the cell can be demonstrated by the addition of a ferritin tracer to the culture medium. Ferritin is picked up during pinocytosis, and the movement of the vesicles can be followed through the cell [9].

Results from these experiments on the effects of insulin on the growth of normal human epithelium grown in vitro show that insulin has a distinct and pronounced effect on the growth and life-span of prostatic epithelium in vitro (Figs. 11 and 12).

Insulin was incorporated into the culture medium at different concentrations, and cells were maintained on these media. Insulin even at a level as low as 0.01 IU/ml slightly increased the growth of prostatic epithelium in vitro, and the growth increased steadily with increase in the level of insulin in the culture medium, reaching a peak at 1.0 IU/ml. Beyond this concentration, growth declined, and toxicity was evident in specimens even at a level of 5.0 IU/ml. This growth-stimulatory effect of insulin is further demonstrated in Figures 11 and 12. Cultures were exposed to insulin for one or 24 hours, followed by pulse labeling with tritiated thymidine. Results show (Fig. 13) that the effect of insulin is rapid and that even after one hour of exposure, the cells incorporated ^{3}H-thymidine at a higher level than the controls. The effects, however, are more pronounced after a 24-hour exposure.

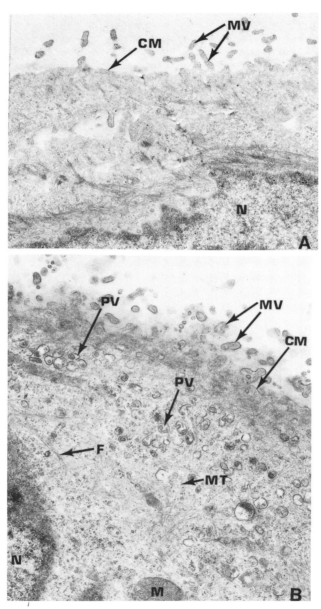

Fig. 10. Effects of insulin on cell membrane and pinocytotic activity. A. Electron micrograph of a portion of a prostatic epithelial cell in culture without insulin. Note few microvilli on the cell surface. (CM = cell membrane; MV = microvilli; N = nucleus; magnification, × 10,459; from Webber [9]). B. Electron micrograph of a prostatic epithelial cell from a culture exposed to insulin, showing a marked increase in pinocytotic activity. Note the large number of microvilli (MV) on the cell surface and pinocytotic vesicles (PV) in the area underlying the cell membrane (CM). (M = mitochondria; F = filaments; MT = microtubule; N = nucleus; magnification, × 12,915; from Webber [9]).

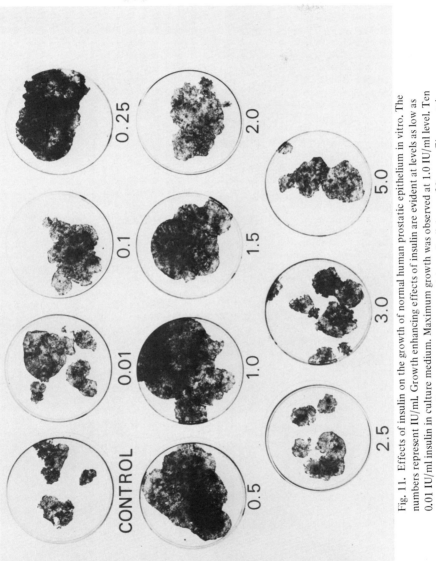

Fig. 11. Effects of insulin on the growth of normal human prostatic epithelium in vitro. The numbers represent IU/mL. Growth enhancing effects of insulin are evident at levels as low as 0.01 IU/ml insulin in culture medium. Maximum growth was observed at 1.0 IU/ml level. Ten replicate cultures for each treatment were prepared (age of cell donor, 20 years; Giemsa stain; from Webber [9]).

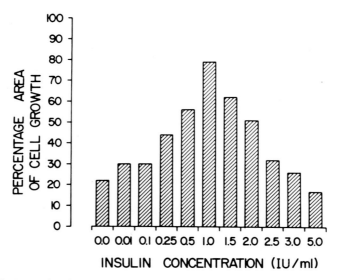

Fig. 12. Histogram showing the effects of insulin on the growth of normal human prostatic epithelium in vitro. Ten different concentrations of insulin were tested. These results show a classic dose response. The growth of cells increases with the increase in the amount of insulin and reaches a peak at 1.0 IU/ml. 5.0 IU/ml insulin and higher levels were toxic (age of cell donor, 20 years; from Webber [9]).

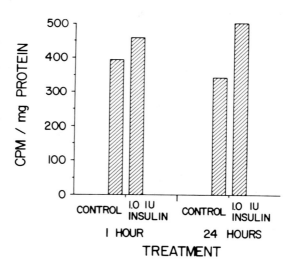

Fig. 13. Short-term effects of insulin on the growth of human prostatic epithelium in vitro. Results show that even after a one-hour exposure to insulin, DNA synthesis increases as compared to control cultures. After a 24-hour exposure, the difference between DNA synthesis in control and insulin exposed cultures is even greater.

Insulin also increases the life-span of human prostatic epithelium in vitro [9]. Cultures maintained on insulin not only show better growth but also they can be maintained in a healthy state for a longer time than cultures without insulin. Results show that after ten days in culture, while the control cultures are already showing signs of declining growth, those maintained on medium containing insulin continue to grow vigorously.

Another interesting and significant observation made in the course of these investigations was that explant cultures maintained on media containing insulin were devoid of fibroblasts, whereas the control cultures had some fibroblast colonies. This observation suggests that insulin may have specific, selective, growth-enhancing effects on prostatic epithelium, and an inhibitory effect on fibroblasts. These observations were confirmed by repeated experiments on several tissue specimens. These results are of particular importance in light of the idea that insulin may have specific effects on growth and differentiation of prostatic epithelium. This matter is being further investigated.

Discussion. Griffith [76] studied the effects of insulin on confluent cultures of W1-38 human embryonic lung fibroblast cells to determine whether it enabled the cells to escape from contact inhibition of growth. Insulin did not overcome contact inhibition and did not permit postconfluence division. It had no effect on RNA synthesis, slightly inhibited DNA synthesis, blocked cell division, and encouraged differentiation. It did, however, enable the cells to take up and utilize nutrients more efficiently, resulting in increased metabolic activity, protein synthesis, and cell size [76].

On the basis of these observations, it appears that these fibroblasts are unresponsive to growth-stimulating effects of insulin. This is interesting in view of the fact that human fibroblasts have been shown [77, 78] to possess specific binding sites for insulin on their cell surface. It is believed that, although fibroblasts have binding sites that interact with insulin, it is possible that these receptor sites are intended really for another chemically related peptide. It is interesting to note that, although insulin stimulated some thymidine incorporation into cultured human fibroblasts, the incorporation was ten times greater in the presence of epidermal growth factor (EGF) [77]. Further, very high concentrations of insulin are required to elicit a response in fibroblasts, indicating the relatively low affinity of the receptors for insulin; hence, these cells are not considered to be primary target cells for insulin.

In conclusion, it can be stated that cultured human fibroblasts arising from lung, skin, and the prostate [9, 76, 79—81] are relatively insensitive to insulin. Thus, either in vivo or while in vitro, they lose their ability to respond to insulin in terms of cyclic AMP metabolism and promotion of growth.

This phenomenon is particularly useful in selectively stimulating growth of prostatic epithelium while inhibiting fibroblasts in mixed cultures. This helps in achieving pure cultures of prostatic epithelium.

The growth-promoting effects of insulin on epithelial cells and its growth-inhibiting effects on fibroblasts can be summarized as follows: Insulin alters the cell membrane permeability and increases glucose and amino acid uptake. It also decreases intracellular levels of cyclic AMP in fibroblasts and stimulates protein, RNA, and DNA synthesis and cell division in target cells [64, 82, 83]. Many cell types have receptor sites on their surface for insulin, and its effects are thus mediated through the cell membrane [82]. It is, however, interesting to note that, although human fibroblasts possess receptor sites where insulin may bind, they are unresponsive to its growth-stimulating effects. Because of this unresponsiveness, our cultures, when exposed to insulin, did not shown any fibroblastic growth.

Effects of Vitamin A

Introduction. It was established over 50 years ago that vitamin A is required for normal differentiation of epithelial cells in many organs [84]. However, the molecular mechanisms whereby vitamin A controls this process are still unknown. It plays an important role in the maintenance of secretory epithelial cells [23]. Vitamin A deficiency usually causes loss of secretory activity, squamous metaplasia, and keratinization, whereas hypervitaminosis results in mucous transformation of epithelial cells [85]. This is also true for prostatic epithelium. In defined medium without vitamin A, prostatic epithelium showed deficiency effects; however, addition of vitamin A completely prevented these changes [23]. When natural medium containing serum and embryo extract was used, glandular structure was preserved. It is possible that in high concentrations of serum (20% or more), some vitamin A may be available to the cells; however, at lower concentrations (10% or less), there is not sufficient vitamin A available to maintain human prostatic epithelium in vitro [14, 86]. Maintenance of dog prostate organ cultures is improved by the addition of vitamin A [22].

Apart from the present studies, no other work appears to have been reported on the effects of vitamin A on growth and maintenance of normal human prostatic epithelium in vitro. Schrodt and Foreman [30] described squamous metaplasia changes in explant cultures of human benign tumors of the prostate and observed the presence of bundles of filaments in the cytoplasm. They did not, however, associate these changes with any deficiency in the culture medium.

Results. Effects of vitamin A on growth of normal prostatic epithelium in vitro were examined. Results show (Fig. 14) that concentrations below 5.0 units/ml stimulate growth. The best growth was observed in cultures containing 0.1 unit/ml vitamin A in culture medium. Levels above 5.0 units/ml are clearly toxic (Fig. 14).

Ultrastructural changes observed in cultures exposed to vitamin A and in control cultures are interesting. Prostatic epithelium, when grown in commercial media, undergoes squamous metaplasia. At the ultrastructural level, these changes manifest themselves in the form of increased number of filaments and filament bundles. However, when vitamin A is added to the culture medium, the cells revert to a more glandular type of ultrastructure with abundant Golgi complex and fewer filaments.

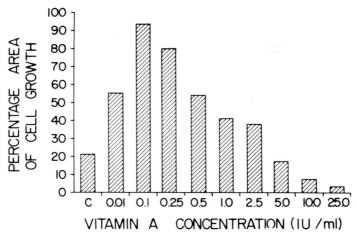

Fig. 14. Histogram showing the effects of vitamin A (retinol acetate) on the growth of normal human prostatic epithelium in vitro. C refers to control cultures. Results show that vitamin A at a level of 0.1 unit/ml stimulates maximum growth of these cells in vitro. 5.0 units/ml and higher levels of vitamin A were toxic (age of cell donor, 21 years; from Webber [6]).

This configuration is similar to the ultrastructure of normal epithelium in vivo. A study of the ultrastructure has therefore been a very useful tool for assessing the physiological well-being of the cell, and changes induced in the ultrastructure can be correlated with the treatment to which the cells are exposed. Effects of vitamin A at the ultrastructural level have been described in detail elsewhere [6].

Discussion. Results presented here show that vitamin A clearly stimulates growth of normal human prostatic epithelium, prevents metaplasia, and regulates the normal course of differentiation. Vitamin A possibly controls the rate of cell multiplication and differentiation in secretory epithelium and restores the normal balance of the two processes [23, 87]. An excess of vitamin A increases the mitotic rate in some cell cultures — eg, prostate, chick heart fibroblasts, and mouse vagina — in vitro [23]. Sporn et al have shown [88] that vitamin A causes a significant increase in cellular RNA content in vitro. They used CMRL 1066 medium without serum to grow epidermis from newborn mice. Addition of retinyl acetate also altered the direction of differentiation.

Few studies have been made on the effects of vitamin A on the ultrastructure of mammalian and chick epithelial cells. When vitamin A was not added to the culture, cells showed extensive tonofilament bundles, desmosomes, keratohyalin granules, and a smooth cell surface. On the addition of vitamin A, most tonofilaments and keratohyalin granules disappeared, desmosomes were short and infrequent, and microvilli appeared on the cell surface [89, 90]. These observations suggest that vitamin A has a direct effect on the cell biosynthesis, and these changes are probably influenced at the gene level.

Effects of Testosterone and 5α-Dihydrotestosterone

Introduction. Prostatic epithelium is under the growth control exerted by testosterone. Testosterone is required for its growth, renewal, maintenance, and secretory activity. Certain testosterone metabolites, particularly 5α-dihydrotestosterone (5α-DHT) actively affect these target cells and control their cell division.

Almost all of the experimental work in vivo and in vitro, on the effects of testosterone on the prostate, has been done on mice and rats [65, 87, 91–93]. Lasnitzki [65] was one of the earliest investigators to make detailed studies on the effects of testosterone in organ cultures of mouse prostate. In the absence of testosterone, the cultures showed regression of alveolar epithelium. These regressive changes were prevented if the medium was supplemented with testosterone propionate, which restored the secretory activity and the cell morphology to normal and also induced a mild epithelial hyperplasia. Edwards et al [20] have also recently shown regressive changes in epithelium when testosterone is omitted from the culture medium.

In vitro studies on the effects of testosterone on the human prostate are recent and few [26, 30, 31, 37, 94]. All of these studies were made on benign or malignant epithelium, primarily, to determine tumor sensitivity for therapeutic purposes. Studies on the use of testosterone or its metabolites for growth and maintenance of normal prostatic epithelial cells were not made. Hence, the present observations on normal human prostatic epithelium may be considered pioneer studies.

Results. Incorporation of testosterone into the culture medium at levels over a wide range did not have a marked stimulatory effect on the growth of normal prostatic epithelium. It also did not increase the life-span of the cells. However, 5α-DHT had a distinct and a marked stimulatory effect on prostatic epithelium. Dose response data are presented in Figure 15. Results consistently show that 0.1 μg/ml 5α-DHT in culture medium induces optimum growth of prostatic epithelial cells. Concentrations above 10 μg/ml were clearly toxic. This toxicity is indicated at the ultrastructural level by a large number of autophagosomes [95].

Discussion. Results show that testosterone, when incorporated into the culture medium, did not appreciably increase growth of normal human prostatic epithelium under the culture conditions provided. Although stimulatory effects of testosterone have been demonstrated on the rat and mouse prostate [20, 65], other investigators [21, 96], did not observe any growth-promoting effects or improvement in the maintenance of normal morphology in organ cultures of dog prostate.

On the other hand, when 5α-DHT was added to the culture medium, an increase in cell growth occurred. Many studies support the present observations made on the effects of 5α-DHT on prostatic epithelium. The mode of action of testosterone has unfolded only recently [97]. Testosterone is rapidly converted

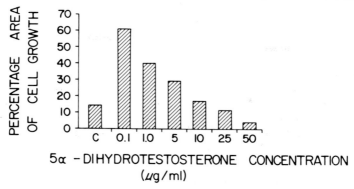

Fig. 15. Histogram showing the effects of 5α-dihydrotestosterone on the growth of normal human prostatic epithelium in vitro. 0.1 μg/ml DHT stimulated maximum growth of these cells in vitro. With increasing levels, growth declined and levels above 25 μg/ml DHT in culture medium were toxic (from Webber and Bouldin [95]).

to 5α-DHT in prostatic epithelial cells. It is the active metabolite of testosterone, and is a potent androgen and mitogen for target cells. It induces cell proliferation in animal and human prostatic epithelium. The mechanism of mitogenic action of 5α-DHT has been linked to the nuclear receptors in target cells [98].

The interaction of testosterone and insulin is an interesting phenomenon and can be demonstrated by some experiments done by Lostroh [99]. In organ cultures of prostate from orchiectomized mice, insulin was able to stimulate extensive repair. This repair was similar to that obtained in vivo when testosterone was given to orchiectomized mice. However, in vitro, testosterone was unable to induce repair unless insulin was present in the culture medium.

Effects of Other Growth Factors

Effects of epidermal growth factor (EGF) and polyamines have also been investigated. Due to limited space these cannot be discussed in detail here. It will suffice to say that EGF enhanced the growth of prostatic epithelium at levels of 1 to 10 ng/ml. Beyond this level, there was no further enhancement. EGF also increased the life-span of prostatic epithelial cultures.

Another area of major interest to us is growth regulation of prostatic epithelium by polyamines and their possible role in the process of cellular aging as related to oncogenesis and the etiology of benign and malignant disease of the prostate. It should be noted that prostate produces large amounts of two polyamines, spermine and spermidine. We are investigating the effects of putrescine and spermine on the growth of prostatic epithelium in vitro. This work has already produced two significant findings. One is the observation that spermine selectively enhances growth and life-span of prostatic epithelium in mixed cultures when it is added to culture medium containing both fetal bovine and horse serum. At the same time, growth of fibroblasts is inhibited, as shown in Figure 16. Bovine serum contains diamine oxidase, which oxidizes spermine to rather unstable aminoaldehydes which decompose releasing stable acrolein. Acrolein is toxic to cells. Hence, it is possible that the observed toxicity of spermine to fibroblasts is really due to oxidation products of spermine. The important point here is that the prostatic epithelial cells are resistant to the toxicity of these oxidation products. In fact, they show some growth stimulation by spermine. This phenomenon can be used in the selection of epithelial cells from mixed cultures. Details of investigations on the effects of spermine and putrescine are discussed elsewhere [100].

CHARACTERIZATION

Once the cells have been isolated and established in vitro, it is necessary to prove that these cells are indeed of prostatic epithelial origin. Efforts have been made to characterize prostatic epithelial cells on the basis of a variety of their unique physiologic, secretory, and morphologic characteristics. Characterization of prostatic epithelial cells is the subject of a detailed discussion elsewhere in this volume (see Merchant), therefore, only a few specific comments are appropriate here. Our methods for characterization of prostatic epithelium by cytochemical localization of prostatic acid phosphatase were described earlier [5, 101, 102]. One of these methods is based on the greater resistance to inhibition of prostatic acid phosphatase by 10% neutral buffered formaldehyde, than other acid phosphatases. Results show [5] that even after 24-hour immersion in cold 10% formalin, the acid phosphatase activity is still present in cells. On the basis of these results, it can be stated that the cells isolated by our collagenase method or grown from explants are indeed of prostatic epithelial origin.

COMMENTS, CONCLUSIONS, AND FUTURE RESEARCH

Having established methods for isolation of prostatic epithelium and defined many of its growth requirements in vitro, and having established that the cells being grown in culture are indeed of prostatic epithelial origin, a further point still needs clarification. Prostatic epithelial cells are specialized, hormone-responsive, secretory cells. Generally, such cells have a limited potential for division, unless they have been reverted to a de-differentiated state. This raises the question as to the source of cells that contribute to the growth in culture.

When prostatic epithelial cells are first placed in culture, two types of cells can be seen — large cells, often with vacuolated cytoplasm, and small cells. The large cells are the differentiated cells which form the layer of cells closest the the lumen of acini. These cells are incapable of division and are generally lost as the culture grows older. The small cells are the basal cells and contribute primarily to the growth of prostatic eptihelium in vitro. The basal cells of the prostate are undifferentiated

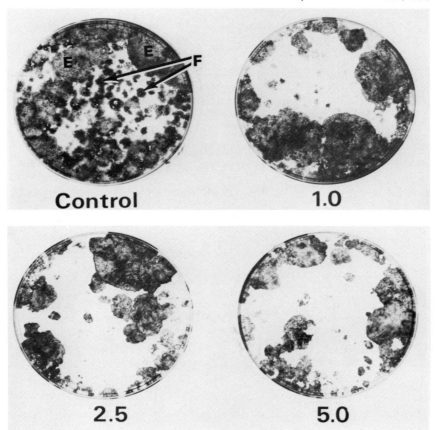

Fig. 16. Effects of spermine and its oxidation products on the growth of prostatic epithelium and fibroblasts. Numbers represent μg/ml of spermine in culture medium. The control cultures contain both epithelial cells (E) and fibroblasts (F). Addition of spermine to the culture medium containing both fetal bovine and horse serum results in elimination of fibroblasts. Cultures containing 2.5 μg/ml spermine are completely fibroblast-free. Higher levels show toxic effects.

and have the ability to divide. These cells represent reserve cells and are involved in the replacement of normal glandular epithelium in vivo [103]. Recent investigations by Dermer [104] show that, in organ culture, the differentiated secretory cells do not incorporate thymidine, indicating their inability to divide. However, the basal cells show signs of proliferation and are responsible for replacing dying and sloughed secretory cells. The presence of these basal cells if fortunate in that actively growing cultures of prostatic epithelium could not be obtained without the presence of the undifferentiated basal cells.

In conclusion, the findings presented here may be summarized as follows:

1) Isolation of normal, viable, postpubertal, human prostatic epithelium has been accomplished. Vigorously growing cultures can be obtained from isolated acini.

2) Medium RPMI 1640 containing a combination of horse and fetal bovine serum supports good growth and maintenance of these cells in vitro.

3) Insulin selectively enhances growth of prostatic epithelium but inhibits growth of fibroblasts. This effect is useful for selection of epithelial cells. Insulin is an important growth regulator for prostatic epithelium, and it potentiates the effects of testosterone.

4) Vitamin A is necessary for growth and maintenance of normal ultrastructural morphology of prostatic epithelium, and it selectively enhances growth of these cells.

5) 5α-Dihydrotestosterone induces cell division in prostatic epithelium in culture; however, testosterone has no appreciable effect under the culture conditions provided.

6) Epidermal growth factor increases growth and life-span of prostatic epithelium in culture. Spermine also selectively enhances growth and life-span of prostatic epithelium but indirectly inhibits growth of fibroblasts.

7) Cells grown from explants and isolated acini have been characterized by cytochemical localization of prostatic acid phosphatase. The test is based on the greater stability of prostatic acid phosphatase in neutral buffered formalin than other acid phosphatases.

Studies described in this paper were all made on primary cultures. Efforts are now being made to subculture these cells. Plating cells on feeder cultures has been particularly successful. Subcultivation will be greatly facilitated by what we now know about the growth requirements of these cells in vitro. Studies on the importance of stromal—epithelial interaction are also in progress.

The next goal in the development of this model system is to develop a totally defined medium. The need and usefulness of chemically defined media for normal, diploid human cells has been well expressed by Ham [105], who is a pioneer in developing chemically defined media for many types of animal and human cells. It must be kept in mind that we are dealing with postpubertal, hormone-responsive cells. Thus, media that may support growth of fetal or neonatal prostatic epithelium will not necessarily be adequate for the adult epithelium. The importance of using epithelium from postpubertal, sexually mature donors has already been emphasized. In the past, we have used media containing large amounts of serum, this being the major undefined component. This medium, however, supported good growth and has been extremely useful in establishing several growth requirements of normal human prostatic epithelium. The goal is to completely replace the serum with growth factors that have already been tested and other agents. These experiments are underway, and some progress has already been made. We have now been able to replace most of the serum with a supplement of several growth factors. A considerable amount of work still needs to be done to develop a completely chemically defined medium. However, one must keep in mind that chemically defined media should be designed not just for rapid growth but also for maintenance.

It is hoped that studies using the described in vitro cell model will make it possible to examine the early steps in human prostatic carcinogenesis; the carcinogen—target cell interaction; metabolic activation of specific carcinogens; and the role of multiple agents and co-carcinogens in transformation. Such human cell models can also be used for screening suspected carcinogenic and toxic environmental agents. Other promising areas for future research, using this cell model are: cell nutrition, metabolism, growth, and aging in hormone-dependent cells.

ACKNOWLEDGMENTS

The author wishes to thank Lucy Jankowsky, Thomas Bouldin, and Robert McGrew for their assistance in accomplishing this work; Dr. Robert Donohue for securing normal tissue; the Veterans' Administration Hospital for the use of their electron microscopy facility; the Department of Molecular Cellular and Developmental Biology for the use of their scanning electron microscope; Richard Carter for his help in the preparation of photographs; and Fidelia Malz and Carol Williams for their help in the preparation of this manuscript.

This work was supported by the Division of Cancer Cause and Prevention, National Cancer Institute, DHEW contract NO1-CP-65849.

REFERENCES

1. Merchant DJ: Prostatic tissue cell growth and assessment. Semin Oncol 3:131–140, 1976.
2. Walsh PC: Benign prostatic hyperplasia: Etiological considerations. In Marberger H, Haschek H, Schirmer HKA, Colston JAC, Witkin E (eds): "Prostatic Disease, Progress in Clinical and Biological Research." New York: Alan R. Liss, Inc., vol 6, 1976, pp 1–8.
3. Franks LM: The natural history of prostatic cancer. In Marberger H, Haschek H, Schirmer HKA, Colston JAC, Witkin E (eds): "Prostatic Disease, Progress in Clinical and Biological Research." New York: Alan R. Liss, Inc., vol 6, 1976, pp 103–109.
4. Lechner JF, Narayan KS, Ohnuki Y, Babcock MS, Jones LW, Kaighn ME: Replicative epithelial cell cultures from normal human prostate gland: Brief communication. J Natl Cancer Inst 60:797–801, 1978.
5. Webber MM: Normal and benign human prostatic epithelium in culture. I. Isolation. In Vitro (in press).
6. Webber MM: Growth and maintenance of normal human prostatic epithelium in vitro. IV. Effects of vitamin A (in preparation).
7. Webber MM, Donohue RE, Jankowsky L: Growth and maintenance of normal human prostatic epithelium in vitro. I. Effects of serum (in preparation).

8. Webber MM, Jankowsky L: Growth and maintenance of normal human prostatic epithelium in vitro. II. Effects of different media and glutamine (in preparation).

9. Webber MM: Growth and maintenance of normal human prostatic epithelium in vitor. III. Effects of insulin (in preparation).

10. Stoner GD, Harris CC, Bostwick DG, Jones RT, Trump BF, Kingsbury EW, Fineman E, Newkirk C: Isolation and characterization of epithelial cells from bovine pancreatic duct. In Vitro 14:581–590, 1978.

11. Stonington OG, Hemmingsen H: Culture of cells as a monolayer derived from the epithelium of the human prostate: A new cell growth technique. J Urol 106:393–400, 1971.

12. Webber MM: Effects of serum on the growth of prostatic cells in vitro. J Urol 112:798–801, 1974.

13. Webber MM, Stonington OG: Hypocellularity in organ culture of human prostate – Application in epithelial cell isolation. J Urol 114:246–248, 1975.

14. Webber MM, Stonington OG, Poché PA: Epithelial outgrowth from suspension cultures of human prostatic tissue. In Vitro 10:196–205, 1974.

15. Hay RJ: The pancreatic epithelial cell in vitro: A possible model system for studies in carcinogenesis. Cancer Res 35:2289–2291, 1975.

16. Kirk D, King RJB, Heyes J, Peachey L, Hirsch PJ, Taylor RWT: Normal human endometrium in cell culture. I. Separation and characterization of epithelial and stromal components in vitro. In Vitro 14:651–662, 1978.

17. Buehring GC: Culture of human mammary epithelial cells: Keeping abreast with a new method. J Natl Cancer Inst 49:1433–1434, 1972.

18. Waymouth C: To disaggregate or not to disaggregate. Injury and cell disaggregation, transient or permanent? In Vitro 10:97–111, 1974.

19. Chopra DP, Wilkoff LJ: Induction of hyperplasia and anaplasia by carcinogens in organ cultures of mouse prostate. In Vitro 13:260–267, 1977.

20. Edwards WD, Bates RR, Yuspa SH: Organ cultures of rodent prostate: Effects of polyamines and testosterone. Invest Urol 14:1–5, 1976.

21. Fisher TV, Burkel WE, Kahn RH, Herwig KR: Effect of testosterone on long-term organ cultures of canine prostate. In Vitro 11:382–392, 1976.

22. Herwig KR, Fischer TV, Burkel WE, Kahn RH: Organ culture of canine prostate. Invest Urol 15:291–294, 1978.

23. Lasnitzki I: Growth patterns of the mouse prostate glands in organ cultures and its response to sex hormones, vitamins A and 3-methylcholanthrene. In Vollmer EP (ed): "Biology of the Prostate and Related Tissues." Natl Cancer Inst Monogr 12:381–403, 1963.

24. Norris JS, Bowden C, Kohler PO: Description of a new hamster ventral prostate cell line containing androgen receptors. In Vitro 13:108–114, 1977.

25. Allgower M: The cultivation of human prostate adenomata in vitro. Exp Cell Res (Suppl 1):456–459, 1949.

26. Brehmer B, Marquardt H, Madsen PO: Growth and hormonal response of cells derived from carcinoma and hyperplasia of the prostate in monolayer cell culture. A possible in vitro model for clinical chemotherapy. J Urol 108:890–896, 1972.

27. Ioachim HL: Tissue culture of human tumors: Use and prospects. In Summers S (ed): "Pathology Annual." New York: Appleton-Century-Crofts, 5:217–256, 1970.

28. Röhl L: Prostatic hyperplasia and carcinoma studies with tissue culture technique. Acta Chir Scand (Suppl) 40:1–88, 1959.

29. Rose NR, Choe BK, Pontes JE: Cultivation of epithelial cells from the prostate. Cancer Chemother Rep 59:147–149, 1975.

30. Schrodt GR, Foreman CD: In vitro maintenance of human hyperplastic prostate tissue. Invest Urol 9:85–94, 1971.
31. Schroeder FH, Mackensen SJ: Human prostatic adenoma and carcinoma in cell culture. Invest Urol 12:176–181, 1974.
32. Shipman PAM, Littlewood V, Riches AC, Thomas GH: Differences in proliferative activity of rat and human prostate in culture. Br J Cancer 31:570–580, 1975.
33. Stone KR, Paulson DF, Bonar RA, Reich C: In vitro culture of epithelial cells derived from urogenital tissue. Urol Res 2:149–153, 1975.
34. Bregman RU, Bregman ET: Tissue culture of benign and malignant human genitourinary tumors. J Urol 86:642–649, 1961.
35. Stone KR, Stone MP, Paulson DF: In vitro cultivation of prostatic epithelium. Invest Urol 14:79–82, 1976.
36. Jones RE, Sanford EJ, Rohner TJ, Rapp F: In vitro viral transformation of human prostatic carcinoma. J Urol 115:82–85, 1976.
37. Schroeder FH, Sato G, Gittes RF: Human prostatic adenocarcinoma. Growth in monolayer tissue culture. J Urol 106:734–739, 1971.
38. Webber MM, Batts AF: Cultivation of human prostatic epithelium – Present status. In Vitro 13:143, 1977.
39. Gross J: Collagenases of animal origin. In Mandl I (ed): "Collagenase; First Interdisciplinary Symposium on Collagenase." New York: Gordon and Breach Science Publishers, 1972, pp 33–36.
40. Mandl I: Collagenase comes of age. In Mandl I (ed): "Collagenase; First Interdisciplinary Symposium on Collagenase." New York: Gordon and Breach Science Publishers, 1972, pp 1–15.
41. Lasfargues EY: Cultivation and behavior in vitro of the normal mammary epithelium of the adult mouse. Anat Rec 127:117–129, 1957.
42. Schwartz SM: Selection and characterization of bovine aortic endothelial cells. In Vitro 14:966–980, 1978.
43. Acosta D, Anuforo DC, Smith RV: Primary monolayer cultures of postnatal rat liver cells with extended differentiated functions. In Vitro 14:428–436, 1978.
44. Leiter EH, Coleman DL, Waymouth C: Cell culture of the endocrine pancreas of the mouse in chemically defined media. In Vitro 9:421–433, 1974.
45. White MT, Hu ASL, Hammamoto ST, Nandi S: In vitro analysis of proliferating epithelial cell populations from the mouse mammary gland: Fibroblast-free growth and serial passage. In Vitro 14:271–281, 1978.
46. Mandl I: Collagenases and elastases. Adv Enzymol 23:163–264, 1961.
47. Webber MM, Bouldin TR: Ultrastructure of human prostatic epithelium – Secretion granules or virus particles? Invest Urol 14:482–487, 1977.
48. Porter KR, Todaro GJ, Fonte V: A scanning electron microscope study of surface features of viral and spontaneous transformants of mouse BALB/3T3 cells. J Cell Biol 59:633–642, 1973.
49. Poché PA, Webber MM, Jankowsky L: A rapid method for in situ staining of prostatic and other tissue culture cells. Stain Technol 49:229–233, 1974.
50. Lasfargues EY, Moore DH: A method for the continuous cultivation of mammary epithelium. In Vitro 7:21–25, 1971.
51. Gilbert SF, Migeon BR: D-valine as a selective agent for normal human and rodent epithelial cells in culture. Cell 5:11–17, 1975.
52. Soukupova M, Huevkovsky P, Chvapil M, Hruza Z: Effect of collagenase on the behavior of cells from young and old donors in culture. Exp Gerontol 3:135–139, 1968.

53. Webber MM, Webber PJ: The use of a television scanning densitometer for measuring growth in stained cell cultures. Stain Technol (submitted for publication).
54. Puck TT, Cieciura SJ, Fisher HW: Clonal growth in vitro of human cells with fibroblastic morphology. Comparison of growth and genetic characteristics of single epithelioid and fibroblast-like cells from a variety of human organs. J Exp Med 106:145–158, 1957.
55. Schröder FH, Jellinghaus W: Prostatic adenoma and carcinoma in cell culture and hetero-transplantation. In Marberger H, Haschek H, Schirmer HKA, Colston JAC, Witkin E (eds): "Prostatic Disease, Progress in Clinical and Biological Research." New York: Alan R. Liss, Inc., vol 6, 1976, pp 301–312.
56. Temin HM: Control of multiplication of uninfected rat cells and rat cells converted by murine sarcoma virus. J Cell Physiol 75:107–119, 1970.
57. Trowell OA: The culture of mature organs in a synthetic medium. Exp Cell Res 16: 118–147, 1959.
58. Waymouth C, Reed DE: A reversible morphological change in mouse cells (Strain L. Clone NCTC 929) under the influence of insulin. Tex Rep Biol Med 23:413–419, 1965.
59. Blaker GJ, Birch JR, Pirt SJ: The glucose, insulin and glutamine requirements of sus-pension cultures of HeLa cells in a defined culture medium. J Cell Sci 9:529–537, 1971.
60. Flaxman BA, Lasfargues EY: Hormone-independent DNA synthesis in epithelial cells of adult human mammary gland in organ cultures. Proc Soc Exp Biol Med 143:371–374, 1973.
61. Donaldson LJ, Thomas GH: Uptake of (^{125}I) iodo-deoxyuridine in cultured rat and human prostate: Effects of insulin and testosterone. J Endocrinol 69:85–92, 1976.
62. Franks LM: The growth of mouse prostate during culture in vitro in chemically defined and natural media, and after transplantation in vivo. Exp Cell Res 22:56–72, 1961.
63. Ichihara I: Some ultrastructural effects of testosterone and insulin on the ventral prostate of rats in organ culture. Cell Tiss Res 181:327–337, 1977.
64. Johansson R: RNA, protein and DNA synthesis stimulated by testosterone, insulin and prolactin in the rat ventral prostate cultured in chemically defined medium. Acta Endo-crinol 80:761–774, 1975.
65. Lasnitzki I: The action of hormones on cell and organ cultures. In Willmer EN (ed): "Cells and Tissues in Culture." New York: Academic Press, vol 1, 1965, pp 591–658.
66. Lostroh AJ: Regulation by testosterone and insulin of citrate secretion and protein syn-thesis in explanted mouse prostates. Proc Natl Acad Sci USA 60:1312–1318, 1968.
67. Tisell LE, Andersson H, Angervall L: A morphologic study of the prostatic lobes and the seminal vesicles of castrated rats injected with oestradiol and/or insulin. Urol Res 4: 63–69, 1976.
68. Mierzejewski K, Rozengurt E: Stimulation of DNA synthesis and cell division in a chemi-cally defined medium: Effect of epidermal growth factor, insulin and vitamin B$_{12}$ on resting cultures of 3T6 cells. Biochem Biophys Res Commun 73:271–278, 1976.
69. Rillema JA, Linebaugh BE: Characteristics of the insulin stimulation of DNA, RNA and protein metabolism in cultured human mammary carcinoma cells. Biochim Biophys Acta 475:74–80, 1977.
70. Gospodarowicz D, Moran JS: Stimulation of division of sparse and confluent 3T3 cell populations by a fibroblast growth factor, dexamethasone and insulin. Proc Natl Acad Sci USA 71:4584–4588, 1974.
71. Paul J, Pearson ES: The action of insulin on the metabolism of cell cultures. J Endo-crinol 21:287–294, 1960.
72. Ross EJ: Insulin and the permeability of cell membranes to glucose. Nature 171:125, 1953.

73. Barnett RJ, Ball EG: Metabolic and ultrastructural changes induced in adipose tissue by insulin. J Biophys Biochem Cytol 8:83−101, 1960.
74. Hunt EL, Bailey DW: The effects of alloxan diabetes on the reproductive system of young male rats. Acta Endocrinol 38:432−440, 1961.
75. Sufrin G, Prutkin L: Experimental diabetes and the response of the sex accessory organs of the castrate male rat to testosterone proprionate. Invest Urol 11:361−369, 1974.
76. Griffith JB: The effect of insulin on the growth and metabolism of the human diploid cell, W1-38. J Cell Sci 7:575−585, 1970.
77. Hollenberg MD, Cuatrecasas P: Human fibroblast receptors related to deoxyribonucleic acid synthesis and amino acid uptake. J Biol Chem 250:3845−3853, 1975.
78. Rechler MM, Podskalny JM: Insulin receptors in cultured human fibroblasts. Diabetes 25: 250−255, 1976.
79. Hollenberg MD, Fryklund L: Insulin and somatomedins A and B: Comparison of biological activities in cultured human skin-derived fibroblasts. Life Sci 21:943−950, 1977.
80. Kelley LA, Butcher RW: The effects of epinephrine and prostaglandin E, on cyclic adenosine 3′:5′monophosphate levels in W1-38 fibroblasts. J Biol Chem 249:3098−3102, 1974.
81. Rosenthal JW, Goldstein S: The effect of insulin on basal and hormone-induced elevations of cyclic AMP content in cultured human fibroblasts. J Cell Physiol 85:235−242, 1975.
82. Cuatrecasas P: Insulin receptors, cell membranes and hormone action. Biochem Pharmacol 23:2353−2361, 1974.
83. Hsueh HW: Serum and insulin initiation of DNA synthesis in mammary gland epithelium in vitro. J Cell Physiol 83:297−308, 1974.
84. Wolbach GB, Howe PR: Tissue changes following deprivation of fat soluble A vitamin. J Exp Med 47:753−777, 1925.
85. Fell HB, Rinaldini L: The effects of vitamins A and C on cells and tissues in culture. In Willmer EN (ed): "Cells and Tissues in Culture." New York: Academic Press, vol 1, 1965, pp 659−699.
86. Webber MM: Ultrastructural changes in human prostatic epithelium grown in vitro. J Ultrastruct Res 50:89−102, 1975.
87. Lasnitzki I: The influence of A hypervitaminosis on the effect of 20-methylcholanthrene on mouse prostate gland in vitro. Br J Cancer 9:434−441, 1955.
88. Sporn MB, Dunlop NM, Yuspa SH: Retinyl acetate: Effect on cellular content of RNA in epidermis in cell culture in chemically defined medium. Science 182:722−723, 1973.
89. Fitton JF, Fell HB: Epidermal fine structure in embryonic chicken skin during atypical differentiation induced by vitamin A in culture. Dev Biol 7:394−419, 1963.
90. Peck GL, Elias PM, Wetzel B: Influence of vitamin A on differentiating epithelia. In Seji M, Bernstein IA (eds): "Biochemistry of Cutaneous Epidermal Differentiation." Baltimore: University Park Press, 1977, pp 110−126.
91. Franks LM, Barton AA: The effect of testosterone on the ultrastructure of the mouse prostate in vivo and in organ culture. Exp Cell Res 19:35−50, 1960.
92. Györkey F: The effects of sex hormones on the histochemistry of mouse prostate organ cultures. Invest Urol 2:154−172, 1964.
93. Helminen HJ, Ericson JL: Ultrastructural studies on prostatic involution in the rat. Changes in the secretory pathways. J Ultrastruct Res 40:152−166, 1972.
94. McMahon MJ, Butler AVJ, Thomas GH: Morphological responses of prostatic carcinoma to testosterone in organ culture. Br J Cancer 26:388−394, 1972.
95. Webber MM, Bouldin TR: Growth and maintenance of normal human prostatic epithelium in vitro. V. Effects of testosterone and 5α-dihydrotestosterone (in preparation).

96. Sinowatz F, Pierrepoint CG: Hormonal effects on canine prostatic explants in organ culture. J Endocrinol 72:53–58, 1977.
97. Mawhinney MG, Schwartz FF, Thomas JA, Lloyd JW III: Androgen assimilation by normal and hyperplastic dog prostate glands. Invest Urol 12:17–22, 1974.
98. Liao S, Tymoczko L, Castaneda E, Liang T: Androgen receptors and androgen-dependent initiation of protein synthesis in the prostate. Vitam Horm 33:297–317, 1975.
99. Lostroh AJ: Effect of testosterone and insulin in vitro on maintenance and repair of the secretory epithelium of the mouse prostate. Endocrinology 88:500–503, 1971.
100. Webber MM, Chaproniers-Rickenberg D: Spermine oxidation products are selectively toxic to fibroblasts in cultures of normal human prostatic epithelium. Cell Biology International Reports (submitted for publication).
101. Stonington OG, Szwec N, Webber M: Isolation and identification of the human malignant prostatic epithelial cell in pure monolayer culture. J Urol 114:903–908, 1975.
102. Stonington OG, Szwec N, Webber M: Identification of cultured, human, malignant prostatic epithelial cells. Natl Cancer Inst Monogr 49:31–33, 1978.
103. Kastendieck H, Altenähr E: Role of basal cells in non-malignant lesions of the prostate. Arch Androl 2(Suppl 1):abstr 64.
104. Dermer GB: Basal cell proliferation in benign prostatic hyperplasia. Cancer 41:1857–1862, 1978.
105. Ham RG: Nutritional requirements of primary cultures. A neglected problem of modern biology. In Vitro 10:119–129, 1974.

Nutrition of Prostate Cells

J.F. Lechner, PhD, and M.E. Kaighn, PhD

   The work reported in this paper is part of an overall program to isolate and characterize human prostatic cells from normal, benign prostatic hypertrophy (BPH) and carcinoma tissue. A major goal of this program was to develop a defined medium suitable for culture of prostatic cells and to reduce the serum requirements so that meaningful hormonal studies could be carried out.

   In 1973, when these studies were initiated, very little was known about the nutritional requirements of human cells, especially normal human epithelial cells. As pointed out by Ham [1, 2], much of the information that was available had been derived from studies on highly evolved aneuploid cancer lines such as the human HeLa or the mouse L cells. Subsequently, Ham and co-workers have made significant progress in defining media for normal human fibroblasts [3, 4]. The approach used in their studies employed a clonal growth assay. In brief, the approach was to reduce the serum concentration to a minimal level, then to titrate the growth-promoting activity of the low molecular weight components such as amino acids, vitamins, ions, and trace elements in the medium. This "fine-tuning" of medium components was alternated with progressive reduction in serum levels. This approach has made possible clonal growth of the normal human lung line WI 38 in as little as 25 μg/ml of fetal bovine serum protein [3, 4].

   We have employed a similar but not identical approach with human prostatic cells. Like Ham, we used the clonal growth assay. In our early studies we found that evaluation of plating efficiency permitted us to screen individual lots of serum for toxicity [5, 6]. Rather than survival, growth, as measured by increase in cells per colony, appeared to be a more accurate reflection of the activity of various medium components. With the exception of inclusion of HEPES buffer in medium F12K, we were unable to improve the medium for

Models for Prostate Cancer, pages 217–232
© 1980 Alan R. Liss, Inc., 150 Fifth Ave., New York, NY 10011

prostatic cells [7]. However, by adding several known growth factors [8, 9], dramatic improvement in growth-promoting activity was achieved. The shape of the clonal serum growth-response curve suggested that the application of enzyme kinetics might provide a useful means to compare the activities of various growth-promoting factors. Using this approach, we discovered several interactions between factors [10–12].

Further, this technique has facilitated developing media for different prostatic cell types. Significant differences have been found between normal cell types and between normal and prostatic cancer cells. Details of these findings are the subject of this paper.

MATERIALS AND METHODS
Cells, Culture Medium, and Growth Factors

A normal, human prostate epithelial cell line, NP-2s [13], a foreskin fibro-blastic line, NF2 developed from the same neonate, a benign prostatic epithelial line, HP1-7 [14], and a human tumorigenic adenocarcinoma line PC-3 [15–17] were used in these studies. The growth medium consisted of nutrient medium (PFMR-4) supplemented with 7% fetal bovine serum (FBS). Fetal bovine serum protein (FBSP) concentrations were measured using the Folin technique [18], with bovine serum albumin as reference. Calcium-free serum was prepared by first adding EGTA to a final concentration of 5 mM, then dialyzing the mixture sequentially for two days at 4°C against a total of 1×10^6 volumes of distilled water. Low Ca^{2+} nutrient medium consisted of PFMR-4 prepared without calcium except for that contained in calcium panthenate, 1×10^{-6} M.

Stock solutions of epidermal growth factor (EGF) and fibroblast growth prepared in growth medium. Insulin stocks at 0.1 mg/ml were prepared in 0.01 N HCl. Hydrocortisone (HC) (4-Pregnen-11-β-17-α-21-triol, 3,20-dione, Steroids Incorporated, Wilton, NH) was dissolved in absolute ethanol at 10^{-3} M. The phorbol ester TPA (12-0-decanoyl-phorbol-13-acetate, Consolidated Midland Corp., Brewster, NY) was dissolved in acetone at 1 mg/ml.

Clonal Growth Assay

Four replicate Petri dishes per variable were used. Enzymatically dissociated cells [13, 19] were washed twice with HEPES balanced salts (HBS), then diluted in HBS for clonal plating. Each dish received 300 cells in a final volume of 4 ml of medium. After six to eight days of growth, the clones were fixed in 10% formalin and stained with 0.25% crystal violet.

Clonal Growth Rate

The rate of clonal growth was constant except when culture conditions were highly unfavorable [10]. Therefore, clonal growth rates were used as a measure of mitogen potency. Growth rate (R) was defined as average population doublings per clone per day (PD/day). To measure this the enlarged images of stained clones were projected onto a screen. For each datum point, the number of cells per clone in 16 randomly selected clones were determined manually. Three cells were subtracted from each count, since the average clone which developed in medium without serum or growth factor supplementation consisted of three cells. The average number of cells per clone was converted to population doublings by dividing the $\log_{10}$ cells per clone by $\log_{10} 2$. R was obtained by dividing this value by the number of days of growth. In experiments where growth factor activity was titrated in medium containing a low level of serum, an additional background cell count was subtracted. This value corresponded to the average colony size (cells/clone) that developed in media supplemented with serum alone.

Growth Rate Parameters

Enzyme kinetic parameters were adopted to describe the influence of mitogen concentration on R. The data were analyzed using the Lineweaver-Burk transformation of the Michaelis-Menten equation. The formulations for developing statistically weighted linear regressions of the data were adopted from Ellem and Geirthy [20]. Correlation coefficients were calculated to estimate the closeness of fit of the line to the datum points. The theoretical maximal growth rate (R_{MAX}^T) is defined as the reciprocal of the Y intercept. The substrate concentration at which half-maximal growth occurred $(K_m^{mitogen})$ is the negative reciprocal of the X intercept. Student's t-test was used to evaluate significant differences between the R_{MAX}^T and $K_m^{mitogen}$ values derived from different experimental groups.

RESULTS

Serum Selection and Requirement

Selection of an acceptable lot of FBS was important in achieving sustained growth of normal prostatic epithelial cells [13]. Colony size as well as plating efficiency was used to evaluate each lot. Of 23 individual lots evaluated, 70% were unacceptable (Fig. 1). The average size ranged from 22 cells/colony with the least active serum lot to 111 cells/colony with the most effective serum lot. No significant difference in growth-promoting activity of the various serum lots was observed with the prostatic carcinoma line, PC-3.

As one approach we sought to circumvent serum variability by supplementing the medium with several putative mitogenic factors. To standardize conditions, the FBSP requirements for NP-2s, NF2, and PC-3 were assayed in dose-response experiments. The most effective serum lot was used for these and all subsequent experiments. The rate of cell multiplication was found to be proportional to

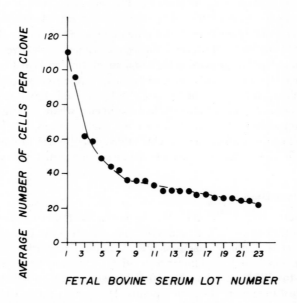

Fig. 1. Clonal growth of NP-2s cells as a function of fetal bovine serum (FBS) lot. Twenty-three individual FBS lots were tested at 7% using the clonal growth assay (see Materials and Methods). After seven days of incubation, the average number of cells per clone was determined. Lot number was plotted in rank order from highest to lowest activity value.

FBSP concentration in a manner analogous to the effect of substrate concentration on an enzyme reaction rate (Fig. 2). Growth rate increased with serum concentration until a maximal velocity was approached. Since growth rate was dependent upon serum concentration, we used the principles of Lineweaver-Burk analysis to determine the K_m^{FBSP} value for each of the three cell lines. K_m^{FBSP} and R_{MAX}^T values were derived using statistically weighted regression analysis of the Lineweaver-Burk transformations. Half-maximal growth rate of PC-3 was attained with 10 μg FBSP per ml, equivalent to 0.025% FBS. The levels of FBSP required for the normal epithelial and fibroblastic cells to proliferate at their half-maximal rates were 2,230 μg (FBSP/ml (5.7$ FBS), and 1,480 μg ıg FBSP/ml (3.8% FBS), respectively. The maximal growth rates of these three cell lines also differed. Expressed as generation time, PC-3 doubled every 28.6 hours, NF2 every 19 hours, and NP-2s every 17.6 hours.

Action of EGF, FGF, and Insulin

It was assumed that maximal rates had been attained with saturation levels of serum. Therefore, low levels were used to permit stimulation of growth rate by

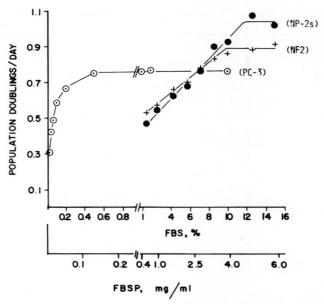

Fig. 2. The effect of FBSP on clonal growth rates. Cells were plated at 300 cells/dish in PFMR-4 medium containing increasing concentrations of FBSP. After seven days of incubation the clonal growth rates were determined (see Materials and Methods). ⊚—⊚, PC-3; ●—●, NP-2s; +—+, NF2. The data are plotted both as percent serum supplement and FBSP, mg/ml

EGF, FGF, or insulin (Table I). Under the conditions used, insulin had no effect on the growth rates of these cell lines. However, both EGF and FGF significantly increased the growth of normal cells. They had no effect on the growth of PC-3. In preliminary experiments, growth of the benign cells (HP1-7) was also markedly enhanced in EGF- and FGF-supplemented media.

The relative mitogenic potencies of EGF and FGF on normal cells were assayed by titration. The data were analyzed by the kinetic method and are summarized in Table II. On a molar basis, EGF was ten times as potent a mitogen as FGF for NP-2s. In contrast, EGF and FGF were equally potent mitogens for NF2 $(P > 0.90)$.

Serum Sparing by EGF and FGF with Hydrocortisone (HC)

The above results showed that both EGF and FGF increased the rate of normal cell division at suboptimal serum levels. The extent to which these two factors could substitute for serum was then determined (Fig. 3). The K_m^{FBSP} values derived by Lineweaver-Burk transformation of the dose-response data are summarized in

TABLE I. Effect of EGF, FGF, and Insulin on Clonal Growth Rate and Clonal Plating Efficiency

Cell line	Addition[a]	R[b]	Plating efficiency[c]
NP-2s	None	0.71 ± 0.13	5
	EGF[d]	1.06 ± 0.15	25
	FGF[e]	0.98 ± 0.11	26
	I[f]	0.76 ± 0.14	7
NF2	None	0.71 ± 0.12	28
	EGF	0.88 ± 0.14	29
	FGF	0.95 ± 0.10	33
	I	0.69 ± 0.10	30
HP1-7	None	0.59 ± 0.11	16
	EGF	0.78 ± 0.13	24
	FGF	0.78 ± 0.18	29
	I	Not tested	Not tested
PC-3	None	0.69 ± 0.13	32
	EGF	0.69 ± 0.11	35
	FGF	0.73 ± 0.11	31
	I	0.71 ± 0.17	34

[a]Media for lines NP-2s, NF2, and HP1-7 contained 2,700 μg FBSP/ml; media for PC-3 contained 150 μg FBSP/ml.
[b]Growth rate, PD/day $\pm$ standard deviation.
[c]Plating efficiency (%) = number of clones/number of cells inoculated.
[d]EGF, 5 ng/ml.
[e]FGF, 30 ng/ml
[f]Insulin, 1 μg/ml.

TABLE II. Half-Maximal Concentrations of EGF and FGF Required for Growth of Normal Cells

Cell line	Growth factor	$K_m^{mitogen}$
NP-2s	EGF	48.0 pM
	FGF	504.5 pM
NF2	EGF	119.1 pM
	FGF	129.1 pM

Table III. Both growth factors reduced the K_m^{FBSP}. On the other hand, R_{MAX}^T was not significantly altered. For each cell line, R_{MAX}^T was the same value regardless of whether it was derived from serum, EGF, or FGF dose-response data.

Hydrocortisone has been reported to potentiate the activity of both EGF [21] and FGF [8]. Both normal cells were cloned in nutrient medium containing 1,000 μg/ml FBSP and increasing concentrations of HC. The addition of HC alone

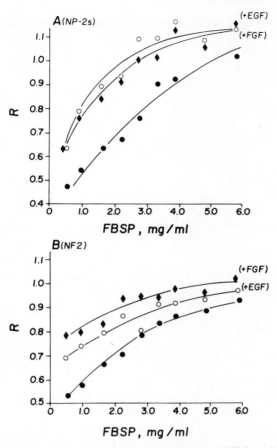

Fig. 3. Influence of growth factors on the clonal growth rate of NP-2s and NF2 as a function of FBSP concentration. A, NP-2s; B, NF2. FBSP without growth factor ●—●; FBSP with EGF (5 ng/ml), ○—○; FBSP with FGF (30 ng/ml), ◆—◆.

TABLE III. Reduction of FBSP Requirements by EGF and FGF

	NP-2s		NF2	
Additive[a]	K_m^{FBSP}[b]	R_{MAX}^T[c]	K_m^{FBSP}	R_{MAX}^T
None	2,230	1.36	1,480	1.26
EGF	627	1.27	490	1.22
FGF	467	1.18	350	1.15

[a]EGF (5ng/ml); FGF (30 ng/ml).
[b]FBSP, μg/ml.
[c]R, PD/day.

TABLE IV. Potentiation of Growth Factor Activity by Hydrocortisone

Cell line	FBSP[a]	HC[b]	EGF[c]	FGF[d]	R[e]
NP-2s	+	−	−	−	0.56
	+	+	−	−	0.61
	+	−	+	−	0.78
	+	+	+	−	0.93
	+	−	−	+	0.91
	+	+	−	+	1.08
NF2	+	−	−	−	0.58
	+	+	−	−	0.58
	+	−	+	−	0.78
	+	+	+	−	0.88
	+	−	−	+	0.76
	+	+	−	+	0.97

[a]FBSP (1,000 μg/ml).
[b]HC (1×10^{-6} M).
[c]EGF (5 ng/ml).
[d]FGF (30 ng/ml).
[e]R (PD/day).

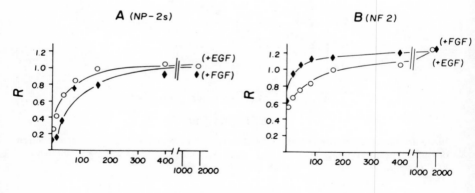

Fig. 4. Reduction in serum requirement by the combination of hydrocortisone with growth factors. A = NP-2s; B = NF2. Cells were cloned in PFMR-4 medium containing HC (1×10^{-6} M) and either EGF (5 ng/ml) or FGF (30 ng/ml) and increasing concentrations of FBSP. EGF, ○—○; FGF, ◆—◆.

did not increase the growth rate of either cell line. On the other hand, HC significantly potentiated growth when combined with either EGF or FGF (Table IV). The combination of either EGF or FGF with hydrocortisone synergistically reduced the serum requirements of NP-2s and NF2 27.5-fold and 40-fold, respectively (Fig. 4, Table V). Further, the R_{MAX}^{T} values observed at lower than 1.5%

TABLE V. Serum Sparing by Factors

Additive[a]	NP-2s	NF-2
None	2,230[b]	1,480
EGF	670	490
FGF	467	350
HC and EGF	84	40
HC and FGF	78	34
Overall reduction	27.5-fold	40-fold

[a]EGF (5 ng/ml); FGF (30 ng/ml); HC (1×10^{-6} M).
[b]K_m^{FBSP} (μg/ml).

TABLE VI. Effect of FBSP on K_m^{EGF}

FBSP (μg/ml)	K_m^{EGF} (pM)
1,000	40
2,000	48
2,500	28
3,000	40

Deviations from the mean K_m^{EGF} value
(39.75 pM) were not significant (P > 0.90).

serum were comparable to those observed in media supplemented with 15% serum but without added factors (Fig. 4; compare with Fig. 2).

Interaction of EGF, FBSP, and HC

Since EGF reduced the K_m^{FBSP} we determined whether FBSP affected the K_m^{EGF}. To do this, the growth-promoting activity was assayed at several EGF concentrations. FBSP did not significantly affect the K_m^{EGF} (Table VI).

We also investigated the possibility that HC potentiated EGF activity by lowering the requirement for EGF. Such a reduction would be reflected in a reduced K_m^{EGF} value. Accordingly, we measured the K_m^{EGF} both with and without HC. The values in the presence (29.5 pM) and the absence (40.4 pM) of HC were not significantly different (P > 0.90).

Effect of EGF on Ca^{2+} Requirement

EGF is known to alter cell permeability and increase the rate of transport of small molecules [22, 23]. Thus, growth factors might stimulate more rapid growth indirectly by correcting medium imbalances and thereby altering optimal

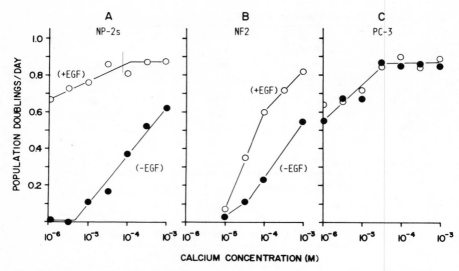

Fig. 5. Interaction of calcium and EGF on the growth rates of normal and tumorigenic cell lines. The growth medium consisted of low Ca^{2+} PFMR-4 supplemented with dialyzed FBS, 2 mg/ml. A = NP-2s; B = NF2; C = PC-3. Control, ●——●; plus EGF (5 ng/ml), ○——○.

concentrations of various medium components. We have begun to test this possibility by measuring the K_m values of several required nutrients in both the presence and the absence of EGF. To date, we have identified at least one such relationship.

The calcium (Ca^{2+}) concentration of the medium markedly affects the growth rate of normal cells, whereas transformed cells are generally much less responsive to this ion [24]. We determined the $K_m^{Ca^{2+}}$ of NP-2s, NF2, and PC-3 cells in both the absence and the presence of EGF. The growth rates of the normal cells were proportional to the concentration of Ca^{2+} (Fig. 5A, B). In contrast, the tumorigenic cell line divided at 2/3 maximal rate even at 10^{-6} M Ca^{2+} (Fig. 5C). Whereas EGF did not affect the Ca^{2+} response of the tumor line, it dramatically altered the Ca^{2+} response of the normal epithelial cells (Fig. 5A). In the presence of 5 ng/ml EGF, the Ca^{2+} dose-response curves of both normal and carcinoma lines were identical. At 10^{-6} M Ca^{2+}, NP-2s cells grew at 75% maximal rate in the presence of EGF and reached a plateau at $10^{-4.5}$ M Ca^{2+}. EGF also influenced the Ca^{2+} dose-response of the fibroblastic cells (Fig. 5B). However, in contrast to the normal epithelial cells, the fibroblasts were unable to divide in medium containing less than 1×10^{-5} M Ca^{2+}.

The $K_m^{Ca^{2+}}$ value for the normal epithelial cells (129 μM) was 120 times greater than that of the tumorigenic line (1.6 μM). In the presence of EGF the $K_m^{Ca^{2+}}$

values of NP-2s (1.1 μM) and PC-3 (1.6 μM) were virtually identical. The $K_m^{Ca^{2+}}$ of the normal fibroblast cells in the absence of EGF was 79 μM. However, EGF reduced this value only one-third (28 μM).

To further investigate the relationship between EGF and Ca^{2+}, we measured growth rate of normal epithelial cells as a function of EGF concentration at a fixed Ca^{2+} level. The K_m^{EGF} was then calculated by regression analysis. This process was repeated for graded concentrations of Ca^{2+}. Within the range tested (2.5 $\times$ 10^{-6} M to 8.0 $\times$ 10^{-4} M), K_m^{EGF} was not significantly changed [12].

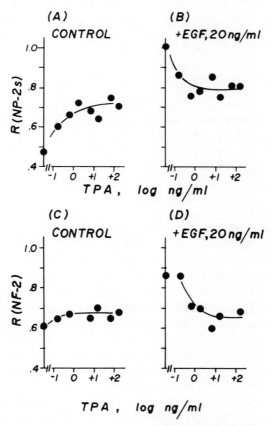

Fig. 6. Interaction of TPA with EGF. Growth rates of NP-2s (A) and NF2 (C) were determined in PFMR-4 medium supplemented with FBSP (1500 μg/ml) both without and with increasing concentrations of TPA. The experiment was repeated (B = NP-2s; D = NF2) with the media further supplemented with EGF (20 ng/ml). TPA stimulated growth of the epithelial (A = NP-2s) but not the fibroblastic (C = NF2) cells. On the other hand, TPA neutralized the EGF-stimulated growth of both cell types (B = NP-2s; D = NF2).

Influence of Tumor-Promoting Phorbol Esters on Growth

The tumor-promoting phorbol ester TPA has been reported to stimulate growth of some mammalian cell lines [25]. On the other hand, TPA has been shown to inhibit EGF-binding [26]. Thus, we measured the growth-promoting effect of TPA on the normal cell lines. Unexpectedly, we found that TPA affected the growth rates of these two genetically identical lines differentially. Whereas the growth rate of the epithelial line was stimulated by TPA (Fig. 6A), the growth rate of the fibroblastic line was not significantly changed (Fig. 6C). Incorporation of EGF (20 ng/ml) into the medium radically altered these dose-response curves. In the absence of TPA, EGF stimulated growth. However, for both cell lines, increasing TPA concentrations progressively neutralized the influence of EGF until the growth rates became comparable to those observed when the media contained only TPA (Fig. 6B, D).

DISCUSSION

Cultured tumor cells are generally distinguished from their normal counterparts by a significantly reduced serum requirement for growth [27, 28]. The evidence suggests that this reduced serum dependence may result from decreased response to growth factors and nutrients [29, 30]. Thus, it should be possible to minimize serum growth dependence of normal cells by identifying and determining the optimal levels of required nutrient and serum components. Our results support this hypothesis. Clonal growth dose-response experiments have been used to determine the optimal concentrations of these factors. This approach has made possible reduction of the serum requirements of normal human prostatic epithelial cells to a level comparable to that of a human prostatic adenocarcinoma line.

By optimizing the concentration of small molecular weight nutrients, Ham and co-workers [3, 4] succeeded in markedly reducing the level of serum required for clonal growth of normal human lung fibroblasts. Initially this approach was used in our laboratory. However, with the exception of including HEPES buffer, we have been unable to reduce serum dependence by variation in the low molecular weight components of nutrient medium F12K [7, 11]. It should be emphasized that complete systematic studies of the kind described by Ham were not done. On the other hand, the results of the serum selection experiments clearly indicated that the normal epithelial cells required unidentified serum factors. The carcinoma line neither responded to nor required these factors. Further, since the majority of the serum lots screened were deficient in growth-promoting activity, it became clear that addition of known serum mitogens (growth factors and hormones) might provide an effective medium for normal prostatic epithelial cells.

Enzyme kinetic analysis provides a useful way to measure a cell's reponse to growth-promoting factors. This approach makes possible derivation of two descriptive and comparative parameters, $K_m^{mitogen}$ and R_{MAX}^T [10, 20, 31]. These parameters permit comparisons of nutrient requirements between cells that grow at intrinsically different rates. We define the $K_m^{mitogen}$ as that concentration of factor (or nutrient) which supports growth at the half-maximal rate. The second characteristic growth parameter, R_{MAX}^T corresponds to the maximal theoretical growth rate.

The epithelial and fibroblastic cell lines, although genetically identical, responded differentially to serum, growth factors, Ca^{2+}, and TPA. Even though the R_{MAX}^T of both lines was virtually identical, the epithelial cells required 1.5 times more serum than did the fibroblasts. Growth factors were ineffective for the carcinoma line. However, saturating levels of either EGF or FGF reduced the serum requirement of both of the normal cell cultures an average of 3.75-fold. Although both lines responded similarly to FGF, significant differences were observed with EGF. The K_m^{FBSP} for the epithelial cells was only 1/10 that for the fibroblastic cells.

Hydrocortisone potentiated the mitogenic activity of both factors. Overall, the serum requirement was reduced 95% by adding HC in combination with either growth factor to PFMR-4 nutrient medium. It had been postulated that the synergistic action of glucocorticoids with growth factors is due to a modulation of the number of EGF surface receptors [21]. We found that hydrocortisone did not significantly change the K_m^{EGF}. In contrast, HC in combination with EGF further reduced the K_m^{EGF}. These results suggest that the amount of EGF required for optimal growth is probably not directly correlated with half-maximal saturation of EGF surface receptors. Further experimentation is necessary to elucidate the mechanism of synergism between HC and EGF.

EGF is known to modulate several cellular properties, including stimulation of cell migration [32], increased division potential [9, 11], alteration of nutrient transport [22], and induction of enzyme activities [23]. We have found that EGF also reduces serum and Ca^{2+} requirements. When the Ca^{2+} requirements of the three cell lines, NP-2s, NF2, and PC-3 were determined, it was found that in the absence of EGF, PC-3 required only 5% as much Ca^{2+} as did the two normal lines. Furthermore, there was a small but significantly different Ca^{2+} requirement between the two normal cell types. EGF markedly altered these Ca^{2+} dose-response results. The Ca^{2+} requirements were decreased 99% and 65% for the epithelial and fibroblastic lines, respectively. On the other hand, Ca^{2+} did not affect the K_m^{EGF}. Thus, the interaction between Ca^{2+} and EGF is analogous to that between FBSP and EGF. In both cases, the interaction is unidirectional. EGF modulates requirements for both Ca^{2+} and FBSP, but neither influences the requirement for EGF.

The tumor-promoting phorbol esters have been reported to stimulate the proliferation of several, but not all, cell types [25, 33]. Interactions between TPA and EGF have been observed. Dicker and Rozengurt [34] reported synergistic growth promotion by EGF and TPA, whereas Lee and Weinstein [26] showed that TPA inhibited the binding of EGF. We found that, in the absence of EGF, the normal epithelial and fibroblastic cell types did not show similar responses to TPA. TPA stimulated proliferation of the epithelial cells. However, when tested under identical conditions, TPA did not influence the growth rate of the fibroblastic line. These latter results are similar to other reported studies using human fibroblasts [34] and suggest a possible correlation between TPA growth stimulation and cell morphology. Our results were quite different when EGF was present. Instead of being mitogenic, TPA abolished EGF growth stimulation. This result was not unexpected, since Lee and Weinstein [26] had shown that TPA inhibited EGF binding.

Our data clearly show that the mitogenic activity of TPA depends on both cell type and growth conditions. In the absence of growth factors it is a mitogen for normal human epithelial cells but not for fibroblastic cells. However, this tumor promoter neutralizes EGF growth stimulation in both cell lines.

CONCLUSIONS

1) Considerable progress has been made toward formulation of completely defined media for prostatic epithelial cultures. Normal and neoplastic lines have significantly different requirements. The carcinoma line, PC-3 multiplies at half-maximal growth rate in nutrient medium PFMR-4 supplemented with only 10 μg/ml FBSP. However, the normal line, NP-2s requires 80 μg/ml FBSP and both EGF or FGF and HC to grow at this same rate. Complete replacement of the residual serum required appears to be a realistic goal. Experiments are in progress either to identify these residual factors or, possibly, to replace them with other known growth factors or lipids.

2) Significant interactions between growth-promoting factors have been revealed by application of enzyme kinetic analysis to clonal dose-response data. For example, in addition to reducing the serum requirement of normal cells, EGF also spares their calcium requirement. Furthermore, whereas HC potentiates EGF activity, it does so by reducing the serum requirement but not the EGF requirement.

3) Another potentially important class of interactions has been found. The tumor promoter TPA stimulates the growth of normal epithelial cells. On the other hand, TPA competitively neutralizes EGF growth promotion.

ACKNOWLEDGMENTS

This work was supported by Public Health Service (PHS) grant R26-CA19826-01 from the National Cancer Institute through the National Prostatic Cancer Project, and PHS contract NO1-CP-65850 from the Division of Cancer Cause and Prevention, National Cancer Institute (NCI). We thank M. Babcock, K. Gaas, M. Marnell, and T. Smith for technical assistance.

REFERENCES

1. Ham RG: Unique requirements for clonal growth. J Natl Cancer Inst 53:1459–1463, 1974.
2. Ham RG: Nutritional requirements of primary cultures. A neglected problem of modern biology. In Vitro 10:119–129, 1974.
3. McKeehan WL, McKeehan KA, Hammond SL, Ham RG: Improved medium for clonal growth of human diploid fibroblasts at low concentrations of serum protein. In Vitro 13:399–416, 1977.
4. McKeehan WL, Genereux DP, Ham RG: Assay and partial purification of factors from serum that control multiplication of human diploid fibroblasts. Biochem Biophys Res Commun 80:1013–1021, 1978.
5. Kaighn ME: Choice, treatment, and storage of sera for the growth of specialized cells. In Vitro Monogr 3:21, 1973.
6. Kaighn ME: "Birth of a Culture" – Source of postpartum anomalies. J Natl Cancer Inst 53:1437–1442, 1974.
7. Kaighn ME: Characteristics of human prostatic cell cultures. Cancer Treat Rep 61: 147–151, 1977.
8. Gospodarowicz D, Moran JS: Growth factors in mammalian cell culture. Annu Rev Biochem 45:531–558, 1976.
9. Rheinwald JG, Green H: Epidermal growth factor and the multiplication of cultured human epidermal keratinocytes. Nature 265:421–424, 1977.
10. Lechner JF, Kaighn ME: Application of the principles of enzyme kinetics to clonal growth rates: An approach for delineating interactions among growth promoting agents. J Cell Physiol (in press).
11. Lechner JF, Babcock MS, Marnell M, Narayan KS, Kaighn ME: Normal human prostate epithelial cell cultures. In Harris C, Trump BF, Stoner GD (eds): "Methods and Perspectives in Cell Biology; Cultured Human Cells and Tissues in Biomedical Research." New York: Academic Press, Vol II, Ch 8 (in press).
12. Lechner JF, Kaighn ME: Reduction of the calcium requirement of normal human epithelial cells by EGF. Exp Cell Res 121:432–435, 1979.
13. Lechner JF, Narayan KS, Ohnuki Y, Babcock MS, Jones LW, Kaighn ME: Replicative epithelial cell cultures from normal human prostate gland. J Natl Cancer Inst 60: 797–801, 1978.
14. Kaighn ME, Babcok MS: Monolayer cultures of human prostatic cells. Cancer Chemother Rep 59:59–63, 1975.
15. Kaighn ME, Lechner JF, Narayan KS, Jones LW: Prostate carcinoma: Tissue culture cell lines. Natl Cancer Inst Monogr 49:17–21, 1978.
16. Kaighn ME, Narayan KS, Ohnuki Y, Lechner JF, Jones LW: Establishment and characterization of a human prostatic carcinoma cell line (PC-3). Invest Urol 17: 16–23, 1979.
17. Ohnuki Y, Marnell M, Babcock MS, Lechner JF, Kaighn ME: Chromosomal analysis of human prostatic adenocarcinoma cell lines. Cancer Res (in press).
18. Lowry O, Rosebrough NH, Farr AL, Randall RJ: Protein measurement with the Folin phenol reagent. J Biol Chem 193:265–275, 1951.
19. Kaighn ME: Human liver cells. In Kruse PF Jr, Patterson MK Jr (eds): "Tissue Culture. Methods and Applications" New York: Academic Press, 1973, pp 54–58.
20. Ellem KAO, Gierthy JF: Mechanism of regulation of fibroblastic cell replication. IV. An analysis of the serum dependence of cell replication based on Michaelis-Menten kinetics. J Cell Physiol 92:381–400, 1977.

21. Baker JF, Barsh GS, Carney DH, Cunningham DD: Dexamethasone modulates binding and action of epidermal growth factor in serum-free culture. Proc Natl Acad Sci USA 75:1882–1886, 1978.
22. Hollenberg MD, Cuatrecasas P: Insulin and epidermal growth factor. J Biol Chem 250: 3845–3853, 1975.
23. DiPasquale A, White D, McGuire J: Epidermal growth factor stimulates putrescine transport and ornithine decarboxylase activity in cultured human fibroblasts. Exp Cell Res 116:317–323, 1978.
24. Boynton AL, Whitfield JF, Isaacs RJ, Tremblay R: The control of human WI 38 cell proliferation by extracellular calcium and its elimination by SV-40 virus-induced proliferative transformation. J Cell Physiol 92:241–248, 1977.
25. Weinstein IB, Wigler M, Fisher PB, Sisskin E, Pietropaolo C: Cell culture studies on the biologic effects of tumor promoters. In Slaga TJ, Sivak A, Boutwell RK (eds): "Mechanisms of Tumor Promotion and Cocarcinogenesis." New York: Raven Press, 1978, pp 313–333.
26. Lee L, Weinstein IB: Tumor-promoting phorbol esters inhibit binding of epidermal growth factor to cellular receptors. Science 202:313–315, 1978.
27. Risser R, Pollack R: A nonselective analysis of SV40 transformation of mouse 3T3 cells. Virology 59:477–489, 1974.
28. Shields R: Transformation and tumorigenicity. Nature 262:348, 1976.
29. Holley RW: Control of growth of mammalian cells in cell culture. Nature 258:487–490, 1975.
30. Todaro GJ, DeLarco JE: Transformation by murine and feline sacroma viruses specifically blocks binding of epidermal growth factor to cells. Nature 264:26–31, 1976.
31. McKeehan WL, Ham RG: Calcium and magnesium ions and the regulation of multiplication in normal and transformed cells. Nature 275:756–758, 1978.
32. Cohen S, Savage CR Jr: Part II. Recent studies on the chemistry and biology of epidermal growth factor. Recent Prog Hormone Res 30:551–574, 1974.
33. Mondal S, Brankow DW, Heidelberger C: Two-stage chemical oncogenesis in cultures of C3H/10T-1/2 cells. Cancer Res 36:2254–2260, 1976.
34. Dicker P, Rozengurt E: Stimulation of DNA synthesis by tumour promoter and pure mitogenic factors. Nature 276:723–726, 1978.

Characterization of Prostate Cells

Donald J. Merchant, PhD, Alva H. Johnson, PhD, and
Sara M. Clarke, PhD

The usefulness of any in vitro model system is dependent upon adequate characterization. The minimal amount and kinds of characterization required will depend upon the particular system and the questions to be asked.

As the science of cell and organ culture has developed over the past three to four decades certain basic procedures have been accepted as fundamental to the integrity of the field. Thus the ability to certify species of origin and to assure freedom from contamination by aerobic and anaerobic bacteria, fungi, protozoa, mycoplasma, and common viruses are considered fundamental to the use of cell cultures for any experimental purposes.

The major additional criteria required for any model system that is to be used in the study of prostatic cancer are: 1) evidence that the cells or tissue are of prostatic origin; 2) evidence that the cell population is derived from acinar epithelial cells or, in special situations where a mixed population is desired, that acinar-derived cells predominate; and 3) the ability to differentiate between acinar cells of normal, BPH or carcinoma origin. Obviously, depending upon the use to be made of the model system, additional criteria may be necessary. However, it is beyond the scope of this presentation to review each of these specific situations, and the balance of the chapter is devoted to the questions of organ and cell specificity and the recognition of benign and malignant acinar cells and their distinction from normal cells.

ORGAN SPECIFICITY

It long has been recognized that certain enzymes and metabolic products are present in the prostate and in its secretion in relatively high concentrations as compared to other tissues. These include, as examples, acid phosphatase, 5α reductase, citric acid, and zinc [1−6]. The ability to demonstrate continued production and/or concentration of one or more of these compounds at significant levels in vitro would be strongly suggestive but not proof that the tissue was of prostatic origin. On the other hand, failure to maintain significant levels may reflect only a modulation with the loss of phenotypic expression.

Models for Prostate Cancer, pages 233−237

A finding of great significance has been the demonstration of an immunologically specific prostatic acid phosphatase [7, 8] . Since the enzyme is secreted in prostatic fluid and can be demonstrated in the blood, it is necessary to demonstrate its presence within acinar cells to confirm the prostate origin of the cells or tissue. The ability to detect the enzyme by rapid and sensitive immunofluorescent techniques is an added advantage. It still is not possible to interpret the absence of the enzyme or a reduced level of it as evidence that the cells are not of prostatic origin, however, as we know little about factors governing its expression.

CELL SPECIFICITY

In the case of cell lines, either cloned or uncloned, it is imperative to know that the cells were derived from acinar or basal cells rather than from fibroblasts, endothelium, muscle cells, or other cellular components. In the case of primary cell cultures, the cell population should be predominantly, if not exclusively, derived from the acinar or basal cells.

Although our knowledge of prostatic biology is very incomplete [9], the preponderance of evidence suggests that basal cells divide in vivo, and through maturation some of the daughter cells become differentiated, secretory acinar cells. It is a working hypothesis in our laboratory that only the basal cells are capable of division and that, therefore, these cells are the precursors of the epithelial cells grown in culture.

From the earliest days of tissue culture it was recognized that cells of any tissue origin in vivo may undergo extensive and varied morphologic modulation in vitro in response to a range of environmental influences. As a result, characterization of cells as "epithelial" or "fibroblastic" solely on the basis of morphologic features is extremely hazardous. Nevertheless, the initial pattern of outgrowth from explants of the prostate tend to be quite characteristic and distinctly different for such cells as the acinar epithelial cells, connective tissue fibroblasts, and muscle cells, which make up th major components of the prostate.

Over the past two and one-half years we have cultured cells from 61 different prostatic specimens. The technique used has been explant culture in which 1 mm^3 fragments are allowed to attach to the surface of plastic tissue culture flasks or Petri dishes. These are fed a medium consisting of RPMI 1640 containing 20% fetal calf serum, 2.5 pg/ml of testosterone, and penicillin, streptomycin, and fungizone. The growth obtained from approximately 500 explants prepared from these specimens has consisted of epithelial sheets in more than 90% of instances. Moreover, the pattern of growth has been so highly reproducible that photographs easily could be transposed without knowing it if great care were not taked in labeling and storing them.

To assure that the fragments of tissue that are put in culture are predominantly glandular, we trim the tissue to yield strips measuring 1 × 2 × 4 mm. These strips are then divided lengthwise to provide two pieces 1 × 1 × 4 mm, which are mirror images. With the fragments in their original positions relative to one another, each strip is cut into four explants measuring 1 mm^3. Each pair of explants that faced each other in the original tissue is dispersed, so that one explant is cultured and its "twin" is fixed, sectioned, mounted, and stained. In this way we can evaluate the tissue of origin for any outgrowth. Our preliminary results suggest that the epithelial outgrowth observed is due to division and migration of basal cells. When differentiated acinar cells are dislodged, they may remain viable in the medium surrounding the explant for long intervals, but they have never been observed to spread out or to divide.

A number of investigators have used transmission electron microscopy to examine the presumed epithelial cells they have grown from the prostate, and they have reported finding desmosomes, which they cite as confirmation of the epithelial origin of the cells [10–12]. Franks has pointed out that some literature reports claiming the finding of desmosomes actually have shown only intermediate junctions, which may be present in mesenchymal cells as well as epithelial cells [13]. It appears, however, that the proper use of transmission electron microscopy, and perhaps scanning electron microscopy as well, will play an important role in cell identification.

In an effort to approach the characterization of acinar cells by a different route, and using methods with a high degree of specificity, we have initiated a program to look for specific antigen markers in prostatic fluid. Based on the assumption that the chief function of acinar cells is to produce and secrete prostatic fluid, it would seem logical to examine it for acinar cell-specific antigens. The fluid consists of a mixture of products synthesized by the cells, enzymes involved in synthesis, and cellular break-down products resulting from apocrine secretion and sloughing of differentiated cells.

We are using prostatic fluid as a source of antigens. This material is being fractionated on discontinuous gradient acrylamide columns. Using a variety of modifications of the basic fractionation procedure, coupled with immunologic methods, we expect to purify multiple antigens, to prepare specific antisera and, using indirect immunofluorescence procedures, to detect the localization of antibody on acinar cells in frozen sections of the prostate. A battery of antibodies shown to be specific to prostatic acinar cells could be used to "fingerprint" cells grown in culture. An acrylamide gel electrophoretic separation of a prostatic fluid sample has separated in excess of 11 different proteins.

Success in developing multiple specific antibodies for prostatic acinar cells would make possible simultaneous identification of organ and cellular origin.

DIFFERENTIATION OF NORMAL FROM BENIGN AND MALIGNANT CELLS

By far the most difficult task in characterization of prostatic cells in vitro is the differentiation of normal, benign, and malignant acinar cells. It is safe to say that we have no direct methods available and that the indirect methods cannot provide a definitive answer.

The only truly satisfactory method for assessing malignancy is by the production of tumors in a suitable host. Unfortunately we have no syngeneic host for studying prostatic cancer, and the only model available is the athymic or nude mouse. This has been reviewed elsewhere in this volume by Dr. Gittes [14], and it is obvious that this model has yielded variable results in the hands of different investigators.

A number of characteristics have been attributed to neoplastic cells grown in vitro which appear to correlate closely with their ability to produce tumors. Though these are, at best, only correlates and there are many exceptions, at least two show a sufficient record of correlation to be useful. They are the cells' ability to grow in soft agar and the loss of contact inhibition. The degree of aneuploidy also is a useful but less reliable criterion. Differentiation of normal from benign cells is even more difficult.

A hopeful approach to differentiation would be the finding of antigens specific to the benign and/or the malignant state. Several investigations are underway with the aim of isolating and identifying such antigens, but no positive results have been reported. It is possible that an extension of our studies of prostatic fluid to include specimens from BPH and carcinoma tissue as well as normal tissue might provide differential markers.

SUMMARY

It is obvious from this brief review that the weakest link in the successful application of in vitro models to answer questions related to prostatic cancer is the lack of adequate markers to permit characterization of the cells with regard to organ and tissue origin and their neoplastic status. In our opinion there is little to be gained in defining markers for other purposes until we can manage these basic areas of recognition.

ACKNOWLEDGMENTS

Department of Microbiology and Immunology, Eastern Virginia Medical School, PO Box 1980, Norfolk, VA 23501.

This work was supported by NIH grants 5-R26-CA16540-03 and DRGI-R26-CA23699-01.

The authors wish to acknowledge the technical help of Lynn Ellis and Suzanne Harris in the experimental work reported.

REFERENCES

1. Whitmore WF: Comments on zinc in the human and canine prostates. NCI Monogr 12: 337–340, 1963.
2. Mawson CA, Fischer MI: The occurrence of zinc in the human prostate gland. Can J Med Sci 30:336–339, 1952.
3. Byar DP: Zinc in male sex accessory organs: Distribution and hormone response. In Brandes D (ed): "Male Accessory Sex Organs." New York: Academic Press, 1974, ch 6.
4. Farnsworth WE, Brown JR: Testosterone metabolism in the prostate. Natl Cancer Inst Monogr 12:323–325, 1963.
5. Murphy GP, Joiner JR, Saroff J: Prostatic cancer. Urology 8:357–362, 1976.
6. Mann T: Biochemistry of the prostate gland and its secretion. Natl Cancer Inst Monogr 12:235–251, 1963.
7. Choe BK, Pontes EJ, McDonald I, Rose NR: Purification and characterization of human prostatic acid phosphatase. Prep Biochem 8:73–89, 1978.
8. Catane R, Madajewicz S, Wajsman ZI, Chu TM, Mittelman A, Murphy GP: Prostatic cancer. Immunochemical detection of prostatic acid phosphatase in serum and bone marrow. NY State J Med 78:1060–1061, 1978. .
9. Merchant DJ: Requirements of in vitro model systems (this volume).
10. Kaighn ME, Lechner JF, Narayan KS, Jones LW: Prostate carcinoma: Tissue culture cell lines. Natl Cancer Inst Monogr 49:17–21, 1978.
11. Stone KR, Mickey DD, Wunderli H, Mickey GH, Paulson DF: Isolation of a human prostate carcinoma cell line (DU 145). Int J Cancer 21:274–281, 1978.
12. Webber MM: Ultrastructural changes in human prostatic epithelium grown in vitro. J Ultrastruct Res 50:89–102, 1975.
13. Franks LM: Primary cultures of human prostate. In Harris CC, Trump BF, Stoner GD (eds): "Methods and Perspectives in Cell Biology." Vol II. (in press).
14. Gittes RF: The nude mouse. Its use as a tumor-bearing model of the prostate (this volume).

Establishment of Cultures from the Prostate - Technical Aspects: Summary

Betty Rosoff, PhD

The preceeding chapters in this section discuss the technical problems of establishing cell cultures from the prostate. The contributors have addressed themselves essentially to four aspects of the problem. These are: sources of the tissue, the type of culture established, the nutrition media, and the cell markers. The progress in recent years in each of these areas is reflected in the exciting de-developments of the conference from which this volume derived.

1) The source of tissue is the key to establishing cultures that can be useful for the study of normal BPH and carcinoma of the prostate. Dr. McNeal has proposed a new scheme for the regional anatomy of the prostate that could be helpful in tissue sampling. He has distinguished between a peripheral zone that is the area where carcinoma arises, transitional and periurethral zones where BPH occurs, and the central zone in which there is no known pathology arising. He suggests that the histology of the gland is not homogeneous. For example, central zone cells differ appreciably when compared to peripheral and transitional cells. There are also changes with age and, therefore, samples of tissue must be fully characterized. While there is some difference of opinion on the validity of this particular scheme, certainly further studies of the anatomy and histology of the postpubertal gland will be important in the source of tissue. If normal prostate is cultured to study carcinogenesis, then it should be obtained from the peripheral zone. If cultures of carcinoma cells are needed for screening treatment drugs, then they will not be found in the transitional or central zone.

Another aspect that requires reexamination is the homology between species and the regional anatomy of the prostate. Dr. Price [1] has suggested that the dorsal and lateral lobes of the rat corresponded to the same area in man. Dr. McNeal suggests that in the Rhesus monkey the cranial lobe is homologous to the central zone of man and the caudal lobe to the peripheral zone. Further studies of homology seem necessary in order to be able to use various animals for sources of tissue for tissue culture and for other areas of prostatic research.

Models for Prostate Cancer, pages 239—241

2) The type of culture that is used is the next question that was addressed. Since we are interested in acinar epithelial cells, should we grow them as primary cell explants with the stroma present of should we digest away the stroma and have pure epithelial cell cultures? Dr. Malinin uses explants and found the growth similar to the parent tissue. He seemed to get preferential epithelial growth because these cells grew before the fibroblasts were able to grow Dr. Webber successfully stripped the stroma with collagenase and obtained a pure epithelial cell culture. In the discussion, Dr. Coffey suggests that stroma might be important in the morphology of the epithelial growth. There might be differences in stroma, and indeed the connective tissue of the host might play a role in determining the development of the epithelial tissue and whether the tissue develops normally or pathologically. While we can learn from pure epithelial cultures, we might have to put them back together with the stroma to understand more of the in vivo situation.

The epithelial cells that grow in culture are not the acinar cells of the mature glandular tissue but rather the basal cells because these are the only ones capable of division. Both Dr. Webber and Dr. Merchant felt that these cells, which are the precursors of the acini cells in vivo, perform the same function in vitro. This is probably one of the explanations for the difficulty in growing adult normal prostate compared with fetal prostate and for the fact that carcinoma and BPH tissue grow better in culture than normal adult prostatic tissue.

3) One of the problems in culturing prostate tissue has been in finding the right media for initiation and maintenance of cell growth. Starting with various combinations of bovine and horse serum, different growth factors were added in an attempt to reduce the serum requirements and eventually develop a chemically defined medium. Some of the hormones and growth factors tested were hydrocortisone, testosterone, dihydrotestosterone, insulin, fibroblast growth factor, epithelial growth factor, phorbol esters and vitamin A. The effectiveness of each of these in promoting growth vary with the cell lines. In addition, there was clearly a bimodal effect, that is, insulin showed a dose-dependent growth effect up to one international unit per ml, and then with higher levels growth declined. The same effect was seen with vitamin A, and both these factors seemed to selectively stimulate epithelial growth over fibroblastic growth.

This bimodal effect was seen in some experiments in our laboratories [2], where using an animal model, the Dunning tumor R3327-H, we found that a prolactin stimulant, perphenazine, inhibited the growth of the tumor at the dose level administered. Other reports have shown that prolactin at a different dose level enhances prostate and prostate tumor growth and is synergistic with testosterone. Consequently, quantitative measures of the amount of added factors, and their effects on growth are very important. Measurement of clonal growth rate either manually or using a densitometer seems an effective way of determining the right media for proper growth. It is important to note that there seem to be different requirements for maximum growth of adult prostate, fetal prostate, and carcinomatous prostate tissue, leading to the conclusion that possibly different defined media might be necessary for each type of tissue.

4) The final and probably the most important aspect of this discussion is the characterization of the cells that are growing in culture. How do we know that we are growing the parent cells? Do changes take place under the culture conditions? How can we study carcinogenesis and normal cell cultures and effects of treatment in pathological cell lines unless we have specific markers that are peculiar to the prostatic epithelial cells? Morphology is important, but when Dr. Merchant looked at a large number of cultures, he found that the cells were remarkably similar in appearance from culture to culture. Dr. Malinin found many differences. Dr. Webber uses cytochemical localization of acid phosphatase as a marker.

The other aspect of distinguishing between normal and malignant cells is more difficult. Some methods that were used by the discussants are loss of contact inhibition, ability to grow in soft agar, and ability to produce a tumor in a nude mouse. Maybe trying to isolate tumor-specific antigens should be the line of investigation. Certainly the value of these in vitro models will be significantly increased with the development of such specific markers.

The technical problems are being overcome, and we can now grow and maintain prostatic cells in culture. The defined medium is on the way, and in the near future all of these cell culture models will be available to study the etiology and treatment of adenocarcinoma of the prostate.

REFERENCES

1. Price D: Comparative aspects of development and structure in the prostate. In Vollmer EP (ed): "Workshop on the Biology of the Prostate and Related Tissues." NCI Monograph 12, 1963, pp 1−27.
2. Rosoff B: Unpublished observations.

The Dunning Tumors

David M. Lubaroff, PhD, Larry Canfield, and Craig W. Reynolds, PhD

In 1963 Dr. W.F. Dunning published the first report of a spontaneous tumor of the rat prostate she had observed two years earlier [1]. The tumor was found to occupy a large portion of the abdomen in a retired male breeder of the inbred Copenhagen rat. Dr. Dunning successfully transplanted the tumor in the flank of syngeneic Copenhagen recipients as well as (Copenhagen × Fischer) F_1 hybrids. Histologically, the tumor, now termed R3327, resembled a papillary adeno-carcinoma. The glandular formation of the tumor was reported to resemble the dorsal-type glands of the prostate by Dunning's colleagues, Drs. Gwen and Gould. Additional evidence that the R3327 originated in the dorsal component of the dorsolateral prostatic lobe, as cited in this original publication, was positive periodic-acid Schiff stain, negative dithizone stain and electrophoretic pattern; all supposedly characteristic of dorsal lobe secretions.

The subject of which lobe this tumor originated from has attracted additional attention. One laboratory has published biochemical evidence for a dorsolateral prostate derivation [2], whereas another contends that enzymatic profiles of the R3327 tumor would support an origin in either the dorsolateral or anterior lobe [3]. The former study, published by Smolev and the investigators at the Brady Urological Institute, measured the enzymatic activity of amino-peptidase, gamma-glutamyl transpeptidase, acid phosphatase, alkaline phosphatase, and beta-glucuronidase in the R3327 tumor, dorsolateral and ventral prostates, seminal vesicle, kidney, and liver of the Copenhagen rat. The results obtained by these authors clearly showed that the only tissue examined that had an activity profile similar to the R3327 was the dorsolateral prostatic lobe. Contrary to those results, Müntzing and his colleagues reported that the enzymatic activities in R3327 tumor tissue and various prostatic lobes could not provide conclusive evidence that this

Models for Prostate Cancer, pages 243–263

tumor originated from the dorsal prostate. Both histochemical and biochemical results indicated that the Dunning adenocarcinoma could equally well have originated from the anterior as from the dorsal prostate. Although evidence that this tumor was derived from the dorsal lobe would make it more like the majority of human prostatic adenocarcinomas than if it were anterior or ventral lobe-derived, the absence of such strong evidence does not diminish the usefulness of the model system.

For a period of 11 years after Dunning's original publication, the tumor system was absent from the literature. In 1974 Dr. Dunning and her collaborators, led by Voigt, published the first of what turned out to be an avalanche of papers describing the R3327 tumor as a model for human prostatic adenocarcinoma [4].

DESCRIPTION AND CHARACTERIZATION OF THE DUNNING R3327 TUMOR

The original description by Dunning of this rat prostatic tumor was that of a well-differentiated adenocarcinoma [1]. The tumor apparently remained unchanged for the first five transfer generations. After the fifth, a rapidly growing variant was discovered, which was classified as an androgen-insensitive squamous cell carcinoma [5]. The discovery of this variant and others during the course of the investigation emphasized the importance of constantly monitoring the histologic picture and sensitivity to androgenic hormones of the tumor during serial transplantation.

Two laboratories, at Iowa and Johns Hopkins, began work at approximately the same time on the R3327 tumor [2, 6–9]. Although these two groups were using the model for different experiments, they were interested in presenting the Dunning tumor as an equivalent cancer to that found in human prostatic adeno-carcinoma. The goal of the research was to have a system, controlled in as many ways as possible, that could be used to study the precise mechanisms of cause, diagnosis, and treatment of human cancer of the prostate. The investigators, working with the well-differentiated adenocarcinoma, showed it to be capable of growing both in the flank and in the dorsolateral lobe of the recipient Copenhagen [6–8] or (Copenhagen × Fischer) F_1 hybrid rats [2, 9]. For subcutaneous tumor induction, tissue mince or freshly prepared tumor cells could be used, whereas cells were required for intraprostatic tumor induction. Depending upon whether tumor tissue mince or cells were inoculated, and the size of the inoculum, palpable tumors could be obtained in six to eight weeks. The tumors grew slowly, often taking six months or longer to reach a maximum size. They also were found to grow much slower in females [5, 6] and castrated males [2, 5] than in intact males.

The gross appearance of the tumor was one of a homogeneous, white, glistening tissue. Histologic examination of both subcutaneous and intraprostatic tumors revealed a well-differentiated adenocarcinoma forming glands with acid-staining secretions within the acini. This glandular pattern of the R3327 tumor is similar to the histologic picture found in well-differentiated human prostatic adenocarcinomas [2, 6]. The tumor also had connective tissue stroma within it and occasional areas of osteometaplasia, particularly in older tumors. The osteometaplastic lesions were found only in subcutaneous tumors and not in those induced in the prostate. The reason for this is unknown, but perhaps the fact that intraprostatic tumors were generally not left in the experimental animals for as long a time as were the subcutaneous tumors played an important role. The intraprostatic tumors were, in general, smaller than those in the flank. Perhaps the environment of the prostatic lobes, with their high enzyme content, was not conducive to the formation of boney structures.

In our laboratory, we wished to approximate closely the course of human disease and therefore studied tumors produced in the dorsolateral prostatic lobe of recipient rats. Early lesions were confined to the injected lobe but soon spread outside the capsule of the prostate, invading the surrounding tissues, and then metastasizing to the draining lymph nodes [6]. With continued growth of tumor in these animals, metastatic lesions were often found in the lungs. Metastases were also found, although not as frequently, in the liver, on the diaphragm, on the xyphoid process, on the intercostal muscles, and in mediastinal lymph nodes. The pattern of growth and spread of prostatic adenocarcinomas in humans is the same as seen with the R3327 — that is, first confined within the capsule, then extending outside the capsule, involving lymph nodes, and, finally, causing distant metastasis. The classification of various stages of the human disease by Flocks [10] was based upon this type of growth and spread. A similar type of spread was also noted in rats bearing long-term subcutaneous tumors. Although no prostatic capsule was involved, the tumor was found to spread to the draining axillary lymph nodes and then to the lungs. To date the only site of metastasis seen in human cancer of the prostate not observed in the Dunning tumor has been the bone.

It is interesting to speculate at this point on the reason for this apparent difference in incidence of boney metastasis in rats versus humans. Although we cannot detect metastatic lesions in the bones of the Copenhagen rat bearing large tumors, we are not willing to state with certainty that these lesions may not be present. To date our methods of detection have been by x-ray and by examining bone marrow aspirates of autopsied rats. No abnormalities in the bone were found in any of the rats studied by x-ray. Our examinations of bone marrow cell preparations were less than rewarding. No obvious signs of neoplastic cells were found in the animals studied. To direct our attention first to radiologic studies, it is entirely possible that tumor cells may have traveled to the bones but were only microfoci when the x-rays were taken. These lesions would not have had sufficient time to produce osteoblastic or osteolytic lesions of the type routinely seen in metastatic human prostatic cancer [11]. If this were the case, then one would have to examine animals bearing tumors of longer duration. The failure to detect metastatic tumor cells in bone marrow cell suspensions may also be the result of two few cells at too early a time after tumor implantation. If only microfoci of malignant cells were present in the marrow they might go undetected in a random sample of marrow aspirates.

Now that we have discussed reasons for not detecting metastatic lesions that may be present, let us address ourselves to the possibility that, in fact, the Dunning R3327 tumor *does not* metastasize to the bone. The obvious question is, why? There is some controversy in the literature on the mode of spread of boney metastases. As summarized by Mostofi and Price [12], there are three current theories to explain the spread of tumor to the bone. Warren and his colleagues suggested that perineural lymphatic spread was an important auxiliary route for this spread [13]. Batson proposed that the vertebral venous plexus was the usual route of spread [14]. The third theory would seem to combine lymphatic and venous spread, with tumor arising in the lung first, before reaching the bone [15]. If spread is primarily via a specialized venous network, as proposed by Batson, it is possible that, in the absence of these structures in subcutaneous space of the flank or surrounding the dorsolateral prostate, osseous metastases may not occur. Definitive data are lacking to indicate whether the vertebral venous plexus is present in the Norway rat. If metastatic lung disease must precede lesions in the bone, as proposed by Willis, our examination of tumor-bearing rats may have been too early.

It is evident from the publications by individuals studying the Dunning R3327 tumor that, in spite of the lack of definitive evidence for metastatic bone lesions, this is an excellent model for detailed and controlled studies of human cancer of the prostate.

To this point, we have described a well-differentiated adenocarcinoma, similar to the tumor originally described by Dunning [1]. However, a tumor that possesses a single histologic picture may not be the best model for a complete study of human cancer. This is particularly true of prostatic cancer, inasmuch as the disease in man may present itself in many different ways. The variability seen relates to the degree of cellular differentiation, rate of growth, and sensitivity to hormonal influences, just to name a few factors.

Evidence has accumulated that the Dunning R3327 tumor also displays the variability seen in human carcinoma of the prostate. Reports from a number of different laboratories have documented the existence of many sublines of the original tumor. [2, 5, 6, 16–19]. The first report of a variant derived from the original Dunning tumor was that of Voigt et al, who described the androgen-insensitive squamous cell line designated R3327-A [5]. However, Claflin noted that Dunning had isolated eight sublines, which she termed A through H [16], although no publication can be found in the literature. The R3327-A subline, as mentioned earlier, was discovered in recipient rats at the fifth transplant generation with a shortened survival time of the host [5]. This tumor grew much more rapidly than did the original adenocarcinoma and the rate of growth was identical in both male and female recipients, as well as in castrated males. These results indicated a loss of sensitivity to adrogenic hormones, confirmed when Voigt and colleagues demonstrated that this subline showed very little 5 alpha-reduction of testosterone as compared with values obtained for the prostate itself and the androgen-sensitive R3327 tumor [5].

Another rapidly growing tumor, demonstrating cellular anaplasia, was described by Smolev [2] and by Lubaroff [5]. This subline, designated R3327-AT by Smolev and R3327/150 by us, grew to an extremely large size within three weeks of injection into recipient rats, reaching a size rarely attained by the well-differentiated tumor, even at 15 weeks. The tumors ulcerated through the skin and often had central necrotic areas. The histology demonstrated an absence of cellular organization, the tumor cells growing in sheets with no gland formation. The tumor grew with equal speed in male and female rats, again indicating an absence of androgen sensitivity.

Other sublines include the R3327-HI [17] and R3327-C-F [18]. The former resembles the original Dunning tumor in that it is slow growing and demonstrates a well-differentiated picture on histologic examination. It differs from the original in that it is hormone-insensitive, growing at the same rate in intact or castrated males. The R3327-C-F subline has been described as being histologically different from other R3327 tumors [18]. This tumor is well differentiated and androgen sensitive, growing better in normal males than in castrates or in females, and displays organized glandular structures when examined by light microscopy. The features that distinguish the R3327-C-F from other tumors is the lumpy, encapsulated appearance of the tumors at autopsy, as well as the presence of large, abnormal fibroblasts in the stroma and of lymphocytes in the epithelium.

Our laboratory has isolated four distinct sublines, distinguished from one another by the rat number from which the tumors were derived [19]. The original well-differentiated adenocarcinoma line has been designated R3327/130 and has all the characteristics of the original Dunning tumor as described earlier. A second subline, designated R3327/133, is still a moderately well-differentiated tumor with glands present, although fewer in number than in the 130 line. This tumor grows at a slightly faster rate and, although it will grow faster in males than females, the difference in rate is not as large as in the 130. The R3327/141 subline represents an undifferentiated tumor that grows rapidly and equally well in males and females. The microscopic appearance was of a tumor with no gland formation. Finally, the R3327/150 subline, as described earlier, is an anaplastic tumor, growing extremely fast, killing the recipient rats in a few short weeks.

It is evident that many sublines of the Dunning R3327 tumor exist in a number of different laboratories. How each relates to every other and which of those described are identical is unknown at this time. Perhaps some organized collaboration between the laboratories possessing the lines is in order to characterize each subline and standardize the nomenclature. A few points are worthy of comment here. First and foremost, the heterogeneity of the tumor with continual production of new lines may be criticized by some, labeling this tumor as unfit for experimentation. On the contrary, this property supports the contention that, in fact, the Dunning R3327 prostatic tumor is an excellent model system for study of the human disease. The sublines, once fully characterized, may be shown to correspond to the many different types of prostatic cancer of man from the well-differentiated adenocarcinoma to the wildly anaplastic cancer. Handelsman, in a paper titled "The Limitation of Model Systems in Prostatic Cancer" [20], stated ". . . a *specific* model may not be a prerequisite for a *useful* model for human tumors. Focusing on the issue of prostatic tumor models, one would readily admit that it would be nice to have hints of antitumor activity in a model realistically mimicking the variability of responses encountered clinically." With what we know of the properties of the various R3327 sublines thus far, this tumor system seems to fit the need set down by Handelsman.

The variability seen in the Dunning tumor brings us to the second point we wish to make. That is, the need for careful monitoring of each tumor-bearing rat. In our laboratory the subcutaneous tumors in rats used to maintain each line are biopsied at the time they reach $1,000-2,000$ mm^3 in size and their histologic identity to the prototype of that line verified. In addition, each tumor is transferred to both male and female recipients and measured every two weeks to monitor growth rate and androgen sensitivity.

We have begun examining the mechanism of tumor heterogeneity using a tissue culture line derived from the well-differentiated adenocarcinoma [8, 21]. The culture is a pure epithelial line with morphological characteristics of neoplastic cells. These include the large size of the nucleus relative to the amount of cytoplasm, many nucleoli within the nucleus, the presence of high number of mitotic figures, and the formation of multinucleated giant cells. The cultured cells, upon subcutaneous or intraprostatic injection into recipient Copenhagen rats, produced tumors similar to the original Dunning adenocarcinoma. Within a short time in culture, tumors produced by the cultured cells demonstrated a heterogeneity similar to that seen with the in vivo maintained tumors. This was evidenced by rate of growth, size of tumors produced, and sensitivity of androgens (by growth in males and females).

A heterogeneity of the cell populations within the R3327 tumors was described by the John Hopkins group with respect to hormone sensitivity [2, 9]. Cell kinetic studies indicated that $70-90\%$ of the total tumor cells are hormonally sensitive, and $8-30\%$ are hormone insensitive [9]. It is not clear whether the observed differences in the properties of the tumors are due to the presence of multiple populations of cells within the tumor, each with separate but fixed properties, or to a single population with changing or highly mutable properties. We have isolated 11 different cloned sublines by limiting dilution in microtiter tissue culture plates. In early experiments one of the uncloned cultures and two

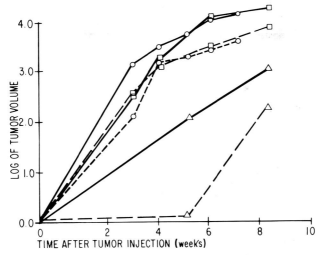

Fig. 1. Growth of subcutaneous tumors induced by uncloned and cloned R3327/TC cells. o—o male, uncloned; o– – –o female, uncloned; □—□ male, clone 5; □– – –□ female, clone 5; △——△ male, clone 9; △– – –△ female, clone 9.

sublines were injected into male and female Copenhagen rats (Fig. 1). The uncloned line and clone 5 grew as undifferentiated tumors with rapid growth, equal in both males and females. Clone 9, on the other hand, grew as a typical differentiated adenocarcinoma. Similar growth curves are now being generated for all the cloned sublines.

We have also examined the cultured sublines with respect to their antigenic characteristics. In a chromium-release cytotoxic assay, each cloned line was tested against xenoantibody produced in the rabbit and alloantibody produced either against the major histocompatibility antigen of the Copenhagen rat or against the uncloned R3327 tissue culture cells. The results in Table I indicate a difference in the susceptibility of cells from each clone to lysis by the various antisera and complement. Whether this is the result of differences in the number and concentration of antigens on the cell surface or a physical resistance to lysis is not known at this time. Certainly, precedent for the latter exists in the literature [22]. Boyle et al have demonstrated that different guinea pig hepatoma cell lines vary in their susceptibility to lysis by antibody and complement independent of antigen concentration.

Our early results would support the concept that tumor heterogeneity, at least as it relates to the Dunning tumor, may be due to separate cell populations within the tumor. Further work obviously is necessary to confirm this. If such proves to be the case, it is extremely important to determine whether the properties of each clone remain constant without modulation.

TABLE I. R3327/TC Antigenic Reactivity

	% Cytotoxicity*		
Clone	Lewis anti-DA	F344 anti-R3327/TC	Rabbit anti-R3327/TC (unabsorbed)
7	61	26	68
9	53	36	68
8	51	23	76
5	47	33	51
10	42	15	37
2	30	ND	35
6	23	13	32
11	23	7	39
3	10	4	15
1	6	3	41
4	2	3	27

*^{51}Cr monolayer Ab + C assay.

ULTRASTRUCTURE

A detailed examination of the Dunning tumor cells has been carried out by Feuchter, who used both transmission and scanning electron microscopy [23]. The author used the epithelial tissue culture line of the R3327 and compared the adenocarcinoma cells to cultures derived from the prostates of normal Copenhagen rats. In contrast to normal cells, which become extensively spread after several days in vitro, the R3327 cells remain as slightly rounded polygonal cells and do not flatten with age. When the tumor cells reach confluence, multiple layers do not form, as with most malignant cell lines. Rather, after seven to ten days in culture, focal areas of the monolayer detach from the culture vessel. Fluid accumulates in the pockets between the cells and dish such that dome-shape blisters of cells are formed. After a few days the blisters progress to form spheroidal aggregates of cells, which remain attached to the underlying cells. These spheroids are cyst-like in appearance and are composed of a single layer of cells surrounding a hollow, fluid-filled space. They are similar in size and morphology to the acinus-like structures formed by the tumor in vivo.

Scanning electron micrographs showed the cell surface of the R3327 grown in vitro and in vivo to be identical. The most prominent surface features of the malignant cells are large numbers of microvilli and ruffles. By transmission electron microscopy, the cell cytoplasm contains an abundance of free polyribosomes as well as lipid droplets and dense bodies, the latter two structures in the vicinity of the cell's euchromatic nucleus. The mitochondria are vesicular in shape, with incomplete, distorted cristae and large irregular granules. The most obvious morphologic deviation from normal is a lack of large bundles of microfilaments in the malignant cells. In normal cells the microfilamentous bundles form one of the major organelles.

Feuchter also studied human prostatic adenocarcinoma from surgical specimens and from the HPC-36 cell line derived from a human cancer of the prostate [24]. The morphology of the human and rat tumor cells was found to be almost identical when compared by light, scanning, and transmission microscopy. Cell surfaces have numerous microvilli and ruffles, the cytoplasm contains bizarre mitochondria with the distorted cristae and granules, and there is a conspicuous absence of microfilaments. Here again we have further evidence for the relatedness of the Dunning R3327 and human prostatic adenocarcinomas.

HORMONAL STUDIES

Because of the important role steroid hormones play in prostatic carcinoma, they were the subject of the early experiments in which the Dunning tumor was used as a model of human cancer of the prostate [4, 5]. Voigt and Dunning demonstrated that, like the prostate gland and other androgen-sensitive organs of the genital tract, the R3327 tumor metabolizes testosterone by 5-alpha reduction [4]. This is in contrast to oxidative metabolism carried out in tissues such as the muscle and liver. The authors were also the first to show a difference in growth of the tumor in normal males as compared to females and castrated males. In contrast, the squamous carcinoma variant R3327-A, was found *not* to metabolize testosterone by the pathway of 5-alpha reduction [5]. Also, when the R3327 tumors were studied for the presence of receptor proteins in the cytosol, only the androgen-sensitive, not the androgen-insensitive, tumors were positive. The androgen-sensitive tumor was found to possess receptor proteins for estradiol as well. Other Dunning tumor lines were examined for their androgen sensitivity by measuring levels of a series of enzymes [17]. The hormone-sensitive R3327-H, hormone-insensitive R3327-HI, and anaplastic R3327-AT were the three tumor lines studied along with normal male accessory glands. The highest levels of 5-alpha reductase, 7-alpha hydroxylase, and alkaline phosphatase were found in the cytoplasm of the R3327-H tumor, with sequentially lower values in the R3327-HI and R3327-AT tumors, respectively. In contrast, the enzymes 3-alpha hydroxy-steroid dehydrogenase and lactic dehydrogenase were lowest in the well-differentiated tumor and highest in the anaplastic tumor.

Subsequent publications from other laboratories have verified the presence of both androgen and estrogen receptors on the R3327 adenocarcinoma [25, 26]. In addition, a relationship between the presence of these hormone receptors and degree of tumor differentiation was again documented [25]. No receptors for progesterone were detectable in the cytosol of the androgen-sensitive tumor [26]. However, in tumor-bearing rats that had been castrated and showed a subsequent

reduction in tumor size, followed by relapse, high-affinity receptors for progesterone were detected. The presence of separate tumor cell populations with
different receptors on their surfaces, supports the concept of cellular heterogeneity within each tumor. The emergence of a population of tumor cells in
castrates was the basis on which the estimates were made that approximately
8–30% of R3327 cells are insensitive to androgenic action [9]. Again, the
question arises as to whether the separate populations are present in the original
tumor or arise in an environment that allows their induction. It is our hope that
experiments with the cloned cell lines will answer the question.

CHEMOTHERAPY

Thus far only two reports have appeared in the literature that describe use of
the Dunning R3327 tumor for chemotherapy studies [27, 28]. Block et al carried
out a large study on the effectiveness of various chemotherapeutic agents alone
and in combination against the R3327 tumor [27]. In general, the authors found
a consistency in the response of the rat tumor with the literature reported on
human tumors [29]. L-asparaginase, CCNU, and actinomycin D had no effect on
established tumors. Hydroxyurea and 5-fluorouracil (5FU) treated rats had tumors
slightly smaller than control animals (57.7 mg and 60.9 mg, respectively, vs
74.8 mg). Chemotherapeutic regimes with a pronounced effect were, listed in
order of effectiveness: Cis-platinum, cyclophosphamide (CTX), CTX plus
Adriamycin, diethylstilbestrol (DES), Adriamycin, CTX plus Adriamycin plus
5FU, and DES plus CTX. Orchiectomy alone was as effective as cyclophosphamide.

When comparing the effectiveness of each treatment regime to what had been
published for man at the time of their report, Block et al pointed to similarities
for cyclophosphamide, orchiectomy, and DES [27, 29, 30]. Only Adriamycin
had an effect on the R3327 tumor, whereas it has not been reported to be an
adequate drug for the treatment of human prostatic adenocarcinoma.

These results are encouraging for the future use of the Dunning tumor to screen
chemotherapeutic agents, alone or in combination, in order to give the urologist
an effective means in the treatment of this disease. However, a possible weakness
in the report just discussed is the use of a fast-growing subline, R3327-G. Although
this line has been reported to have maintained its hormone dependence, the rapid
growth may reduce its usefulness as a "representative" model system. Caution
must be exerted in the interpretation of results obtained with this tumor line. It
is hoped that investigations of many lines, with the variety of histologic types and
hormone sensitivities available, will be employed in the future.

In another study, this time utilizing the original well-differentiated slowly
growing Dunning tumor, Müntzing and colleagues studied the effectiveness of
Estracyt (estramustine phosphate) on established tumors [28]. The authors were
able to demonstrate that the drug was capable of retarding growth of tumors when

compared to saline-injected controls. The effectiveness of Estracyt was found to be even more pronounced in orchiectomized rats given androgens. From these results Estracyt was thought to have potential clinical use for the treatment of human prostatic cancer.

IMMUNOLOGIC STUDIES

In the past two years a number of investigators have published papers on studies of the immunology of prostatic cancer in which the Dunning R3327 tumor was used [16, 31–39]. Our work and how it relates to human cancer of the prostate is discussed in detail later in this chapter. Published results in other laboratories have demonstrated that specific immune responses to the R3327 tumor can be measured. These include lymphocyte transformation in the presence of tumor extracts [32], nonspecific cytotoxicity of chicken erythrocytes by mitogens [32] or tumor antigens [16], inhibition of tumor cell cultures by serum from tumor-bearing rats [33], and "non-specific" immunotherapy with pyran in combination with other treatment modalities [31].

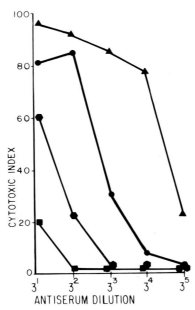

Fig. 2. Cytotoxicity of unabsorbed and absorbed rabbit anti-R3327 serum against ^{51}Cr-labeled R3327/TC cells. ▲——▲ unabsorbed; ●——● absorbed with Lewis lymphocytes; ●——● absorbed with Lewis and Copenhagen lymphocytes; ■——■ absorbed with above plus normal prostate.

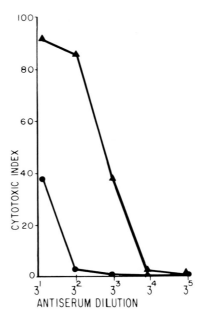

Fig. 3. Cytotoxicity of unabsorbed and absorbed rabbit anti-R3327 serum against ^{51}Cr-labeled Copenhagen lymphocytes. ▲——▲ unabsorbed; ●——● absorbed with Lewis lymphocytes.

Our interest in the Dunning tumor as a model system dates back to 1973, when we became intrigued with reports in the literature of remission of primary and metastatic tumor following treatment of the primary by cryosurgery [35–40]. These results have prompted a great deal of research into possible immunologic mechanisms mediating tumor cell destruction. Independent studies have shown that freezing of normal urogenital tissues in experimental animals can engender specific immune responses directed against the target organ [41–51]. It is conceivable, then, that tumor-specific immune responses could also be produced, the end result being the immunologic elimination of metastatic tumor.

In order to proceed with our studies, it was necessary to demonstrate that immune responses could be produced by, and directed to, the R3327 antigens using "conventional" immunization procedures. Species-, histocompatibility-, organ-, and tumor-associated antigens were detected by rabbit antisera produced following immunization with the R3327 tumor cells (Figs. 2 and 3) [34]. Unabsorbed rabbit antiserum killed virtually all tumor target cells and Copenhagen lymphocytes. Antibodies to species-specific antigens were removed by absorption with Lewis strain cells (lymphocytes, liver, and skin). Lewis rat tissues were chosen, since they would contain only the species antigens and not the histocom-

TABLE II. Cytotoxic Antibody Responses Against the R3327/TC Cells

Antiserum	Cytotoxic Index
Allogeneic responses	
Lewis anti DA	45.6 ± 20.4
NBR anti-R3327/TC	54.7 ± 22.8
LBN anti-R3327/TC	5.3 ± 3.6
F344 anti-R3327/TC	17.1 ± 13.1
Syngeneic Response	
COP anti-R3327/TC	1.27 ± 3.4

patibility antigens of the Copenhagen rat. Further absorption with Copenhagen lymphocytes removed all antibodies to the histocompatibility antigens, since the serum now killed none of the target Copenhagen cells (Fig. 3) but still destroyed 60% of the tumor cells (Fig. 2). The activity remaining in the serum was directed against organ-specific antigens of the prostate and tumor antigens, since absorption with prostate tissue reduced R3327 cell killing to 20%. Only absorption with the tumor cells eliminated reactivity to the R3327 targets.

Alloantigens could be demonstrated on the tumor cells by antisera raised against the major histocompatibility antigens of the Copenhagen rat (Lewis anti-DA) as well as antisera produced by immunization of various rat strains with the R3327 cells (Table II). Both the Lewis and NBR strains produced positive antisera, while the F344 and LBN were very weakly reactive. It is possible that the latter rat strains were genetically incapable of responding to the antigens on the R3327 tumor.

Syngeneic immunizations of Copenhagen rats (COP) with R3327 cells have failed to produce positive antisera. Using a variety of immunization procedures, we have not been able to detect antibody in vitro either by complement-dependent cytotoxicity or complement-independent Staph A binding.

We have been able to produce cell-mediated immunologic reactions to the Dunning tumor directed against histocompatibility and syngeneic tumor antigens. NBR, LBN, COP, and COP × DA F_1 hybrid rats were immunized with 1×10^7 R3327 tissue-cultured cells (R3327/TC) emulsified in complete Freund's adjuvant (CFA). Eight days afterwards, draining lymph nodes and spleens were removed and tested for cytotoxic activity against R3327/TC target cells. Figure 4 shows that good allogeneic responses were obtained with Lewis and NBR lymph node cells but not with LBN. The reactivity Lewis and NBR lymphocytes produced against R3327 antigens with no response detected in lymph node cell populations of LBN rats correlated with the pattern of responsiveness seen with humoral antibodies. Syngeneic, cell-mediated, cytotoxic responses to tumor antigens were detected in spleen cells of immunized Copenhagen rats but not in

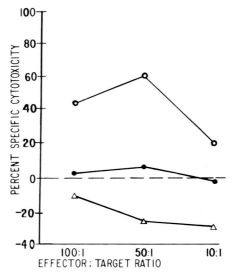

Fig. 4. Cell-mediated cytotoxicity. Allogeneic responses to R3327. ○———○ NBR anti-R3327/TC;
●———● LBN anti-R3327/TC; △———△ normal NBR.

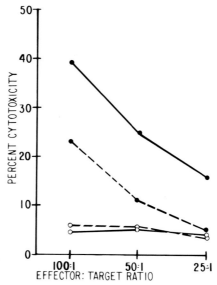

Fig. 5. Cell-mediated cytotoxicity of spleen and lymph node lymphocytes from Copenhagen rats immunized against R3327/TC cells. Target cells were ^{51}Cr-labeled R3327/TC cells.
●———● immunized spleen cells; ●– – – ● normal spleen cells; ○———○ immunized lymph node cells; ○– – –○ normal lymph node cells.

lymph node cells (Fig. 5). In addition to the presence of cytolytic cells, Copenhagen spleens also contained a population of natural killer cells, as demonstrated by the high background killing detected in immunized rats. These cells were not readily found in the lymph nodes of Lewis, NBR, or LBN rats.

The compartmentalization of allogeneic and syngeneic immune responses seen in these experiments is an interesting one and may be of importance in future clinical applications. Tumor-immune cells were found in the spleen and were absent from lymph nodes draining the site of immunization, whereas cells cytotoxic for alloantigens were found in the lymph nodes. This difference may be the result of separate T cell populations mediating the two responses. Shiko et al have shown that the cytotoxic responses for alloantigens in mice and phenotypically different from cells mediating tumor immune responses [52, 53]. We have begun experiments to determine whether different lymphocyte subpopulations mediate responses to the two antigens in this rat system. Using antisera to rat lymphocyte antigens developed in our laboratory [54–57], the cells reactive to alloantigens have already been described [58]. A second hypothesis to explain the spleen-lymph node difference in rat allogeneic and syngeneic responses is the presence of tumor-specific suppressor cells in lymph nodes and their absence from spleen.

Another technique employed to study cell-mediated immune responses to the R3327 antigens was the proliferative response of lymphocytes following antigenic stimulation, based upon similar work reported by Glaser et al [59]. Lymphocyte suspensions were prepared from spleens of Copenhagen rats immunized with R3327 cells and mixed with mitomycin C-treated target cells. After incubation and a pulse label with tritiated thymidine, the mixture was analyzed by liquid scintillation counting to measure the amount of isotope incorporation. These results (Table III) show an eightfold stimulation over controls, another indication of tumor-specific immune responses.

A degree of protective immunity can be produced against the Dunning tumor by injection of tumor cells in CFA. Figure 6 summarizes the results obtained when rats were immunized either with 1×10^7, 1×10^6, or 1×10^5 cells (controls

TABLE III. Mixed Lymphocyte–Tumor Interaction: Copenhagen Tumor Cells Plus R3327-TC Cells

Incubation mixture	Activity (mean cpm)	Stimulation index
Tumor cells alone*	31.4	—
Lymphocytes alone	60.0 ± 31.6	—
Lymphocytes plus tumor cells*	486.8 ± 176.2	8.11

*Mitomycin-c treated.

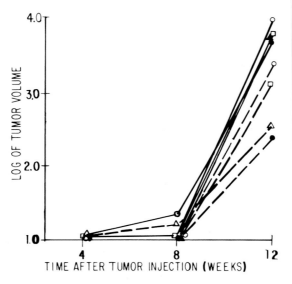

Fig. 6. Protection against R3327 tumor production following immunization with fresh tumor cells in CFA. Tumors produced in the prostate by injection of either 10^7 or 10^6 cells. ○——○ control, 10^7 challenge; ○− − −○ control, 10^6 challenge; ●——● 10^7 immunized, 10^7 challenged; ●− − −● 10^7 immunized, 10^6 challenged; ▲——▲ 10^6 immunized, 10^7 challenged; △− − −△ 10^6 immunized, 10^6 challenged; □——□ 10^5 immunized, 10^7 challenged; □− − −□ 10^5 immunized, 10^6 challenged.

received balanced salt solution in CFA), followed two weeks later by a challenge into the dorsolateral lobe of the prostate of either 1×10^7 or 1×10^6 cells. Animals immunized either with 1×10^7 or 1×10^6 cells and challenged with 1×10^6 cells had significantly smaller tumors than did controls. None of the rats challenged with 1×10^7 cells displayed any protective immunity, nor did any rats immunized with 1×10^5 cells, irrespective of the challenge dose.

In order to proceed further with our studies on whether cryosurgery is responsible for the disappearance of metastatic lesions via the production of immune responses toward prostatic tumor antigens, it was necessary to demonstrate the ability of cryosurgery to destroy the primary tumor. Copenhagen rats bearing intraprostatic tumors of varying sizes following the inoculation of R3327 cells were treated by cryosurgery. A trocar probe was applied to the exposed tumor-bearing prostate and cooled by liquid nitrogen to $-170°C$. This temperature was held for 30 seconds, and the tumor was thawed by switching to the heat cycle. The results of these experiments (Table IV) demonstrate that rat tumors smaller than 1,000 mm^3 could be completely destroyed by this cryosurgical treatment. Tumors larger than 1,000 mm^3 were too much tumor mass to obtain total

TABLE IV. Cryodestruction

Time after cryo-surgery (weeks)	Tumors less than 1,000 mm³				Tumors more than 1,000 mm³			
	Decrease in size		Increase in size		Decrease in size		Increase in size	
	% of total	% change	% of total	% change	% of total	% change	% of total	% change
2	45.0	−46.9	55.0	+133.6	65.0	−35.0	35.0	+179.6
4	88.9	−75.4	11.1	+ 33.8	0	−	100	+199.2
6	85.7	−66.7	14.3	+ 50	0	−	100	+342.3
8	100	−59.4	0.0	−				
13	100	−58.2	0.0	−				
15	100	−84.2	0.0	−				

destruction by a single freeze. Apparently enough viable tissue remained after cryosurgery, producing more tumor. Perhaps these would be more completely destroyed by multiple cryosurgical procedures.

Upon autopsy of the rats during the experiments, we observed that very small tumors were completely destroyed in a relatively short time (two to four weeks), leaving a nodule consisting of fibrous connective tissue and inflammatory cells. Larger tumors (but still less than 1,000 mm³) when examined within two to four weeks of cryosurgery were usually soft and filled with necrotic material. Autopsy performed later than four weeks failed to show any viable tumor.

Our next experiment attempted to incorporate the success in affording some protective immunity by CFA-tumor cell immunization with cryodestruction. In essence, we wished to determine if we could augment the cryosurgery and perhaps produce protection by use of an adjuvant. We chose the widely used immuno-therapeutic agent BCG (kindly donated by Dr. Ray Crispin, University of Illinois). For technical reasons these early experiments used tumors induced in the flank rather than in the prostate. Copenhagen rats bearing subcutaneous tumors were divided into groups according to the size of the tumors. These were: 1–350 mm³, 351–800 mm³, 801–1,500 mm³, and 1,501–3,00 mm³. Each group was further subdivided into the following subgroups: BCG only, cryosurgery only, BCG followed by cryosurgery 24 hours later, and no treatment. The BCG was given by intralesional injection of 5×10^6 organisms. Data obtained from these early experiments indicated that the combination of BCG and cryosurgery was better in reducing or eliminating tumor than cryosurgery alone, particularly when treating large tumors. In general, small tumors were controlled equally well by BCG + cryosurgery or by cryosurgery alone. BCG alone was ineffective in all cases. At five months after treatment, tumors were removed from rats bearing detectable tumors. Those animals, as well as animals that had their tumors completely destroyed by previous treatment, were challenged six weeks later with 1×10^6 R3327 tumor cells in the opposite flank. At eight weeks after rechallenge, 75% of the rats treated by BCG and cryosurgery did not grow tumors whereas *all* rats in other groups had tumors. These preliminary results would indicate a protective immunity produced against the R3327 by the combination treatment of BCG and cryosurgery.

We have shown that immune responses can be produced against antigens on the R3327 tumor cells by conventional immunization techniques and, like the human prostatic tumors, the R3327 can be destroyed by cryosurgery. The next task is to determine whether immune responses can be induced in tumor antigens by cryosurgery. Encouraging results were obtained in the experiment combining cryosurgery and BCG injection. With success in these investigations, we will be able to determine whether the immune response plays a role in post-cryosurgical remissions of metastatic disease. It is also hoped that we may be able to augment the response to deal with the tumor load more efficiently. Use of the R3327 tumor in these experiments appears promising.

SUMMARY

We have described the Dunning tumor, R3327, as a most useful model system in studies of human prostatic cancer. The tumor resembles the human disease in its histologic picture, ultrastructure, and most of its metastatic capabilities. The one exception to the latter is the apparent absence of metastatic lesions in the bone. Like the variability seen in human cancer of the prostate, the R3327 has been shown to develop multiple sublines, each with different histologic pictures, growth rate, and androgen dependence. Thus far the literature is replete with reports of the Dunning tumor as a model in hormonal, chemotherapeutic, and immunologic experiments. When we look at the results obtained in the five years since the Dunning tumor has been resurrected, we can be encouraged with what the future of prostatic cancer research holds with the use of this system.

REFERENCES

1. Dunning WF: Prostate cancer in the rat. Natl Cancer Inst Monogr 12:351–369, 1963.
2. Smolev JK, Heston WDW, Scott WW, Coffey DS: Characterization of the Dunning R-3327-H prostatic adenocarcinoma: An appropriate animal model for prostatic cancer. Cancer Treat Rep 61:273–287, 1977.
3. Müntzing J, Saroff J, Sandberg AA, Murphy GP: Enzyme activity and distribution in rat prostatic adenocarcinoma. Urology 11:278–282, 1978.
4. Voigt W, Dunning WF: In vivo metabolism of testosterone-^{3}H in R-3327, an androgen-sensitive rat prostatic adenocarcinoma. Cancer Res 34:1447–1450, 1974.
5. Voigt W, Feldman M, Dunning WF: 5-Alpha-dihydrotestosterone-binding proteins and androgen sensitivity in prostatic cancers of Copenhagen rats. Cancer Res 35:1840–1846, 1975.

6. Lubaroff DM, Canfield L, Feldbush TL, Bonney WW: R3327 adenocarcinoma of the Copenhagen rat as a model for the study of immunologic aspects of prostatic cancer. J Natl Cancer Inst 58:1677–1689, 1977.

7. Lubaroff DM, Culp DA: Experience with an animal model of prostatic carcinoma. Trans Am Assoc GU Surg 69:72–77, 1978.

8. Lubaroff DM, Canfield L, Rasmussen GT, Reynolds CW: An animal model for the study of prostate carcinoma. Natl Cancer Inst Monogr 49:275–281, 1978.

9. Smolev JK, Coffey DS, Scott WW: Experimental models for the study of prostatic adenocarcinoma. J Urol 118:216–220, 1977.

10. Flocks RH: Carcinoma of the prostate. J Urol 101:714–749, 1969.

11. Jorgens J: The radiographic characteristics of carcinoma of the prostate. Surg Clin North Am 45:1427–1440, 1965.

12. Mostofi FK, Price EG: In: "Tumors of the Male Genital System." Washington, DC: Armed Forces Institute of Pathology, 1973.

13. Warren S, Harris PN, Graves RC: Osseous metastasis of carcinoma of the prostate with special reference to the perineural lymphatics. Arch Pathol 22:139–160, 1936.

14. Batson OV: The function of the vertebral veins and their role in the spread of metastases. Am Surg 112:138–149, 1940.

15. Willis RA: Carcinoma of the prostate. In: "Pathology of Tumors." London: Butterworth, 1948, pp 585–595.

16. Claflin AJ, McKinney EC, Fletcher MA: The Dunning R3327 prostate adenocarcinoma in the Fischer-Copenhagen F_1 rat: A useful model for immunological studies. Oncology 34:105–109, 1977.

17. Isaacs JT, Heston WDW, Weissman RM, Coffey DS: Animal models of the hormone-sensitive and insensitive prostatic adenocarcinomas, Dunning R3327-H, R-3327-HI, and R-3327-AT. Cancer Res 38:4353–4349, 1978.

18. Seman G, Myers G, Bowen JM, Dmochowski L: Histology and ultrastructure of the R3327 C-F transplantable prostate tumor of Copenhagen-Fischer rats. Invest Urol 16:231–236, 1978.

19. Lubaroff DM, Canfield L, Rasmussen GT, Reynolds CW: Heterogeneity of the Dunning R3327 prostatic tumor. (In preparation).

20. Handelsman H: The limitations of model systems in prostatic cancer. Oncology 34:96–99, 1977.

21. Lubaroff DM, Reynolds CW, Rasmussen GT: R3327 prostatic adenocarcinoma: Development of a tissue culture line and its use in the production of tumors. (In press).

22. Boyle MDP, Ohanian SH, Borsos T: Lysis of tumor cells by antibody and complement. III lack of correlation between antigen movement and cell lysis. J Immunol 115:473–475, 1975.

23. Feuchter FA: Surface membranes of normal and malignant prostatic epithelial cells. PhD thesis, University of Iowa, 1979.

24. Lubaroff DM: Development of an epithelial tissue culture line from human prostatic adenocarcinoma. J Urol 118:612–615, 1977.

25. Markland FS, Chopp RT, Cosgrove MD, Howard EB: Characterization of steroid hormone receptors in the Dunning R-3327 rat prostatic adenocarcinoma. Cancer Res 38:2818–2826, 1978.

26. Heston WDW, Menon M, Tananis C, Walsh PC: Androgen, estrogen and progesterone receptors of the R3327H Copenhagen rat prostatic tumor. Cancer Lett 6:45–50, 1979.

27. Block NL, Camuzzi F, Denefrio J, Troner M, Claflin A, Stover D, Politano V: Chemotherapy of the transplantable adenocarcinoma (R-3327) of the Copenhagen rat. Oncology 34:110–113, 1977.

28. Müntzing J, Kirdani RY, Saroff J, Murphy GP, Sandberg AA: Inhibitory effects of Estracyt on R-3327 rat prostatic carcinoma. Urology 10:439–445, 1977.
29. Yogoda A: Non-hormonal cytotoxic agents in the treatment of prostatic adenocarcinoma. Cancer 32:1131–1140, 1973.
30. The Veterans Administration Cooperative Urological Research Group. Treatment and survival of patients with cancer of the prostate. Surg Gyncol Obstet 124:1011–1017, 1967.
31. Weissman RM, Coffey DS, Scott WW: Cell kinetic studies of prostatic cancer: Adjuvant therapy in animal models. Oncology 34:133–137, 1977.
32. Lopez DM, Voigt W: Adenocarcinoma R-3327 of the Copenhagen rat as a suitable model for immunological studies of prostate cancer. Cancer Res 37:2057–2061, 1977.
33. Rao BR, Nakeff A, Eaton C, Heston WDW: Establishment and characterization of an in vitro clonogenic assay for the R-3327-AT Copenhagen rat prostatic tumor. Cancer Res 38:4431–4439, 1978.
34. Lubaroff DM, Reynolds CW, Culp DA: Immunologic studies of prostatic cancer using the R3327 rat model. Trans Am Assoc GU Surg (in press).
35. Ablin RJ, Soanes WA, Gonder MJ: Clinical and experimental considerations of the immunologic response to prostatic and other accessory gland tissues of reproduction. Urol Int 25:511–539, 1970.
36. Soanes WA, Gonder MJ, Ablin RJ, Maser MD, Jagodzinski RV: Clinical and experimental aspects of prostatic cryosurgery. J Cryosurg 2:23–29, 1969.
37. Soanes WA, Ablin RJ, Gonder MJ: Remission of metastatic lesions following cryosurgery in prostatic cancer: Immunologic considerations. J Urol 104:154–159, 1970.
38. Flocks RH, Nelson CMK, Boatman DL: Perineal cryosurgery for prostatic carcinoma. J Urol 108:933–935, 1972.
39. Gursel EO, Roberts MS, Veenema RJ: Regression of prostatic cancer following sequential cryotherapy to the prostate. J Urol 108:928–932, 1972.
40. Horan AH: Sequential cryotherapy for prostatic carcinoma: Does it palliate the bone pain? Conn Med 39:81–83, 1975.
41. Jagodzinski RV, Yantorno C, Shulman S: An experimental system for the production of antibodies in response to cryosurgical procedures. Cryobiology 3:456–463, 1967.
42. Shulman S, Yantorno C, Bornson P: Cryo-immunology: A method of immunization to autologous tissue (31817). Proc Soc Exp Biol Med 124:658–661, 1967.
43. Yantorno C, Soanes WA, Gonder MJ, Shulman S: Studies in cryoimmunology. I. The production of antibodies to urogenital tissue in consequence of freezing treatment. Immunology 12:395–410, 1967.
44. Brandt EJ, Riera C, Orsini F, Shulman S: Cryoimmunology: The booster phenomenon. Cryobiology 3:382–385, 1967.
45. Ablin RJ, Witebsky E, Jagodzinski RV, Soanes WA: Secondary immunologic responses as a consequence of the in situ freezing of rabbit adnexal glands tissues of reproduction. Exp Med Surg 29:72–87, 1971.
46. Ablin RJ, Soanes WA: Experimental production of autoimmune aspermatogenic orchitis in the rabbit in consequence of in situ freezing of the testis. Eur Surg Res 4:98–106, 1972.
47. Zappi E, Orsini F, Shulman S: Cryoimmunization-antibody responses after selective and repeated cryostimulations of the coagulating gland and the seminal vesicle of the male rabbit. Invest Urol 10:171–177, 1972.
48. Zappi E, Shulman S: Cryo-immunology antibody response to epididymitis freezing in the rabbit. Invest Urol 10:226–229, 1972.

49. Drylie DM, Hahn GS: Stimulation of prostatic antibodies by cryosurgery. J Urol 110:324–325, 1973.
50. Stoll HW, Barnes GW, Ansell JS: The autoimmune response to male reproductive tissues of rabbits. I. Simplified cryosurgical procedures for inducing antibody to accessory tissue. Invest Urol 12:108–115, 1974.
51. Stoll HW, Barnes GW, Ansell JS: The autoimmune response to male reproductive tissues of rabbits. II. The secondary response as an indicator of cryosensitization to accessory tissue. Invest Urol 12:116–122, 1974.
52. Shiku H, Kisielow P, Bean MA, Takahashi T, Boyse EA, Oettgen HF, Old LJ: Expression of T-cell differentiation antigens on effector cells in cell-mediated cytotoxicity in vitro—Evidence for functional heterogeneity related to the surface phenotype of T cells. J Exp Med 141:227–241, 1975.
53. Shiku H, Takahashi T, Bean MA, Old LJ, Oettgen HF: Ly phenotype of cytotoxic T cells for syngeneic tumor. J Exp Med 144:1116–1120, 1976.
54. Lubaroff DM: Alloantigenic marker on rat thymus and thymus-derived cells. Trans Proc 5:115–118, 1973.
55. Lubaroff DM: Antigenic markers on rat lymphocytes. I. Characterization of ART, an alloantigenic marker on rat thymus and thymus-derived cells. Cell Immunol 29:147–158, 1977.
56. Report of the First International Workshop on Alloantigenic Systems in the Rat. Trans Proc 10:271–285, 1978.
57. Lubaroff DM, Greiner DL, Reynolds CW: Investigations of T-lymphocyte subpopulations in the rat using alloantigenic markers. Trans Proc 11:1092–1094, 1979.
58. Greiner DM, Reynolds CW, Lubaroff DM: Antigenic markers on rat lymphocyte, IV. (in press).
59. Glaser M, Herberman RB, Kirchner H, Djeu JY: Study of the cellular immune response to gross virus-induced lymphoma by the mixed lymphocyte-tumor interaction. Cancer Res 34:2165–2171, 1974.

The Nb Rat Prostatic Adenocarcinoma Model System

Joseph R. Drago, MD, Laurence B. Goldman, MD, and
Robert E. Maurer, MD

Radical surgery and radiotherapy have not significantly improved the prognosis for most patients with advanced carcinoma of the prostate. Only a small number of patients with prostatic adenocarcinoma seek medical care at a time when the disease is locally either resectable or amenable to radiotherapy, either external or internal. These treatment modalities have had little to offer patients with disseminated prostatic carcinoma, which represent the bulk of patients with this disease who come to urologists for further therapy. With advances in the initial treatment of localized neoplasms of the prostate, the use of chemotherapeutic agents has been adjunct to local treatment and may become more widespread. At present, however, the primary modality for treatment of metastatic disease is hormonal manipulation — either estrogen or orchiectomy. However, recent reports have given cause for cautious optimism in the treatment of patients with metastatic disease with chemotherapy. There have been, however, few clinical data on the efficacy of the available neoplastic agents for prostatic carcinoma. The primary difficulty in performing large clinical studies with the numerous drugs available is obvious. If cytotoxic chemotherapeutic agents are to have any chance of success (or increased success), the best agents or combinations of agents must be determined, and newer agents must be monitored as they become available for experimental investigation. One avenue for obtaining and evaluating this information may lie in the use of appropriate animal model systems for the trial and screening of chemotherapeutic agents now available and for the screening of agents that are becoming available almost on a daily basis. In using such animal model systems, large numbers of subjects are available in which investigators are able to make statistically significant comparisons of the efficacy of the multitude of agents available.

The data base and methodology for evaluation of potentially useful hormonal and chemotherapeutic programs in the treatment of prostatic adenocarcinoma

Models for Prostate Cancer, pages 265–291

has not been significantly altered for more than a decade and remains hampered for several reasons [1–4]. In particular, the natural history of prostatic carcinoma is variable and unpredictable, with major significant options involving the utility and effectiveness of treatment at different stages of disease [5–9]. Moreover, the often dramatic clinical response of hormonal manipulation has led to reliance on this mode of therapy for symptomatic, advanced prostatic carcinoma, despite well-controlled observations that this form of therapy almost invariably is followed by relapse and death [10–14]. Indeed, despite intensive investigations, the mechanism of hormonal escape remains largely unknown and is the subject of many investigations [15–18]. Furthermore, there have been only a few well-controlled, randomized trials of nonhormonal cytotoxic chemotherapy in prostatic carcinoma [19–22]. Finally, and critically, in vitro tumorcidal and tumorstatic assays have not been well established for prostatic carcinoma. Because of these problems, several groups have suggested a need for the development of appropriate animal models with prostate neoplasia [23–30].

This need for an appropriate animal model of prostatic carcinoma is based upon major theoretical and practical considerations and the large number of chemotherapeutic agents now available and in the process of discovery. The majority of these chemotherapeutic agents are extremely cytotoxic, with many side-effects, some of which are lethal. Use of toxic agents that are inactive against a patient's own tumor not only denies him the benefit of appropriate chemotherapy, but also may result in complications that deny him the option of additional chemotherapeutic agents in treatment of the disease. Additionally, although heavy reliance has been placed on studying humans as models, these studies are, nonetheless, subject to the associated problems of clinical trials, limitations of money and manpower, and the magnitude of all too obvious known and unknown variables [31–33]. Indeed, over the past decade, there have been intensive efforts to develop in vitro assays to determine the sensitivity of human tumors to chemotherapeutic agents. At present, there are three major such in vitro sensitivity tests available to estimate, for screening purposes, the therapeutic effectiveness of various drugs: agar plate assays, radioactive tracer studies (monitoring incorporation of thymidine to DNA and uridine C-14 to RNA), and the succinic dehydrogenase inhibition test (SDI test) [33–38]. Although these tests have been extremely useful in ruling out inactive compounds, the correlation between in vitro and in vivo tumor sensitivity testing is often disappointing. Similarly, such procedures often fail to provide significant toxologic data on specific human organelles. Some further limitations of in vitro models for testing anti-tumor agents include (1) failure to detect the activity of the compounds, which become active only after modification by host tissues; (2) failure to detect agents that may act indirectly rather than directly on tumor cells; (3) some compounds may be active in vivo only in large concentrations, which may be overlooked in fixed or low concentrations tested in vitro; (4) intrinsically active compounds may not remain stable for the duration of an in vitro test; and, (5) using microbiological assays, one may frequently detect antibacterial activity for agents completely devoid of antitumor activity [39]. In the case of cultured prostatic carcinoma, some deficiencies have been frequently noteworthy, as pointed out in other chapters in this book.

Carcinoma of the prostate is a disease of unknown etiology, with a median age for tumor diagnosis of 55 to 70 years. It is rarely seen in men younger than 45. Carcinoma of the prostate is the second most common site of cancer causing death in men, and approximately 63,000 new cases are diagnosed annually [41]. Surgical treatment for well-localized disease has been advocated since 1905 and, with the more recent addition of pelvic lymphadenectomy, McCullough reports five- and ten-year survivals of 82% and 62%, respectively [42, 43]. With widespread disease, survival decreases dramatically. This author reports ten-year survival for stage C disease of 29%; 50% of stage D patients, however, are dead within one year of diagnosis [44]. Radiation therapy is another accepted mode of treatment of localized disease [45]. Only 20% of patients with prostatic carcinoma, however, have with stage A or B disease at the time of diagnosis [46]. The remaining 80% are candidates for palliation. While dramatic results in patients with widespread metastases and bone pain have been reported with the use of estrogen, hormonal therapy has little effect on prolongation of life [14, 47]. These patients almost invariably relapse with an "autonomous," hormonally independent tumor.

Clinical experimental trials using nonhormonal cytotoxic chemotherapeutic agents in prostate carcinoma have been limited. This is due, in part, to lack of appropriate animal models with prostatic neoplasia. Because of these limitations, it has been suggested, as mentioned, that further attention be directed at rodent animal model systems. The ideal animal model for prostatic carcinoma should include tumors with spontaneous appearance in aged animals, with histological and biochemical profiles comparable to human disease. In additional, these tumors should metastasize, be hormonally dependent, obstruct the urinary tract, and demonstrate response to "appropriate" therapy. Finally, and of paramount importance, these tumors should be transplantable into large numbers of syngeneic animals with characteristics and parameters that can be monitored thoroughly for diagnostic and therapeutic applications. Unfortunately, this perfect animal model system does not exist, although spontaneous prostatic carcinoma has been described in a few select strains [23, 30, 48]. These tumor systems suffer from an extremely low frequency rate of appearance, a histologic picture oftentimes dissimilar to human disease, and, in some systems, tumor transplantation is achieved only with great difficulty. Other reasons for the lack of development of animal model systems for use in the study of prostatic cancer tumor biology include "lack of perfect animal model," and the emphasis that has been placed on the response of patients with prostatic carcinoma to hormonal manipulation.

Although other animal species than rodents develop benign prostatic hypertrophy (ie, the dog), prostatic carcinoma is much less common in dogs and is almost nonexistent in other animal species [49] . Several investigators have used the introduction of chemicals into the prostate to develop tumors. For example, Moore and Melchionna injected rat prostates with 1:2 benzpryene in the anterior lobe; however, these tumors did not metastasize. Dunning et al inserted pellets of 20 methylcholanthrene into the prostate of rats, with a resultant tumor that was transplantable and did produce metastases. Other investigators have repeated this study and found epidermoid prostatic carcinoma [50] . In Brendler's study, these tumors were not influenced by hormonal manipulation. Other investigators have similarly produced prostate cancer by injection of chemical agents [24, 51, 52] . Still others have evaluated virus-transformed prostatic tissues and have studied the tumor kinetics in tissue culture plates containing prostatic tissues [53–55] .

Recently, rat rodent prostatic carcinoma models have been the subject of much investigational work; specifically, the Dunning-Copenhagen rat model, the AXC rat model, the germ-free Wistar rat model, and the Nb prostatic rat model have been the subject of intensive investigations [23, 25–29, 48] . These investigations have, for the most part, centered on characterizing the appropriate animal model systems and determining the efficacy of the various forms of therapy available, both hormonal and cytotoxic.

THE DUNNING-COPENHAGEN RAT MODEL

In 1961 a spontaneous tumor of the prostate was observed at autopsy in a Copenhagen male rat from a 54th brother-to-sister generation line, 2331 [30] . The tumor occupied a large portion of the lower abdominal cavity and involved, primarily, the dorsal prostatic gland. This tumor was inoculated into ten rats, four of which were from the same inbred line as the source of the primary tumor, and six of which were F1 hybrids from a Copenhagen-Fisher cross. No metastases were identified from the original tumor. These tumors grew slowly and became palpable after the 60th day in each of the inoculated rats. Histologically, the tumors showed glandular formation, with a great deal of cellular material corresponding to normal dorsal-type glands of the rat prostate that was positive for PAS stain and negative to dithiazanine stain, typical of the dorsal prostate gland. Blood samples did not indicate elevated serum acid phosphatase levels, however. This tumor has been passaged for continued study and has been evaluated for hormonal sensitivity and testosterone metabolism [56, 57] . More recently, Coffey et al have described further morphologic, biochemical, electron microscopic, histologic, and histochemical staining of this tumor [58] . It is of interest that therapeutic agents, including testosterone proprionate, diethylstilbestrol, flutamide and estramustine phosphate, ℓ-asparaginase, actinomycin-D, CCNU, hydroxyurea, 5-fluorouracil, cis-platinum, cyclophosphamide and orchiectomy, Adriamycin and stilbestrol, alone and in combination with other chemotherapeutic agents, have been explored [59, 60]. The results of the therapy reveal that ℓ-asparaginase, CCNU, and actinomycin-D had no effect on tumor growth, whereas, 5-fluorouracil, hydroxyurea, cis-platinum, cyclophosphamide, orchiectomy, cyclophosphamide and Adriamycin, diethylstilbestrol, Adriamycin, cyclophosphamide and Adriamycin plus 5-fluorouracil and diethylstilbestrol, and diethylstilbestrol plus cyclophospha-mide all had a significant effect on retarding tumor growth (P < 0.03). Further-more, Coffey et al described some of the characteristics of the Dunning prostatic adenocarcinoma and anaplastic prostate carcinoma tumor models. The well-differentiated prostatic adenocarcinoma, R3327-H, has the histologic pattern of columnar epithelial cells with microvili lining numerous well-developed acini. The biochemical profile of this tumor reveals it to be similar to the dorsal lateral prostatic tissue. Androgens are required for maximal tumor growth, and this tumor grows best in intact, mature males. Additionally, doubling time for this tumor has been calculated and is approximately every 20 days. Also, this tumor responds to certain forms of therapy, including partial regression, with castration, anti-androgen therapy, or estrogen therapy. However, a small number of cells, approximately 20%, are hormonally insensitive and continue to grow despite hormonal therapy. The anaplastic variant of this tumor is R3327-AT, has a histologic pattern consisting of no acini formation or columnar epithelial structures and a lobar chemical correlation to normal lobes of the rat prostate. It does not require androgens for growth and, in fact, grows equally well in females, intact males, and castrate males.

GERM-FREE WISTAR RAT PROSTATIC CARCINOMA MODEL

Pollard recently reported nine aging, germfree Wistar rats to have a distinct prostatic adenocarcinoma, and no viral agent had been detected in the tumor cells. Investigations on these prostatic carcinomas revealed high white blood cell counts, accumulations of leukocytes in tumor tissues, and an excessive number of leukocytes in the splenic red pulp. In addition, these prostatic carcinomas had metastases. These prostatic carcinomas responded to diethylstilbestrol therapy, with tumor weights of less than one-half of those in saline-treated groups. Furthermore, in the saline-treated group, metastases on the lung surface were larger and over twice as numerous as in the diethylstilbestrol-treated animals. In tissue culture two types of cells were identified. The first was the epithelial type showing mitotoc figures and staining positive for acid phosphatase. The second was connector tissue cells, which were negative for acid phosphatase. These prostatic tumors have been investigated with various therapeutic modalities, including chloroform, halothane, ether, sodium barbiturate, x-rays, cyclophosphamide, Corynebacterium parvum, aspirin, and indomethacin. The latter four agents employed had the effect of retarding the number of metastatic foci [25, 26, 61, 62].

A X C RAT ADENOCARCINOMA MODEL

Shain et al, while in the process of evaluating the sex of aging on certain aspects of the endocrinologic determinants of the rat prostate, observed prostatic lesions in some aged A X C rats. In seven of the 41 animals examined, the occurrence of spontaneous adenocarcinoma of the ventral prostate was observed. The histologic appearance of this tumor is characterized by marked atypia of the proliferating cells, expansion of the affected glands, mitotic figures, and mitoses. These tumors have been the subject of investigations of such factors as steroid hormone regulation of prostatic epithelial cell function, androgen receptors in the aging rat prostate, testosterone metabolism by the ventral and dorsal lateral prostate of the aging rat, and metabolic by-products of testosterone [27, 28, 63, 64].

THE Nb RAT PROSTATIC ADENOCARCINOMA MODEL

Discussion

The Nb rat is an inbred strain developed by R.L. Noble of the Cancer Research Center in Vancouver [29, 65–67]. Dr. Noble has developed this black-hooded rat colony over the past 33 years from original stock derived from Dr. J.B. Cullip's laboratory at McGill University. Recently, the Medical Research Council of Canada, upon evaluating the genetics and degree of inbreeding produced by Dr. Noble, "officially" designated this strain Nb (Noble). The origin of this strain is somewhat clouded, but it probably arouse from a Long-Evans rat. In the breeding program, albino, yellow, and red-hooded offspring are discarded, and only black-hooded rats are mated. The present strain, although random littermate breeding, follows more than 33 backcross generations over the past 22 years. Although the major histocompatibility complex of the Nb rat has not been identified, littermates readily accept reciprocal skin allografts and tumor transplants and do not stimulate each other in mixed lymphocyte reactions.

Of striking importance is that the Nb rat is markedly susceptible to induction of prostatic adenocarcinoma by implantation of hormones in young rats. Using androgen and estrogen implants, the incidence of spontaneous prostatic carcinoma increases from 0.45% to 20%, with a mean duration of treatment for tumor induction of 37 to 70 weeks. Moreover, in animals in which the tumor has been induced, 25% have urinary tract obstruction, 40% have extensive intraperitoneal disease, and 20% have metastatic disease to the liver and lungs. These tumors transplant readily into unconditioned animals. Furthermore, the histologic pattern of this tumor resembles human adenocarcinoma (Fig. 1). The tumor mass is made up of compact solid nests and cords of malignant cells, with little cytoplasm and large hyperchromatic nuclei showing variations in size and shape. Most of the nuclei are round oval in configuration, and mitoses are common. In some areas, the malignant cell nests are less compact, and there is an attempt at gland formation, with

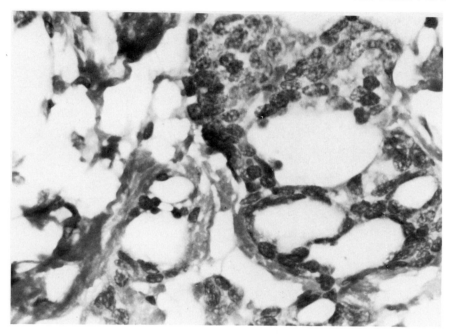

Fig. 1. Nb rat prostatic adenocarcinoma. Note the glandular formation and ductal structures that are present. This well-differentiated adenocarcinoma is of the androgen-dependent tumor line 2 Pr 129 and has remained stable for multiple transplant generations (hematoxylin and eosin stain; magnification, × 525; at this power, note the hyperchromatic nuclei).

rudimentary lumens present. In still other areas, the cords of tumor cells are surrounded by loose to very compact connective tissue, and the cords have easily recognizable ductal fissures and structures. Indeed, these tumors have been repetitively transplanted in Nb rats and histologically have remained stable.

These tumors can be classified as being androgen dependent, autonomous, or estrogen dependent (Table I). This classification depends on which of the hormones is responsible for progression of growth, and the data correlate with the hormonal dependence of the transplants. Some tumors that initially appeared to be estrogen dependent progressed, over the course of several months, to an autonomous situation in which their growth could no longer be influenced by hormonal manipulation. In contrast, of a total of 200 Nb prostate tumors, only one, initially thought to be estrogen dependent, progressed to an androgen-dependent tumor and has remained so for 32 transplant generations. In this discussion attention is directed primarily at the androgen-dependent tumors and the autonomous tumors.

The autonomous Nb prostate carcinoma is composed primarily of large solid

TABLE I. Nb Rat Tumor Model Classification

Tumor	Doubling time (days)	Time to achieve 1 cm³ growth (days)	Acid phosphatase IU/gm tissue (range)	Histology
Androgen dependent				
2 Pr-128	5.3	36	14.1 (12.3–15.7)	Gland formation,
2 Pr-129	7.5	51	12.5 (10.0–15.0)	ductal structures present
Autonomous				
13 Pr	4.3	29	6.4 (5.2–7.1)	Scant gland formation,
102 Pr	6.0	41	7.2 (6.4–7.8)	cords and sheets of
18 Pr	4.6	31	5.4 (4.8–6.1)	malignant cells, moderate mitotic activity
Estrogen dependent				
52 Pr	8.5	58	8.4 (8.0–9.0)	Glandular formation,
114 Pr	7.3	50	4.1 (3.7–5.0)	well differentiated

sheets and masses of malignant cells. The intervening stroma is ill defined and sparse. The masses of neoplastic cells have a moderate amount of pale-staining amphophilic cytoplasm, with poorly defined cell borders, large nuclei, and a large nucleus. The androgen-dependent carcinomas are made up of cords, well-defined trabeculae of malignant cells with glandular, ductal structures and fissures apparent, lined by, for the most part, cuboidal and columnar epithelial cells. There is a modest amount of cytoplasm with ill-defined cell borders. The nuclei are smaller than those seen in the autonomous tumors, and some nuclei contain nucleoli (Fig. 2).

Factors that may be important in the rate of tumor development are the duration of treatment, the steroid dose, and, possibly, the intermittent application of sex hormones. The hormone dependency and autonomy of these tumors parallels the human situation with respect to hormone dependency and eventual progression to autonomy, advanced disease, metastases, and death. Without exception, all tumors are readily transplantable into Nb rats. Over the past several years Dr. Noble has described the appearance of approximately 200 prostate rad adenocarcinomas. However, out laboratory unit has chosen to classify and study only eight such tumors and to concentrate specifically on the five androgen-dependent and autonomous tumors. The other tumors that Dr. Noble initially characterized are maintained in our laboratory tissue bank. Furthermore, the viability and successful transplantation of frozen tissues has been demonstrated and is accomplished without difficulty.

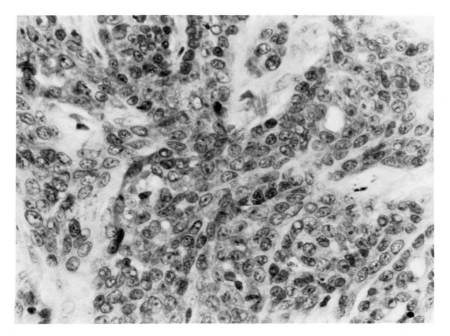

Fig. 2. Nb rat prostatic adenocarcinoma. This section is from autonomous tumor 18 Pr. Note the gland formation, the nests of cords, and the sheets of malignant cells with prominent nucleoli and the hyperchromatic nuclei (hematoxylin and eosin; magnification, × 385).

Since the work of Huggins and Hodges, human prostatic cancer has been shown to be influenced by hormonal manipulation and to be primarily androgen dependent [6]. Thus, the major therapeutic attempts have been directed at suppressing androgenic stimulus to the prostate. The most common way of achieving this goal is by bilateral orchiectomy, estrogen administration, anti-androgen therapy, and/or adrenalectomy. Bilateral orchiectomy directly reduces testosterone production. Estrogens act as potent inhibitors of gonadotrophic secretion and suppress leuteinizing hormone release and testosterone production [7, 11, 16]. Additional effects that have been reported include decreased testicular stored agenesis and in vitro inhibition of DNA polymerase and 5-alpha reductase activity [16]. Adrenalectomy, either medical with aminoglutethimide or surgical, is aimed at reduction of extratesticular androgen sources that have served as stimuli to the prostatic carcinoma. Investigations have revealed that this does have a beneficial effect in some patients [68, 69]; however, the constellation of data indicates that hormonal therapy has only a palliative effect and, therefore, a limited response, with little impact on overall mortality. Hormonal therapy decreases morbidity by decreasing pain and reducing hydronephrosis for a limited time, until the tumor no longer responds to hormonal therapy and becomes autonomous. This animal model system provides an avenue for the study of both hormone-dependent (androgen-dependent) tumors and autonomous tumors. Throughout the multiple transplant generations, in no case has an androgen-dependent tumor progressed to autonomy in our laboratory unit. The versatility of this animal system, with both types of tumors, androgen dependent and autonomous, is apparent. The characterization of these tumors will be presented, including histology, biochemistry, histochemistry, acid phosphatase content, percent of metastases, doubling time, tumor latency, hormone response, presence of receptors, as well as the documentation of the hormone dependence and its method of characterization. Additionally, this animal model system has lent itself nicely to heterotransplantation into nude mice, and hormone-dependent patterns have been similar in the heterotransplants to those observed in the Nb rats. The combination of the Nb rat and nude mouse model to study the Nb rat prostatic carcinoma is applicable for many hormonal and chemotherapeutic manipulations, as is further defined later in this chapter.

The method of inducing the Nb rat prostatic carcinomas consists of implanting steroid pellets [29, 67]. These pellets are made individually in a hand press and, for routine work, consist of approximately 10 mg of a 90% steroid, 10% cholesterol mixture. Pure steroid pellets can be made if the crystal size of the hormones used is large. However, the use of the binding agent, cholesterol, facilitates the making of these pellets. The pellets are the same size, but with different concentrations of hormones. In Dr. Nobel's work, estriol was one of the more insoluble compounds, and a 90% pellet disappeared from its subcutaneous implant site in approximately six to seven months, whereas, stilbestroi dissolved in only three months. An advantage of the pellets is that they can be palpated and removed surgically at any time. In most of Dr. Noble's early experiments, the pellet was inserted into the rat at the time of tumor implant, as he had found that prior pelleting was of no advantage and that removal of the pellet containing steroid did not impart a subsequent hormonal status suitable for tumor takes. Additionally, Dr. Noble's laboratory, using radioactive steroids, has measured the absorption of esterone from similarly made pellets and found that the weight change of the pellet closely reflected the loss of the hormone. Using predominantly estrogen pellets, Dr. Noble was able to induce carcinomas of many organs, including adrenal gland, breast, uterus, ovary, salivary gland, cervix, pituitary gland, and Leydig cell carcinoma.

Grossly recognizable prostatic adnocarcinoma in Nb rats after treatment with steroids in the form of pellets was initially observed by Dr. Noble in several groups. Animals treated with only one testosterone pellet did not develop prostate carcinoma, whereas, in animals treated with two pellets, 16.6% did develop prostate carcinoma, with a mean duration of 57 weeks in some five of 30 animals. Of these initial five tumors, three were easily and readily transplantable and have been passed to established lines. The incidence increased to 20% when three testosterone proprionate pellets were implanted; however, the duration necessary was 64 weeks as an average, with a range of 29 to 90 weeks. In this group, 11 of 55 rats developed tumor; metastases were present in four; and in eight animals transplantable established lines have been observed. The most successful combination of estrone pelleting and testosterone proprionate included one esterone and three testosterone pellets. The mean duration necessary for tumor induction was 46 weeks, with an average in the range of 27 to 62 weeks. In such series, 18% of the animals developed tumors of the prostate. Four animals had metastases present at the time of necropsy, and five tumors of this group have been established and transplanted successfully. Since Dr. Nobel's initial report, he has continued to develop and induce prostate cancers in this species.

Our laboratory unit has chosen to study a small number of tumors extensively. Additionally, we have abandoned the pelleting technique, as described by Noble, and we have switched to the use of Silastic implants as a means of increasing levels of the hormones 17-beta-estradiol and testosterone. We have also used this method in a preliminary sense to induce these tumors hormonally. Initially, all of the tumors that were induced by Dr. Nobel's method were autonomous, with one exception, that being the adenocarcinoma Pr 52, which was characterized by slower growth, and this has been estrogen dependent for 12 generations. However, with continued stimulation of this "estrogen"-dependent tumor with androgens, certain sublines of the tumor have developed, which have demonstrated an androgen-dependent nature. In our laboratory unit, over 32 transplant tumor generations, the androgen-dependent tumor has remained androgen dependent, the autonomous tumors have remained autonomous, and the hormonal manipulation studies with estrogen-dependent tumors have revealed that they have remained estrogen dependent to date.

In order to assess and further define the hormonal relationship and its effect on tumor growth, or early work was directed at assigning and verifying the hormonal influences existent now in some of the tumors that were generously donated to us by Dr. Noble. The specific tumors that were studied (Table I) were subject to experimental manipulations. Estrogen-dependent tumors were implanted into animals in the following subgroups: (1) androgenized animals; (2) normal females; (3) normal males; and, (4) estrogenized males. The results obtained revealed that estrogen-dependent tumors grew statistically significantly better in estrogenized animals than in androgenized animals. Some tumor growth was observed in various animals in each group, but this tumor growth was always less than 0.2 the tumor growth of the estrogenized animals. The androgen-dependent tumors 2 Pr 128 and 2 Pr 129 were subject to similar experiments. Briefly stated, the groups consisted of estrogenized animals, androgenized animals, normal females, and normal males, and this tumor, too, grew statistically significantly better in androgenized hosts ($P < 0.003$). In normal, unmanipulated females the tumor did have some tumor growth, but that was less than 10% of the tumor volume of androgenized animals.

TABLE II. Tumor Growth: Nb Rats*

	Number of tumors growing / Number of tumors implanted
Autonomous tumors 18 Pr, 13 Pr-12, 102 Pr	
Normal males and normal females	343/351
Estrogenized males	72/74
Androgenized males	87/90
Estrogenized females	84/88
Androgenized females	76/79
Androgen-dependent tumors 2 Pr-128, 2 Pr-129	
Normal males	296/302
Estrogenized males	3/115[a]
Castrate males with testosterone implants	125/128
Normal females	2/78[a]
Androgenized females	135/139
Estrogen-dependent tumors 52 Pr, 114 Pr	
Normal females	48/52
Androgenized females	3/66[a]
Castrate females with estrogen implants	49/55
Normal males	3/46[a]
Estrogenized males	31/34

*Tumor volume $\geq$ 20% of control — ie, androgenized hosts control for androgen-dependent tumor study.
[a]$P < 0.01$ when compared to growth in these groups.
NOTE: Evaluation of Nb rats subjected to various hormonal manipulations with the three types of tumors reveals statistical significance, especially in the hormone-dependent types. In this experiment animals were subjected to the hormonal manipulation prior to tumor transplantation. As can be seen, rarely will a tumor take occur in an unandrogenized animal.

The autonomous tumors 18 Pr, 18 Pr 12, and 102 Pr were similarly subjected to transplantation into normal males, normal females, androgenized males, estrogenized males, estrogenized females, and androgenized females, and tumor growth was equal in all groups, without any statistical variation for better tumor growth in either androgenized or estrogenized hosts (Table II; Fig. 3). Histologically, similarities were observed between the donor tumors and the transplanted tumors and have remained stable throughout multiple transplant tumor generations.

We were also interested in heterotransplanting these Nb rat prostatic carcinomas into congenitally athymic (nude) mice, a procedure has been the subject of much recent investigation in tumor cell biology, and in assessing potential therapeutic options for treatment. This animal model has been used as a recipient of heterotransplanted human tumors and has been the source of intense evaluation over the

TUMOR RESPONSE

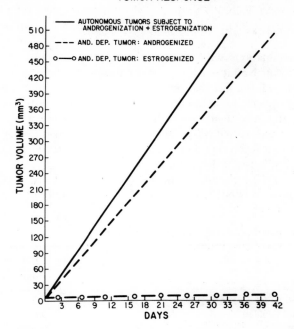

Fig. 3. The autonomous tumors represented herein have been subjected to androgenization and estrogenization. There has been no effect on tumor growth as can be seen. The androgen-dependent tumor 2 Pr-129 is depicted, showing the effects of androgenization on tumor growth. All animals had significant tumor growth during the period of observation. The tumors subjected to estrogenization and/or castration reveal that these animals so estrogenized do not have appreciable tumor growth, especially when contrasted to androgenized animals.

last decade. For those unfamiliar with the congenitally athymic (nude) mouse, a brief description follows.

In 1966 a hairless mutant was discovered in a mouse colony in Scotland [70]. Two years later, it was found to be athymic (nude). (The genes governing hairlessness in thymic agenesis group were found to be either closely linked or identical and are inherited as autosomal recessive traits, genetically symbolized by the designation [71].) Although nude mice contain adequate numbers of T-cell precursors, as demonstrated by immunofluorescence using in vivo absorbed rat antibrain sera, they are, nonetheless, significantly deprived of their thymic-dependent immune system [72, 73]. Indeed, they accept transplants from a variety of sources, both allogeneic and xenogeneic. More than 150 carcinomas have been successfully transplanted into nude mice with a general acceptance rate of approximately 20% to 25% [74]. However, tumors that can be transplanted by serial passage in syngeneic systems are uniformly accepted in nude mice. These transplantage tumors grow locally to form large, uniform masses. Thus, they can be serially measured, needle biopsied, and transplanted from generation to generation.

Hormonal determinations, with regard to the autonomy or hormone dependence of the tumors from the Nb rat prostate, were carried out in the nude mouse. Of particular importance is the fact that these heterotransplanted tumors retained their hormone dependence for autonomy. This, indeed, was statistically significant (P < 0.01) (Table III). Also significant is the finding that the histologic picture of nude mouse heterotransplanted Nb rat prostatic carcinomas was similar to that seen in the Nb rat host receiving tumor transplants, and heterotransplanted carcinomas were similar to the donor tumors [75].

The generation of the congenitally athymic (nude) mouse colony is of interest. The colony used is on an N:NIH(S) background. The availability of these mice

TABLE III. Tumor Growth: Classification for (Nude) Mice*

	Number of tumors growing
	Number of tumors implanted
Autonomous tumors 18 Pr, 13 Pr-12, 102 Pr	
Normal males and females	99/100
Estrogenized males	67/70
Androgenized males	54/56
Estrogenized females	58/60
Androgenized females	69/70
Androgen-dependent tumors 2 Pr-128, 2 Pr-129	
Normal males	51/53
Estrogenized males	4/70[a]
Castrate males with testosterone implants	58/63
Normal females	3/58[a]
Androgenized females	41/45
Estrogen-dependent tumors 52 Pr, 114 Pr	
Normal females	43/45
Androgenized females	2/42[a]
Castrate females with estrogen implants	41/44
Normal males	3/39[a]
Estrogenized males	22/26

*Growth; tumor volume > 60 mm.
[a]P < 0.01 when compared to growth of tumors in these groups; ie, androgen-dependent tumor growth in androgenized hosts is significant when compared to tumor growth in estrogenized hosts.

NOTE: Heterotransplantation of Nb rat tumors into nude mice was done to assess hormonal responsiveness. Note the similar response in the heterotransplants as seen in the Nb rat syngeneic recipients in comparing data with Table II.

results from a vigorously operating program at the National Institutes of Health from 1971 through 1974 [72, 74]. This colony is under the direction of Dr. M. Eric Gershwin at the University of California, Davis. Nude mice were placed on this background because of well-known characteristics of the N:NIH(S) mouse for vigor, fertility, and longevity. These characteristics have continued in these nude mice and permit serial observation and long-term study, including administration of chemotherapeutic agents, without the hazards of runting and early death, as evidenced in most inbred nude colonies. Indeed, under these conditions, this colony of outbred nude mice survives eight to 14 months without signs of runting or cachexia. A longer survival (ie, 12–18 months) would be achieved in a totally unmanipulated system. Nevertheless, the mean survival of 8 to 14 months readily permits serial observations. Finally, this colony is free of mouse hepatitis virus, a frequent problem in other nude mouse colonies. The fertility of these animals permits raising the large numbers of mice necessary for the observations and experiments described later in this chapter. In our laboratory unit mice are raised by mating of nu/+ females with nu/nu males. Approximately three days after delivery, at which time haired n+ mice can readily be distinguished from their nu/nu littermates, the nu/+ offspring are culled to be foster nursed by other nu/+ mothers. This markedly reduces fetal wastage secondary to the more vigorous suckling of nu/+ offspring over their slightly smaller nude litter mates. The weight of nude mice at weaning is within 10% of the weight of the nu/+ littermates. Breeding is performed under specific pathogen-free conditions in a bioclean unit. Experimental mice are removed from the bioclean unit and placed in a Model C laminar flow air station (Germ-Free Labs., Miami, FL). Two males and up to four females are placed in polycarbonate cages fitted with Whatman qualitative filter paper covers, autoclaved, and vitamin supplemented. Purina Lab Chow and water, brought to a pH of 2.8 with HCl, are provided ad libitum.

Transplantation of Tumors

As noted above, one of the advantages of the Nb rat adenocarcinoma is the marked degree of tumor homogeneity. Thus, the tumors can be transplanted into multiple recipients without the attendant hazards of variable tumor transfer. Transplantation of the tumors is performed in a manner similar to that described elsewhere [79]. Briefly, an Nb rat prostatic tumor grows from a 2 mm^3 implant to a 1 cm^3 mass in a period of two and one-half to eight weeks, depending upon the specific tumor (Table I). Similar kinetic data for growth rates an provided for the tumors and their growth in the nude mouse (Table IV). Tumors from our tissue bank or from hosts with tumors growing in vivo are placed directly under the skin, and the skin is closed with a single sterile clip. After suitable mass is achieved, the tumor is resected and minced into 2 mm^3 fragments and transplanted to appropriate recipients. The transplantation procedure is performed under anesthesia and takes approximately 15 to 30 seconds. A skin incision is made with a sterile

TABLE IV. Growth Study in Heterotransplants

Tumor type	Days[a]
Autonomous	42
Androgen-dependent	70
Estrogen-dependent	83

[a]Days to achieve 1 cm^3 tumor volume in nude mice
NOTE: Growth kinetics of heterotransplants. This table depicts the various times necessary for these heterotransplanted tumors to achieve a 500 mm^3 mass (1 cm^3) in congenitally athymic nude mice. Note that there is a difference between the different tumor types that parallels the doubling times previously identified in Table I for Nb rats.

scalpel blade and the tumor is inserted in the subcutaneous pocket. It should be emphasized that all tumors transplanted for studies of chemotherapeutic agents and hormone manipulations have been derived from fresh tissue, not from frozen tissue bank sources. The tissue bank is maintained to permit storage of the large volumes of tumor tissue needed for replicate copies. Thus, at a given time, attention can be focused intensively on an individual tumor. A tumor nodule of 1 cm^3 is sufficient for implantation of 100 to 250 animals. Thus, it is possible to use transplantable tumors from the same transfer generation (ie, standardized replicate tissue). As emphasized, the reproducibility of this method of tissue transplantation is readily demonstrated by a similar growth pattern in multiple littermate recipients. After tumor transplantation, all of the animals are observed twice weekly, with specific tumor measurements begun when palpable masses are demonstrated. This quantitation is performed with a Vernier caliper measurement of length and width of a normally ellipsoid, but occasionally irregularly shaped, tumor mass. Such linear measurements are used to estimate tumor volume and tumor weight, as well as actual tumor weight at the conclusion of the experiment. The formula used for such volume measurements is tumor volume in mm^3 = width^2 × length/2. For comparative purposes, tumor weight is considered to have a unit density of 1.0 and, thus, when the width and the length are in mm, the weight will be in mg. This assumption of unit density is based primarily on a water content of approximately 60% or 70% of these tissues. Rarely, the specific gravity is more likely 1.06 to 1.12. However, since it will vary from tumor to tumor and, since quantitative correlations are made within a given tumor for various chemotherapeutic or radiotherapeutic programs, statistical evaluation is possible.

Characteristics of Individual Tumors: Latency, Histologic Characteristics

Androgen-dependent tumors 2 Pr 129, B 11A, and 2 Pr 128 are among those that had changed characteristics early in Dr. Noble's experience and were the result of prolonged androgenization of a previously estrogen-dependent tumor,

52 Pr. Tumors 2 Pr 128 and 2 Pr 129 have remained androgen-dependent for more than 40 tumor transplant generations. The histologic characteristics of these tumors include moderate gland formation, with mitoses, ductal structures, and fissures apparent. In addition, there are hyperchromatic nuclei, and a large nucleus is present. The mean latency for these tumors to achieve a 10 mm^3 tumor mass from a 2 mm^3 tumor implant is between six and 11 days. The latency period and the histologic characteristics have remained stable throughout many tumor transplant generations.

Tumors 13 Pr 12, 102 Pr, and 18 Pr were the autonomous tumors chosen for study by this laboratory unit. An explanation of our coding system is as follows: Pr represents prostate; the prefix — ie, 13 — is the thirteenth prostatic induced tumor and 12, or the suffix, is the transplant generation that was the source of our tumor from Dr. Noble. These tumors are characterized by a shorter latency period of four to ten days, with the shortest latency being four to seven days in the autonomous tumor 13 Pr 12. The histologic characteristics include abundant mitotic activity with a prominent stromal pattern, large nucleoli, and scant gland formation. The estrogen-dependent tumors are characterized by a longer latnecy period to achieve a 10 mm^3 mass in the order of magnitude of 13 to 17 days and are characterized by marked gland formation with prominent nucleoli and ductal formation. They are similar, histologically, to the androgen-dependent tumor, the distinguishing characteristic being that estrogen is necessary for tumor growth progression.

The growth kinetics of the various tumor types have been studied in terms of the time required for a 2 mm^3 wedge to achieve a 1 cm^3 tutor mass. The autonomous tumors achieve this tumor size generally in a shorter time than do the hormone-dependent tumors. Within each individual tumor line, however, there is stability and reproducibility in terms of the time necessary to achieve this tumor volume, and this has varied less than 10% among the many different tumor transplants observed (Table I). The doubling times of the individual tumors have been calculated with a slight modification of the formula used by Coffey [23] and are as follows: androgen-dependent tumors 2 Pr 128, 5.3 days; 2 Pr 129, 7.5 days; autonomous tumors 13 Pr 12, 4.2–4.4 days; 102 Pr, 6 days; 18 Pr, 4.2–4.6 days; estrogen-dependent tumor 52 Pr, 8.5 days (Table I). Most of these calculations have been made using 2 mm^3 tumor implants. Using injectable cell suspensions, the doubling time calculated is approximately the same, although the latency period is prolonged by one to three days for each tumor evaluated with the cell suspension technique.

Hormone Manipulation

Hormonal manipulation is accomplished using subcutaneous Silastic implants of testosterone and 17-beta estradiol. The dry crystalline hormone is hand packed into medical grade Silastic tubing, which is then sealed with medical adhesive

(Dow Corning Company). The implants are placed through a small incision on the abdominal wall. Serum testosterone and 17-beta estradiol levels were determined in non-tumor-bearing animals by radioimmunoassay [78–80]. Serum testosterone in unmanipulated male animals ranged from 0.75 to 2.8 ng/ml, with the average being 1.63 ng/ml, whereas animals with Silastic testosterone implants had average serum testosterone levels of 11.5 ng/ml, with a range of 3.8 to 21.9 ng/ml. Estradiol levels in normal female rats ranged from 37 to 102 pg/ml, with an average of 59 pg/ml. Estrogen-implanted animals had a serum concentration ranging from 120 to 945 pg/ml, with the average being 369 pg/ml. As can be seen from these determinations, implanted animals had a definitely increased level of testosterone or estradiol. Manipulated Nb rats had serum testosterone and 17-beta estradiol levels reflecting treatment (Table V).

Hormonal induction through the use of 17-beta estradiol and testosterone Silastic implants was carried out in several males. The experiment was designed to see whether prostatic adenocarcinoma could be induced with the use of these implants in the same fashion that Dr. Noble induced such tumors via the pelleting technique. Indeed, with these Silastic steroid-containing implants, this unit has been able to induce prostatic adenocarcinoma in several animals, and these tumors have been successfully transplanted into Nb recipients. They have not, however, been classified in terms of autonomy or hormone dependency. The time of induction has ranged from as short a period as 18 weeks to as long as 36 weeks.

Histochemistry

Six different histochemical staining techniques have been performed on the Nb rat prostate tumors and on the normal prostatic dorsal lobe of the Nb rat. Two main stains were employed for acid phosphatase — the AZO-dye method and the pararosanalin method [81–83]. Other histochemical stains were used in determining the presence of alkaline phosphatase, ATPase, succinic acid dehydrogenase, and glucose-6-dehydrogenase. The amount of stain uptake was graded "blindly" by histochemists and has been assigned a value from 0 to 6, depending upon the intensity of the reactions in each tissue. As can be seen from Table VI, there is a correlation between relative amounts of enzyme activity in the normal prostatic tissues and those in the Nb rat prostatic adenocarcinomas. Additionally, histochemical identification of the enzyme activity of the visceral metastases, as well as pulmonary metastases, demonstrates the presence of acid phosphatase in this qualitative study. There exists, also, a differentiation in the amount of acid phosphatase present in the autonomous tumors versus the androgen-dependent tumors, with the androgen-dependent tumors having more. There is no other differentiation among the other enzymes stained for. The acid phosphatase and succinic dehydrogenase stains reveal a diffuse pattern in both the normal and the prostatic adenocarcinoma, with some localization to the cells themselves, with a concentration of uptake in the granules or organelles presumably representing lysosomes.

TABLE V. Hormone Determination in Nb Rats

Group	ng/ml (range)	
	Testesterone	
Males unmanipulated	1.63	(0.75−2.8)
Males with 1 cm Silastic testosterone implant	11.5	(3.8−21.9)
Castrated males	0.3	(0.1−2.1)
	17-β-estradiol pg/ml (range)	
Females unmanipulated	59	(37−102)
Females with 1 cm Silastic 17-β-estradiol implant	369	(120−945)
Castrated females	21	(11−43)

TABLE VI. Histochemistry Nb Rat Model

Enzyme	Tissue evaluated[a]				
	Normal prostate	Liver	Androgen dependent	Autonomous	Estrogen dependent
Acid phosphatase	++++	++++	+++	++	++
Alkaline phosphatase	++	++++++	++	+++	+++
ATPase	+	+++++	++	++++	+++
Succinic acid dehydrogenase	++	++++++	++	+++	+
Glucose 6-phosphate dehydrogenase	+	++++++	+	+	+

[a]Grading: + = positive; ++++++ = maximum.

These histochemical enzymatic determinations indicate that both the normal prostatic epithelium and prostate cancer of the Nb rat have similar enzymatic distribution, which favors the prostate as the origin of these tumors.

Recent studies by Muntzing et al were carried out to determine the activity distribution of acid phosphatase, alkaline phosphatase, nonspecific esterases, beta-glucuronidase, and aminopeptidase in the transplantable R3327 rat prostate adenocarcinoma from the Dunning-Copenhagen rat prostate model. These were compared with similar determinations in the four prostatic lobes of this rat. The conclusion was that the enzymatic profile of the R3327 adenocarcinoma closely resembles that of anterior and dorsal prostate, suggesting that the origin of this tumor probably is from one of these prostatic lobes, but this was not certain [84].

Quantitative acid phosphatase determinations on the various tumor samples, as well as normal prostatic tissue from the Nb rat, have been performed according to the method of Roy [85]. The results suggest that the androgen-dependent tumor has a higher acid phosphatase content than does the autonomous tumor. Interestingly enough, the rat liver has a higher concentration of acid phosphatase per gram of tissue analyzed than either of the tumor sources. Additionally, the acid phosphatase of a normal rat is in the same range as that of the autonomous Nb rat prostatic adenocarcinomas (Tables I and VII).

Biochemical Parameters

The following laboratory tests have been performed in order to determine baseline levels for Nb rats: hematocrit, hemoglobin, total protein, liver function tests, BUN and creatinine determinations, cholesterol levels, and serum acid phosphatase determinations. These values were obtained for animals with and without a tumor growing in vivo. The same determinations were made on animals with tumors in vivo, subjected to various chemotherapeutic agents and are discussed in a separate chapter (see Hormonal and Chemotherapeutic Considerations of the Nb Rat Model). The normal levels did not vary significantly from the levels obtained in animals with tumors growing in vivo. Note is made of the fact that in neither group were we able to detect any presence of serum acid phosphatase. Additionally, five samples have been analyzed via the radioimmunoassay method, courtesy of Smith Kline Laboratories, and all the values were found to be less than 1 ng/ml of acid phosphatase.

Nuclear Binding of Androgens in Prostatic Tumors

In preliminary work with this model system, Rennie, Bruchovsky and Noble studied the acid phosphatase activity in androgen binding sites and nuclei of the dorsal prostate and in prostatic tumors characterized by androgen-dependent, androgen-stimulated, or autonomous tumor growth [86]. In all tumors, acid phosphatase activity per mg of DNA is 50–65% that found in the dorsal lobe of the prostate. Specific activity of the enzyme is 100–150% higher in androgen-dependent tumors and even higher (300%) in autonomous tumors than in the dorsal lobe of the prostate. In vitro measurements of $(1, 2-^3H)$ dihydrotestosterone binding for nuclear extracts revealed that nuclei from the dorsal prostate have approximately 7,750 specific binding sites, whereas nuclei from the hormone-dependent tumors have 1,080 binding sites. Their preliminary work identifies the difference in nuclear activity of the autonomous and androgen-dependent tumors (Table VIII). The tumors from this laboratory unit have also been evaluated for the presence of cytosol receptors in collaboration with Drs. Richard Santen and Peter Fiel of the

Pennsylvania State University and the presence of cytosol androgen receptors has been found in androgen-dependent tumors to a higher degree than in autonomous tumors. It was possible to separate these groups only qualitatively according to the presence of receptors, marked receptor content, or the absence of receptors. Some of the difficulties involved in determining these receptors include the use of frozen stored tissues, which is currently being abandoned, and assays to be run will be run on fresh tumor samples only.

Hormonal Considerations

The androgen-dependent tumors grow best in the presence of an androgenized environment. Figure 3 is a graphic representation showing the effects of castration, estrogen administration, and androgen administration of androgen-dependent tumors in which no additional form of therapy was administered. Clearly, androgenized animals had a much more rapid progression in tumor growth than either unandrogenized males or castrate males. Similarly, female animals that were castrate and female animals that were castrate plus administration of androgen revealed similar findings, with androgenized females have a more maked tumor growth proliferation than unandrogenized females. The normal females not subject to castration had only small tumor growth in all of the experiments that have been designed and outlined thus far. This represented less than 0.2 of the growth of any of the other hosts, either androgenized or normal males. Autonomous tumors are not affected by hormonal manipulation, testerone or estogen implantation, or castration of oophorectomy. Their tumor group progression is unaffected when compared with saline-controlled groups.

In androgenized animals with tumors growing in vivo that have been previously supplemented with testosterone, we have observed that, upon removal of the testosterone, there was gradual shrinking of the tumor over the next 30 days. This tumor regression was accelerated if, at the time of testosterone implant removal an implant containing 17-beta-estriol was placed. A similar effect was also seen upon removal of testosterone and castration of the animal. It is interesting to note, also, that the combination of estrogenization and chemotherapy caused a more dramatic regression of tumor volume, a finding discussed in detail in a separate chapter (see Hormonal and Chemotherapeutic Considerations of the Nb Rat Model).

Metastases

The percentage of metastatic lesions appearing following subcutaneous tumor implantation of the various Nb rat prostatic adenocarcinomas does differ among the tumor types. Specifically, the autonomous tumors have a much higher rate of pulmonary metastasis and visceral metastasis, including mediastinal and liver metastases, as compared to the androgen-dependent tumors. Approximately 55—60% of saline control animals in which a subcutaneous tumor implant had been placed developed these metastases. This is in sharp contrast to the androgen-

TABLE VII. Acid Phosphatase*

	Specimen	Acid phosphatase (IU/gm tissue) (range)
	Normal prostate	5.2 ± 0.8
	Kidney	4.5 ± 1
	Liver	2.6 ± 5
Androgen dependent	2 Pr 128	14.1 (12.3–15.7)
	2 Pr 129	12.5 (10.0–15.0)
Autonomous	13 Pr	6.4 (5.2–7.1)
	102 Pr	7.2 (6.4–7.8)
	18 Pr	5.4 (4.8–6.1)
Estrogen dependent	52 Pr	8.4 (8.0–9.0)
	114 Pr	4.1 (3.7–5.0)

Metastases	
Pulmonary	Acid phosphatase (IU/gm tissue (range)
A.T.	15 (12.2–18.8)
A.D.	12 (9–14.5)
Liver	
A.T.	24 (15–40)
A.D.	30 (25–44)

The reason(s) for the difference in acid phosphatase content per gram of tissue analyzed for the different primary tumor types versus the metastatic lesions is unclear.

dependent tumors, in which only 18–22% of the animals developed these metastases. These findings have been useful in allowing us to compare additional parameters in regard to therapeutic efficacy. Of special note is the case of chemotherapy, in which one can measure not only the size of the tumor in terms of the chemotherapeutic response but also the decrease number of pulmonary or visceral metastases in response to that chemotherapy. This pattern of metastases has been verified through many experimental programs and is discussed further in the chapter on Hormonal and Chemotherapeutic Considerations of the Nb Rat Model.

SUMMARY

Nb rat prostatic adenocarcinomas have been successfully transplanted into groups of syngeneic Nb rats, as well as into congenitally athymic (nude) mice, with a high frequency of success. This rate of success is one characteristic of this system that allows for experimentation in vivo in large numbers of animals for statistical considerations such as the following: similarity to human prostatic

TABLE VIII. Androgen Receptors

Tumors	Nuclear receptors*
Androgen dependent	1080 ± 200
Autonomous	260 ± 100

Tumors	Cytosol
Androgen dependent	+++
Autonomous	+

*Androgen receptors in Nb rat tumors. The preliminary work on nuclear receptors has been performed by Drs. Rennie and Bruchovsky at the University of Alberta. There are obvious differences in receptor content in the nucleus of the cells analyzed between autonomous tumors and androgen-dependent tumors. Cytoplasmic receptors have been evaluated by this unit and qualitative assessment of androgen receptors has been achieved. The androgen-dependent tumors do have androgen receptors at a higher level than the autonomous tumors. However, the quantitation of the numbers of receptors has varied markedly from one determination to the next. The presence or absence of receptors has been consistent throughout the determination.

adenocarcinoma, histopathologic response to appropriate hormonal therapy in the case of androgen-dependent tumors, histochemical characteristics, presence of metastases, presence of acid phosphatase, preliminary data revealing the presence of receptors and autonomous tumor models that are refractory to hormonal manipulation (analogous to patients with prostatic carcinoma no longer sensitive to hormonal manipulation). Additionally, the stability in tumor growth kinetics, as well as the histologic and biochemical parameters, is an important consideration in this tumor model for chemotherapeutic and hormonal studies and the tumor response to such modalities. Of note is the fact that this tumor model rarely occurs spontaneously in aging rats. This animal model has been successfully used in evaluating chemotherapeutic and hormonal treatment protocols (discussed in the Hormonal and Chemotherapeutic Considerations of the Nb Rat Model chapter). Finally, the combination of the Nb prostatic adenocarcinoma model with the transplantation of these tumors to nude mice will enable us to evaluate chemotherapeutic efficacy in the immunocompetent as well as the immuno-depressed host.

ACKNOWLEDGMENTS

The authors are grateful to P. S. Rennie, MD, and N. Bruchovsky, MD, of the University of Alberta for their collaboration in determining nuclear receptors, and to Peter Fiel, MD, of Pennsylvania State University, Hershey Medical Center, for his assistance with the cytosol assay.

Support for this research was funded by the Elsa U. Pardee Foundation grant 601 and the University of California Cancer Research Coordinating Committee grant 78D10.

REFERENCES

1. Yagoda A: Nonhormonal cytotoxic agents in the treatment of prostatic adenocarcinoma. Cancer 32:1131–1140, 1973.
2. Murphy GP: Prostatic cancer: Progress and perspectives. In Murphy GP (ed): "Perspectives in Cancer Research Treatment." New York: Alan R Liss, Inc, 1973, pp 1–24.
3. Scott WW, Gibbons RP, Johnson DE, et al: Comparison of 5-fluorouracil (NSC-19893) and cyclophosphamide (NSC-26171) in patients with advanced carcinomas of the prostate. Cancer Chemother Rep 59:195–201, 1975.
4. Whitmore WF Jr: The natural history of prostate cancer. Cancer 32:1104–1112, 1973.
5. Prout GR Jr: Diagnosis and staging of prostatic carcinoma. Cancer 32:1096–1103, 1973.
6. Huggins C, Hodges CV: Studies on prostatic cancer: Effective castration of estrogens and androgen injection on serum phosphatases in metastatic carcinoma of the prostate. Cancer Res 1:293–297, 1941.
7. Blackard CE, Byar DT, Jordan WT: Orchiectomy for advanced prostatic carcinoma – A reevaluation. Urology 1:553–560, 1973.
8. Young HH II, Kent JR: Plasma testosterone levels in patients with prostatic carcinoma before and after treatment. J Urol 99:788–792, 1968.
9. Walsh PC, Gittes RF: Inhibition of extratesticular stimuli to prostatic growth in the castrate rat by antiandrogens. Endocrinology 87:624–627, 1970.
10. Robinson MRG, Thomas BS: Effect of hormonal therapy on plasma testosterone levels in prostatic carcinoma. Br Med J 4:391–394, 1971.
11. Franks LM: Estrogen treated prostatic cancer: The variation in responsiveness of the tumor cells. Cancer 13:490–501, 1960.
12. Tavares AS, Coasta J, Costa MJ: Correlation between ploidy and prognosis in prostatic carcinoma. J Urol 109:676–679, 1973.
13. Heaney JA, Chang HC, Daly JJ, Prout GR: Prognosis of clinically undiagnosed prostatic carcinoma and the influence of endocrine therapy. J Urol 118:283–287, 1977.
14. The Veterans Administration Cooperative Urological Research Group: Treatment and survival of patients with cancer of the prostate. Surg Gynecol Obstet 124:1011–1017, 1967.
15. Catalone WJ, Scott WW: Carcinoma of prostate: A review. J Urol 119:1–8, 1978.
16. Walsh PC: Hormonal therapy for prostatic carcinoma. Urol Clin North Am 2:125–140, 1975.
17. Shearer RJ, Hendry WF, Sommerville IF, Fergusson JD: Plasma testosterone: An accurate monitor of hormone treatment in prostatic cancer. Br J Urol 45:668–677, 1973.
18. Correa RJ Jr, Anderson RG, Gibbons RP, Mason JT: Latent carcinoma of the prostate – Why the controversy J Urol 111:644–646, 1974.
19. Scott WW, Johnson DE, Schmidt JD, et al: Chemotherapy of advanced prostatic carcinoma with cyclophosphamide or five fluorouracil: Results of first national randomized study. J Urol 114:909–911, 1975.
20. Schmidt JD, Johnson DE, Scott WW, et al: Chemotherapy of advanced prostatic cancer: Chemotherapy of advanced prostatic cancer. Urology 7:602–610, 1976.
21. Carter SK, Wasserman TH: The chemotherapy of urologic cancer. Cancer 36:729–747, 1975.

22. Flocks RH: Clinical cacner of the prostate; a study of the prostate; a study of 4,000 cases. JAMA 193:559–562, 1965.
23. Smolev KJ, Heston W, Scott WW, et al: Characterization of the Dunning R3327H prostatic adenocarcinoma: An appropriate animal model for prostatic cancer. Cancer Treat Rep 61:273–287, 1977.
24. Fingerhut B, Veenema RJ: An animal model for the study of prostatic adenocarcinoma. Invest Urol 15:42–48, 1977.
25. Pollard M, Chang CF, Burleson GR: Investigations on prostatic adenocarcinomas in rats. Cancer Treat Rep 61:153–156, 1977.
26. Pollard M: Spontaneous prostate adenocarcinomas in aged germ-free Wistar rats. J Natl Cancer Inst 51:1235–1241, 1973.
27. Shain S, McCullough B, Segaloff A: Spontaneous adenocarcinomas of the ventral prostate of aged AXC rats. J Natl Cancer Inst 55:177–180, 1975.
28. Shain S, McCullough B, Nitchuk M, et al: Prostate carcinogenesis in the AXC rat. Oncology 34:114–122, 1977.
29. Noble RL: The development of prostatic adenocarcinoma in the Nb rat following prolonged sex hormone administration. Cancer Res 37:1929–1933, 1977.
30. Dunning WF: Prostate in the rat. Natl Cancer Inst Monogr 12:351–369, 1963.
31. Foley GE, McCarthy RE, Binns VM, et al: A comparative study of the use of microorganisms in the screening of potential antitumor agents. NY Acad Sci Ann 76:413–441, 1958.
32. Holmes HL, Little JM: Tissue culture microtest for predicting response for human cancer to chemotherapy. Lancet 2:985–987, 1974.
33. Johnson RK, Goldin A: The clinical impact of screening and other experimental tumor studies. Cancer Treat Rep 2:1–31, 1975.
34. Knock FE, Galt RM, Oester YT, et al: The use of selected sulfhyohyl inhibitors in a preferential drug attack on cancer. Surg Gynecol Obstet 133:458–466, 1971.
35. DiPaolo J: Analysis of an individual chemotherapy assay system. Natl Cancer Inst Monogr 34:240–245, 1972.
36. Chi-Bom C, Williams A, Krasny J, et al: Inhibition of thymidine phosphorylation and DNA and histone synthesis in Ehrlich ascites carcinoma. Cancer Res 30:2652–2660, 1970.
37. Bickis IJ, Henderson IWD, Quastel JH: Biochemical studies of human tumors. II. In vitro estimation of individual tumor sensitivity to anticancer agents. Cancer 19:103–113, 1966.
38. Kondo T: Prediction of response of tumor and host to cancer chemotherapy. Natl Cancer Inst Monogr 34:251–256, 1972.
39. Handelsman H: The limitations of model systems in prostatic cancer. Oncology 34:96–99, 1977.
40. Noble RL: Contrast in androgen and estrogen induced tumors in Nb rats. Proc Am Assoc Cancer Res 16:186, 1975.
41. Silverberg E: Cancer statistics. Cancer 28:17–32, 1978.
42. McCullough DL, Prout GR Jr, Daly JJ: Carcinoma of the prostate and lymphatic metastases. J Urol 111:65–71, 1974.
43. McLaughlin AT, Saltzstein SL, McCullough DL, Gittes RF: Prostatic carcinoma: Incidence and location of suspected lymphatic metastases. J Urol 115:89–94, 1976.
44. Boxer YR, Kauffman JJ, Goodwin WE: Radical prostatectomy for carcinoma of the prostate: 1951–1976. A review of 239 patients. J Urol 117:208–213, 1977.
45. Bagshaw MA, Pistenna DA, Ray GR, et al: Evaluation of extended field radiotherapy for prostatic neoplasm: 1976 progress report. Cancer Treat Rep 61:297–306, 1977.

46. Parry WL: Prostatic malignancy. In "Urologic Surgery," Ed 2. Hagerstown, Maryland: Harper & Row, Inc., 1975, pp 546–548.
47. Balar JC III, Byer DT, Veterans Administration Cooperative Urologic Research Group: Estrogen treatment for cancer of the prostate – Early results with three doses of diethylstilbestrol and placebo. Cancer 26:257–261, 1970.
48. Drago JR, Ikeda RM, Maurer RE, Goldman LB, Tesluk H: The Nb rat: Prostatic adenocarcinoma model. Invest Urol (in press).
49. Brendler H: Experimental prostatic cancer: Background of the problem. Natl Cancer Inst Monogr 12:343–349, 1963.
50. Moore RA, Melchionna RH: Production of tumors of the prostate of the white rat with 1:2-benzpyrene. Am J Cancer 30:731–741, 1937.
51. Horning ES: Induction of glandular carcinomas of the prostate in the mouse. Lancet 251:829–831, 1946.
52. Heidelberger C, Iype PT: Malignant transformations in vitro by carcinogenic hydrocarbons. Science 155:214–219, 1967.
53. Fairley EE, Taulson BF: Morphologic and biochemical studies of virus (SV-40) transformed prostatic tissue. J Urol 101:735–739, 1969.
54. Jones RE, Sanford EJ, Rohner TJ Jr, Rapp FJ: In vitro viral transformation of human prostatic carcinoma. J Urol 115:82–85, 1976.
55. Sanford EJ, Rohner TJ, Rapp F: Virology of prostatic cancer. Cancer Chemother Rep 59:33–38, 1975.
56. Voight W, Dunning WF: In vivo metabolism of testosterone 3-H in the R3327 and androgen sensitive rat prostatic adenocarcinoma. Cancer Res 34:1447–1450, 1974.
57. Voight W, Feldman N, Dunning WF: 5-Alpha-dihydrotestosterone binding proteins and androgen sensitivity in prostatic cancers of Copenhagen rats. Cancer Res 35:1840–1846, 1975.
58. Sloan W, Heston W, Coffey D: New model for studying the effects of cancer chemotherapeutic agents on growth of the prostate gland. Cancer Chemother Rep 59:185–189, 1975.
59. Block NL, Camuzzi F, Denerfio J, et al: Chemotherapy of the transplantable adenocarcinoma (R3327) of the Copenhagen rat. Oncology 34:124–128, 1977.
60. Weissman RM, Coffey DS, Scott WW: Cell kinetic studies of prostatic cancer: Adjuvant therapy in animal models. Oncology 34:133–138, 1977.
61. Pollard N, Luckert PH: Transplantable metastasizing prostate adenocarcinomas in rats. J Natl Cancer Inst 54:643–649, 1975.
62. Pollard N, Chang CF, Luckert PH: Investigations on prostatic adenocarcinomas in rats. Oncology 34:129–132, 1977.
63. Shain SA, Boesel RW: Saturation analysis of the binding of androgens, antiandrogens and estrogens by the cytoplasmic high affinity androgen receptor of the rat ventral prostate. J Steroid Biochem 6:43–50, 1975.
64. Shain SA, Boesel RW, Axelrod LA: Aging in the rat prostate. Reduction in detectable ventral prostate androgen receptor content. Arch Biochem Biophys 167:247–263, 1975.
65. Noble RL, Collip JB: Regression of estrogen-induced mammary tumors in female rats following removal of stimulus. Can Med Assoc J 44:1–4, 1941.
66. Noble RL: Tumors and hormones. In Pincus G (ed): "Hormones" New York: Academic Press, 1964, vol 5, pp 559–579.
67. Noble RL, Hoover L: A classification of transplantable tumors in Nb rats controlled by estrogen from dormancy to autonomy. Cancer Res 35:2935–2940, 1975.
68. Sanford E, Drago JR, Warner PJ, et al: Aminoglutethimide medical adrenalectomy for advanced prostatic carcinoma. J Urol 115:170–174, 1976.

69. Bhanalaph T, Varkorakis NJ, Murphy GP: Current status of bilateral adrenalectomy for advanced prostatic carcinoma. Ann Surg 179:17–24, 1974.
70. Flanagan SP: Nude: A new hairless gene with pleitrophic effects in the mouse. Genet Res Can 8:295–300, 1966.
71. Pantelouris EN: A thymic development in the mouse. Differentiation 1:457–460, 1973.
72. Gershwin ME, Merchand D, Gelfand N: The natural history and immunobiology of outbred athymic (nude) mice. Clin Immunol Immunopathol 4:324–330, 1975.
73. Loor F, Roelants GE: High frequency T lineage lymphocytes in the nude mouse spleen. Nature 251:229–231, 1973.
74. Komuro K, Boyse EA: Induction of T lymphocytes from precursor cells in vitro by product of the thymus. J Exp Med 138:479–481, 1973.
75. Gershwin ME, Ikeda RM, Kawakami PG, Owens RB: Immunobiology of heterotransplanted human tumors in nude mice. J Natl Cancer Inst 58:1455–1461, 1977.
76. Drago JR, Gershwin ME, Maurer RE, et al: Immunobiology and therapeutic manipulation of heterotransplanted Nb rat prostatic adenocarcinoma into congenitally athymic (nude) mice: I. Hormone dependency and histopathology. J Natl Cancer Inst (in press).
77. Drago JR, Maurer RE, Gershwin ME, et al: Chemotherapy of Nb rat adenocarcinoma of the prostate heterotransplanted into congenitally athymic (nude) mice: Report of 5-fluorouracil and cyclophosphamide. J Surg Res (in press).
78. Kincl FA, Rudelh W: Sustained release hormonal preparations. Acta Endocrinol Suppl:5–30, 1971.
79. Moger WH: Effect of testosterone implants on serum gonadotrophin concentrations in the male rat. Biol Reprod 14:665–670, 1976.
80. Barkle NS, Goldman BD: The effects of castration and silastic implants of testosterone on internal aggression in the mouse. Horm Behav 9:32–37, 1977.
81. Wachstein N, Meisel E: Observations of Gomori's technique for acid phosphatase. J Histochem Cytochem 6:389–395, 1958.
82. Barka T, Anderson TJ: Histochemical methods for acid phosphatase using hexazonium pararosanilin as coupler. J Histochem Cytochem 10:141–148, 1962.
83. Barka T, Anderson TJ: "Histochemistry: Theory, Practice and Bibliography." New York: Paul B Hoeber, 1963.
84. Muntzing J, Saroff J, Sandberg AA, Murphy GP: Enzyme activity and distribution in rat prostatic adenocarcinoma. Urology 11:278–282, 1978.
85. Roy AV, Brower NE, Hayden JE: Sodium thymolphthalein monophosphate: A new acid phosphatase substrate with greater specificity for the prostatic enzyme in serum. Clin Chem 17:1093–1102, 1971.
86. Rennie TS, Bruchovsky N, Nobel RL: Acid phosphatase activity and nuclear binding of androgens in prostatic tumors of Noble rats. Personal communication, RL Noble and TS Rennie, December 1978.

The Pollard Tumors

Morris Pollard

During the last 18 years we have been examining germfree rats and mice for evidence of susceptibilities to "spontaneous" and induced tumors. Most of the tumors that appeared spontaneously in germfree Wistar and Sprague-Dawley rats were benign adenomas of endocrine and endocrine-related glands, and the incidences of such tumors per rat increased with advancing age [1–3]. Germfree Wistar rats older than 30 months had a high incidence of liver tumors, which may be related to contaminants in an all-vegetable diet which they are consuming [3]. At this time, spontaneous carcinoma of the breast has not been observed in germfree rats; however, conventional counterpart rats have developed a significant number of breast carcinomas spontaneously. Germfree and conventional rats and mice have manifested the same comparative spectrums of susceptibility to many of the commonly used carcinogenic agents [4]. These have included 2,3 methylcholanthrene, 7,12 dimethylbenz(a)anthracene, 1,2 dimethylhydrazine, and ionizing irradiations.

Four years ago, while examining aged germfree Wistar rats, we encountered nine rats with adenocarcinomas of the prostate gland; and seven of them had metastasized to other organs, especially the lung [5, 6]. No etiologic agent has been incriminated in these tumors. Similar tumors have not been observed in germfree Lobund Sprague-Dawley rats. Lacking more specific information, we ascribed the development of these tumors to a possible role of the aging process, since our germfree rats live much longer than conventional counterpart rats. However, in fall 1978, similar prostate tumors were observed in two conventional Lobund Wistar rats, which should cause us to reassess the possible role of the germfree environment in the development of prostate neoplasms (Table I). The tumors in the conventional rats caused definite enlargement of the prostate glands, but only one was fresh enough at autopsy to be examined histologically. It was a scirrhotic-type adenocarcinoma with metastatic foci in the lungs.

Among the nine prostate tumors that developed in our germfree Wistar rats, eight were scirrhotic adenocarcinomas, with abundant connective tissue stroma.

Models for Prostate Cancer, pages 293–302

TABLE I. Adenocarcinomas of the Prostate Glands in Lobund Wistar Rats

Rat number	Microbial status	Age (months)	Body weight (gm)	White blood cells (mm^3)
1	Germfree	22	302	15,700
2	Germfree	32	484	26,000
3[a]	Germfree	37	378	–
4	Germfree	39	385	71,000
5	Germfree	35	465	8,400
6	Germfree	37	388	4,000
7	Germfree	31	381	26,000
8	Germfree	38	424	4,200
9	Germfree	38	629	11,800
10[a]	Conventional	24	Degenerated	
11[a]	Conventional	25	284	Degenerated

[a]Dead on arrival in laboratory.
[b]Spleen, liver, peritoneum, lymph nodes, lungs.

The ninth tumor was soft and highly cellular with relatively little stroma. Three transplantable tumor lines have been derived from the tumors of three germfree rats [7]; two are scirrhous, and the third is soft and cellular with little stroma (Table II). The tumor lines are designated prostate adenocarcinoma I (PA-I), PA-II, and PA-III, respectively. The tumor cells have been propagated in vitro as cell monolayers [8]. The cells have been cloned, further characterized, and are now being propagated as cell lines that can be stored at $-70°C$. The tumor cells were examined for immunogenic properties, and the results were negative. Examinations of the tumor cells by several procedures, including electron microscopy, have not revealed microbial flora [9]. After inoculation of each of the in vitro propagated cell lines into Lobund Wistar rats, the same type of metastasizing tumor is reconstituted as in the rat from which the cells had been derived.

MATERIALS AND METHODS

Tumor Lines

Three transplantable prostate adenocarcinomas have been developed as model tumor systems. They are designated PA-I, PA-II, and PA-III. They can be differentiated on the basis of morphology, histology, and patterns of metastasis (Table II). As model systems they are being applied to studies on biochemical characteristics of the tumor cells, on agents that modulate tumor growth, on the patterns of metastasis and endogenous factors that regulate this phenomenon, and on inducible host responses that regulate tumor growth and metastasis.

Hema-tocrit (%)	Spleen weight (gm)	Prostate tumor weight (gm)	Tumor metastases
27	0.31	ND	Lungs
38	1.5	12.0	None
–	0.75	7.0	Multiple organs[b]
38	1.4	34.0	Multiple organs[b]
42	1.09	6.0	Multiple organs[b]
27	1.00	20.8	Multiple organs[b]
24	1.73	13.2	Multiple organs[b]
48	0.8	ND	Lungs
34	1.4	ND	None
–	–	23	Lungs

Rats

Only rats of the Lobund Wistar strain are susceptible to the prostate tumors, and males are more susceptible than females. They have been randomly propagated in this laboratory through 36 generations. They are (1) fed a sterilized vegetable diet L-485 (Tek-lad) and tap water; (2) bedded on sterilized corncobs (Sanicel) in plastic boxes; and (3) housed in air-conditioned rooms with 12-hour light cycles. They are usually inoculated with tumor cells at age eight weeks and maintained until examined at autopsy at age 14 weeks. They show no evidence of spontaneous neoplasms within the parameters of this experimental period.

Tumor Transplantation

1) PA-I and PA-III are passaged by excising aseptically the subcutaneous tumor tissue, mincing it with scissors, suspending the dispersed cells in sterile Medium 199, and inoculating them subcutaneously in the dorsal lumbar region (0.5 ml), or into a hind footpad (0.1 cc) of weanling male Lobund Wistar rats.

2) PA-II is passaged by excising aseptically a swollen lymph node (usually an axillary node), mincing the tissue with scissors, suspending and dispersing the tumor cells in Medium 199, and inoculating them subcutaneously into the dorsal lumbar region (0.5 ml) or into a hind footpad (0.1 ml). In rats with advanced tumor growth and a high white blood cell count, blood can be withdrawn from the exposed heart of anesthetized rats into a syringe coated with heparin. The blood is inoculated IV (0.2 ml) into weanling Lobund Wistar rats, which 40 days later are killed and examined for tumors.

3) An alternate procedure for production of the three tumor types in rats in-

TABLE II. Characteristics of Transplantable Rat Prostate Adenocarcinomas I, II, and III*

	I	II	III	Reference
1. Original tumor	Spontaneous	Spontaneous	Spontaneous	[5, 6]
2. Appearance				
Gross	Scirrhous	Soft	Scirrhous	[7]
Microscopic				
Epithelium	Glandular	Undifferentiated	Glandular	[7]
Stroma	Extensive	Sparse	Extensive	[7]
3. Metastasis	100%	100%	100%	[10]
Route	Lymphatics	Lymphatics and blood	Lymphatics	[10]
Target organs	Lungs	Lung and visceral organs	Lungs	[10]
Effects of				
Na barbiturate	Enhanced	Enhanced	Enhanced	[11, 12]
Heparin	Enhanced	ND	Enhanced	[14]
C parvum	Retarded	ND	Retarded	[11, 12]
Diethylstilbestrol	None	Enhanced	None	[6]
Indomethacin	Retarded	ND	Retarded	[11]
Cyclophosphamide	Oncolytic	Oncolytic	Oncolytic	[15]
4. Host response	Leukemoid (myelocytic)	Leukocytosis (tumor cells)	None	[10]
5. Immunogenic	No	No	No	
6. Preparation in vitro	Monolayer growth	Monolayer growth	Monolayer growth	[8]
7. Microbial flora	None	None	None	[9]

*Only in Lobund Wistar rats.

volves the in vitro propagation of the tumor cells as monolayers in plastic bottles with Eagle's minimum essential medium (MEM) plus 10% heat-inactivated fetal calf serum with penicillin and streptomycin. The cells, in confluent cultures, are suspended and dispersed in the tissue culture medium by rapid syringing, and 10^5 viable cells are inoculated subcutaneously into the dorsal lumbar region or into the footpad. The cells can be stored in tissue culture medium with 10% glycerol at $-70°C$.

Autopsy Procedure

Each rat is weighed, anesthetized by inhaled diethyl ether, and exsanguinated from the exposed heart. The blood is examined for hematocrit level, white blood cell count, and in smear for differential blood cell counts. Organs of each rat are examined for gross changes, weighed, and sections thereof are fixed overnight in Bouin's solution and then stored in 70% ethanol. The lungs are inflated by injecting Bouin's solution by syringe through the trachea, and 24 hours later they are stored in 70% ethanol. The tissues are embedded in paraffin, sectioned, and stained with hematoxylin and eosin. Tissues that are examined microscopically include lung, liver, spleen, kidney, lymph nodes, thymus, and bone marrow.

Applications

Metastasis. In order to determine the route(s) of tumor dissemination from the primary implant site to distant organs in relation to time, each swollen lymph node was examined for comparative weight with the contralateral lymph node, and, along with individual organs, they were examined for histological evidence of tumor invasion. Blood-borne tumor cells were detected by exsanguinating the anesthetized tumor-bearing rat from the exposed heart with a syringe coated with heparin. Usually, 1.5 ml or less of blood was inoculated IV into each of two weanling rats, which 40 days later were examined at autopsy for tumor lesions.

Modulating factors. Rats were inoculated with 10^5 tumor cells subcutaneously in the dorsal lumbar area or into the pad of a hindfoot. Thereafter, groups of them were subjected to a number of treatment schedules to determine if inoculation of tumor cells induced changes in the expected patterns of disease.

Promotion of tumor growth and metastasis. After rats were inoculated with tumor cells, they were fed ad libitum the regular diet plus water that contained 0.1% sodium barbiturate. Control rats were administered the same protocol without sodium barbiturate. Both groups of rats were examined 40 days later for extent and rate of metastasis. This was based on counts of focal tumors that developed on the surfaces of the lungs; by weights of liver, spleen, and lymph nodes; and by histological examinations of these organs for establishment of tumor foci in them.

Retardation of tumor growth and metastasis.

1) Following the inoculation of tumor cells, groups of rats were injected intra-peritoneally with graded doses of freshly prepared cyclophosphamide (25 mg/kg body weight) at weekly intervals, either continuously or at scheduled intervals during the time course of disease. The rats were examined 40 days later to compare the rate and extent of lesions compared to those in the untreated control rats. In addition, groups of treated rats were examined at intervals after cessation of cyclophosphamide treatments.

2) After inoculation of tumor cells, groups of rats were administered aspirin (acetylsalicylic acid) ad libitum in the drinking water (625 mg/liter water) and a control group of rats was fed water without aspirin. Forty days later they were examined for tumor lesions.

3) After inoculation of tumor cells, groups of rats were fed daily by gavage indomethacin (0.25 mg/kg body weight/day) in 1% cornstarch. Control rats were administered 1% cornstarch in water. Forty days later the rats were examined for weights of primary tumor, of lymph nodes, liver, spleen, and numbers of tumor foci in the lungs. These data were compared with data derived from tumor-bearing rats that were not treated with indomethacin.

4) Simultaneously with inoculation of tumor cells into rats, groups were inoculated IV with 2 mg killed Corynebacterium parvum* and control rats were inoculated with physiological saline. In addition, groups of rats were inoculated four times with C parvum at weekly intervals. They were examined for lesions at 40 days after onset of the experiment.

RESULTS

Metastasis

PA-I and III tumors. The patterns of metastatic spread of the three PA tumors were analyzed in Lobund Wistar rats [10]. After PA-I and PA-III tumor cells were inoculated into a hind footpad, they spread sequentially in a predictable pattern, through the draining chain of ipsilateral lymph nodes (popliteal, para-aortic, renal) to the lungs, in and on which they developed as distinct, round, solid, focal tumors. The tumor-infiltrated lymph nodes were significantly larger and heavier than the contralateral lymph nodes. Tumor cells first appeared in the cortical sinus areas, and then they proliferated directly into the lymph node, which they eventually replaced. An alternate pathway was observed through which tumor cells spread from the inoculated footpad, through the ipsilateral popliteal and inguinal lymph nodes, and through a subcutaneous channel along the lateral wall, to the axillary lymph node, to the lungs. The lymphatic channels were lined (perfused) with tumor cells, and detached clumps of these cells were observed in the lumina of the lymphatic vessels. Tumor cells were not observed in blood vessels, and rarely in visceral organs other than the lungs. Tumor cells were not demonstrable

*Strain CN6 134, Burroughs Wellcome Co., Triangle Park, NC.

in the blood of the tumor-bearing rats which had been inoculated IV into weanling Lobund Wistar rats. The usual interval from inoculation to autopsy of the test rats was 40 days.

PA-II tumors. Following inoculation of tumor cells into a hind footpad, they spread in a predictable pattern through lymphatic and hematogenous channels to many of the visceral organs [10]. On the basis of periodic examinations of the circulating blood for tumor cells, the blood of tumor-bearing rats was negative for tumor cells for 14 days after onset; thereafter tumor cells were detected in the blood. The tumor cells spread initially to the draining popliteal lymph node and then through the blood to contralateral lymph nodes, and to lungs, liver, spleen, bone marrow, and kidneys. Frequently, the lymph nodes weighed as much as 2–4 gm; the lymphatic tissue was completely replaced by tumor cells. In the initial stages of metastatic spread into organs such as the lungs and liver, the tumor cells were visibly adherent to the walls of blood vessels, and they were observed multiplying through the vessel wall into the parenchyma. The livers and spleens were very much enlarged, and infiltrated with tumor cells: This started in the livers and lungs as perivascular accumulations of tumor cells which proliferated into the parenchyma. Accumulations of tumor cells were observed in the subcapsular red pulp of the spleens. As little as 0.025 ml of blood from rats with advanced metastatic PA-II disease induced tumors in IV inoculated recipients. The white blood cell counts in such animals were often as high as $70,000/mm^3$; however, many of these cells could be identified morphologically as PA-II cells. PA-II cells have a distinctive appearance: The cells are relatively large and round, with distinct, clear cytoplasm. They were detected microscopically in the visceral organs in bone marrow and in lymph nodes, as well as in blood smears.

Modulation of Metastasis

The modifying effects of test agents on tumor metastasis were measured on the basis of rate and extent of spread from the implant site (hind footpad) to the lungs. This was demonstrable with PA-I and III cells, which demonstrated a pathway through sequences of lymph nodes (which were enlarged) to the lungs in which they produced distinct round focal tumors which could be counted.

1) Enhancement of metastasis was demonstrated in rats with PA-I and III cells, which were administered sodium barbiturate (0.1%) in the drinking water. The drug-consuming rats were heavier in body, liver, primary tumor, lymph nodes, and in numbers of tumors in the lungs than the control rats, which consumed drug-free water [11, 12]. When sodium barbiturate was administered to rats with PA-II cells, the results were not easy to assess because this tumor cell produced, characteristically, extensive diffuse lesions in the lungs, and in other visceral organs. However, the rate and extent of metastasis of PA-II was obviously enhanced in rats that consumed sodium (Na) barbiturate. Thus, although Na barbiturate treatments produced no changes in the gross and microscopic appearances of the metastasized tumors, such tumors were increased in number and in size.

An oncolytic agent in serum, very low density lipoprotein (VLDL), was demonstrated and characterized in vitro on PA-III cells [13]. The tumor cells were propagated as islands (colonies) which were destroyed quantitatively by VLDL and not by other fractions of serum. The in vitro oncolytic effect was demonstrated on several tumor cell lines from species other than the rat. The role(s) of VLDL in host surveillance, as regards metastasis, was investigated in rats that had been inoculated with PA-III cells. In this regard, tumor-bearing rats were inoculated IV repeatedly with heparin, and controls were inoculated with physiological saline [14]. The rate and extent of metastasis were significantly enhanced in the heparin-treated rats. The levels of VLDL in the serums of the latter rats were markedly reduced, a finding that has been attributed to the intravascular production of lipoprotein lipase by heparin. This was further demonstrated by in vitro destruction of VLDL through incubation with serum collected from donor rats shortly after they had been treated with heparin.

2) The metastatic patterns of PA-I, II, and III were suppressed in rats which had been treated early with cyclophosphamide (CPA). Also, in rats with metastatic lesions, CPA caused clearly defined oncolytic changes throughout the body. The tumors were altered: The cell contents were considerably reduced and replaced by amorphous eosinophilic material. However, after the CPA treatments had been terminated tumor growth was usually resumed [15]. In some of the rats that had been treated continuously with smaller doses of CPA, tumors emerged which were resistant to the oncolytic effects of CPA.

Rats with PA-III were administered aspirin in the drinking water during the entire period of observation (40 days). Control rats were fed drinking water without the drug. At autopsy, the aspirin-treated rats had fewer metastatic tumors in the lungs than the control rats [11, 12]. The aspirin-treated rats showed no evidence of toxicity from the effects of the drug.

Rats with PA-III were fed indomethacin by gavage at daily intervals for the entire experimental period. Control rats were administered the carrier (1% cornstarch). When the rats were autopsied after 40 days, the indomethacin-treated rats had fewer metastatic lung tumors than the control rats [11, 12]. The gross and histological characteristics of the tumors were not altered by treatments with aspirin and indomethacin.

Rats with PA-I and III that had been inoculated with C parvum developed reduced numbers of tumor foci in the lungs, compared with the rats that had been inoculated with saline. The numbers of tumor foci in the lungs were further reduced in rats that had been inoculated with four doses of C parvum [11, 12]. This treatment did not modify the size and character of the primary tumor.

DISCUSSION

The phenomenon of metastasis is an important and frustrating complication of cancer in man [16]. The search for model tumor systems in animals has been hampered in that relatively few of them are carcinomas, and few of them metastasize spontaneously and predictably. In many of the reported investigations on metastasis, the test tumors have had to be inoculated intravenously into animals, which actually constituted an artifact. The three prostate carcinomas described in this report (PA-I, II, and III) spread in all inoculated rats from the implant site to distant organs, without special manipulations, and the spread patterns are predictable and reproducible. Two cell lines (PA-I and PA-III) spread only through lymphatic channels to the lungs, in which they produce multiple foci of tumors. PA-II cells spread through lymphatic and blood channels and produce tumors in multiple visceral organs. Thus, with the same experimental protocol (same animal strain, same organ-related carcinoma, same site of implantation, same dose of in vitro propagated cells), the phenomenon of metastasis as regards routes of spread and organotropisms appeared to be governed by some unique characteristic of the tumor cell.

The rate and the extent of metastasis have been modified through administrations of chemical agents to the tumor-bearing host. Ths spread patterns of PA-I, II, and III were accelerated through treatments with sodium barbiturate, and administrations of heparin resulted in accelerations of PA-III spread. The spread patterns of the PA tumors were retarded by treatments of tumor-bearing rats with orally administered aspirin and indomethacin, and with IV inoculated C parvum. The exact mechanisms responsible for accelerating or for retarding the rate and extent of metastasis have not yet been identified.

Thus, whether a malignant tumor metastasizes or remains localized, or whether it manifests specific organotropism, these characteristics are unique to the tumor cell, which also determined its route(s) of dissemination through lymphatic channels, or in addition, through blood channels. However, with tumor cells that do metastasize, the rate and extent of spread can be modulated (accelerated or retarded) experimentally through administration of specified agents to the tumor-bearing host.

Treatments of rats with PA-I, II, and III with cyclophosphamide (CPA) resulted in marked involution of the tumors, but not in cures: The tumors were reactivated following cessation of treatments [15]. Also, tumor-bearing rats that were treated with marginal doses of CPA eventually produced tumors that no longer responded to this drug.

These investigations are far from definitive. The experiments reported herein only provide access to better defined and refined inquiries, which it is hoped will ultimately yield fruit — namely, control measures. Specifically, we need answers to questions such as 1) why some tumor cell lines metastasize and others do not; 2) why some tumor cell lines spread via lymph channels and others via the blood or both; 3) why some metastasizing tumor cell lines spread to the lungs and others to multiple visceral organs. If answers can be secured through experiments in animals, they may be applicable to the problems of metastasis in man.

ACKNOWLEDGMENTS

This work was supported in part by funds from U.S. Public Health Service grant RR00294 from the Animal Resources Branch, and grant CA17559 from the National Cancer Institute, and the Ambrose and Gladys Bowyer Foundation.

REFERENCES

1. Pollard M: Senescence in germfree rats. Gerontologia 17:333–338, 1971.
2. Pollard M: Spontaneous and induced neoplasms in germfree rats. In "Environment and Cancer." Baltimore: Williams & Wilkins Co, 1972, pp 394–406.
3. Pollard M, Luckert PH: Spontaneous liver tumors in aged germfree Wistar rats. Lab Anim Sci 29:74–77, 1979.
4. Pollard M: Carcinogenesis in germ-free animals. Prog Immunobiol Standard 5:226–230, 1972.
5. Pollard M: Spontaneous prostate adenocarcinomas in aged germfree Wistar rats. J Natl Cancer Inst 51:1235–1241, 1973.
6. Pollard M: Prostate adenocarcinomas in Wistar rats. Rush-Presbyterian-St. Luke's Med Bull 14:17–22, 1975.
7. Pollard M, Luckert P: Transplantable metastasizing adenocarcinomas in rats. J Natl Cancer Inst 54:643–649, 1975.
8. Chang CF, Pollard M: In vitro propagation of prostate adenocarcinoma cells from rats. Invest Urol 14:331–334, 1977.
9. Celesk RA, Pollard M: Ultrastructural cytology of prostate carcinoma cells from Wistar rats. Invest Urol 14:95–99, 1976.
10. Pollard M, Luckert PH: Patterns of spontaneous metastasis manifested by three rat prostate adenocarcinomas. J Surg Oncol (in press).
11. Pollard M, Chang CF, Luckert PH: Investigations on prostate adenocarcinomas in rats. Oncology 34:129–132, 1977.
12. Pollard M, Burleson GR, Luckert PH: Factors which modify the rate and extent of spontaneous metastases of tumors in rats. In Day SB et al (eds): "Cancer Invasion and Metastasis: Biologic Mechanisms and Therapy." New York: Raven Press, 1977, pp 349–358.
13. Chan SY, Pollard M: In vitro effects of lipoprotein-associated cytotoxic factor on rat prostate adenocarcinoma cells. Cancer Res 38:2956–2962, 1978.
14. Chan SY, Pollard M: Unpublished information.
15. Pollard M, Luckert PH: Chemotherapy of metastatic prostate adenocarcinomas in germfree rats. Cancer Treat Rep 60:619–621, 1976.
16. Fidler IJ, Gersten DM, Hart IR: The biology of cancer invasion and metastasis. In Klein G, Weinhouse S (eds): "Advances in Cancer Research." New York: Academic Press, 1978, pp 149–250.

Characterization of Animal Tumors: Summary

Arthur E. Bogden, PhD

The session on animal models was opened by Dr. Coffey with a most convincing argument for the validity of the animal tumor model in cancer research. His rationale included, for example, classic examples of the use of animal tumor model systems in elucidating mechanisms of growth and metastasis fundamental to and characteristic of most cancers. The presentation was climaxed by a listing of the properties of human prostate cancer desired in an animal model.

Subsequently, Drs. Lubaroff, Drago, and Pollard elegantly presented the pros and cons of their model systems. It is evident that, with the unique biological characteristics inherent in the three transplantation-established rodent tumor models, plus the potential for use of the in vitro established human prostate tumor cell lines as transplantable xenograft systems in the athymic nude mouse, most of the desirable characteristics listed by Dr. Coffey can, as an aggregate, be met. Rather than attempt to repeat each presentation in summary form, I will make general comparisons by pointing out salient features of each tumor model, indicating similarities as well as differences, and how these tumor systems fit into tumor model categories.

There is no question that in vitro cell culture systems can be exquisitely defined to elucidate biological phenomena and to answer very specific biological questions. In the final analysis, however, much of what is learned in vitro must be tested or confirmed in vivo. What are the basic tumor model systems that can be manipulated experimentally to define phenomena in the biologically complete, and definitely more complex, intact organism?

Models for Prostate Cancer, pages 303–310

The growing acceptance that cancer encompasses a disparate group of diseases in which malignant cells tend to retain certain unique characteristics of the tissue or organ of their origin has been paralleled by an increasing interest in experimental animal model systems that not only are representative of human malignancies histologically, but also originate in the organ or tissues and have the growth and metastasizing characteristics of the particular neoplastic disease for which they serve as a model.

Clearly, in a field that is as vital and complex as cancer therapy, animal experimentalists must have the help of clinicians in developing animal model tumor systems that will predict the clinical success of combinations of new and existing chemotherapeutic agents and treatment modalities. Recognizing the limitations to our knowledge of the mechanisms fundamental to the nature of malignancy as well as to the interaction of drugs with the malignant cell further cautions that the increasing clinical emphasis on the use of combinations of chemotherapeutic agents and therapeutic modalities must have a basis for such selections other than clinical empiricism.

Webster's definition of a model as "a description or analogy used to help visualize something that cannot be directly observed," or as "an example for imitation or emulation," points up the critical consideration in selection of model systems for cancer research — that there is no one animal model for the disparate group of diseases identified as cancer. The age-old argument concerning which animal tumor is the best model for "human cancer" is a fruitless argument because no single human cancer is a proper model for all human cancer, whether it is of breast, lung, colon, or prostate origin.

Most commonly, intact animal systems serve as models of human diseases at what might be appropriately be termed the clinical level, as contrasted to the cellular or molecular levels discussed in the previous sessions. Nonetheless, one should not lose sight of the fact that animal tumor models are assay systems and, as such, must have well-defined and reproducible growth patterns and reactivities so that modifications in such parameters resulting from experimental manipulations can be correctly interpreted. It is an axiom that when attempting to define an unknown, experimental variables must be identified and controlled. In experimental prostatic cancer, the need for tumors with well-defined growth and metastatic patterns as well as responsiveness to chemotherapy, to ionizing radiation, and to immunotherapy is, so far, best met by the syngeneic prostate tumor system that has been established and stabilized in serial transplantation. The heterogeneity that one encounters with autochthonous tumors, animal and human, is also reflected in syngeneic tumor systems, except that the differences are found among established tumor lines rather than among tumors within a line. With careful monitoring, one finds that the characteristics peculiar to a particular tumor line are reproducible in each of the tumors of that line, transplant generation after transplant generation, whether ten animals or a thousand animals are implanted at any particular passage.

Both Dr. Lubaroff and Dr. Coffey have stressed that maintaining the stability of the histologically more complex prostatic adenocarcinoma while in serial transplantation requires intensive monitoring of a number of factors, as well as a "bit of art." The foremost prerequisite is that the tumor will have originated in a member of a highly inbred strain of animals. The purpose of inbred strains, the members of which serve as recipients for syngeneic tumor grafts, is to have available for experimentation a large population of genetically identical animals in which the relationship of each animal to a neoplasm arising in one of its members mimics the autochthonous tumor-host relationship. Thus, malignant tumors should be 100% transplantable in syngeneic hosts, producing progressive and eventually lethal growths.

In large-scale commercial breeding programs, where numerous production breeder lines are maintained, it is essential that such lines be checked periodically for immunogenetic drift from designated parental or reference strains. Such monitoring is carried out under the auspices of the Mammalian Genetics and Animal Production Section of the Division of Cancer Treatment, National Cancer Institute. All rat and mouse strains being bred and maintained under contract with the National Cancer Institute are monitored as a routine quality-control procedure. It behooves the investigator working with syngeneic transplantable systems to know the source and quality of his experimental animals.

Unlike the homogeneous cell populations making up leukemias or fibrosarcomas, prostatic adenocarcinomas are generally differentiated, having definite histological structures such as acini, which may or may not be arranged as papillary extensions of tumor growth, and maintain fairly constant epithelial/stromal ratios. Such characteristics must be monitored histologically. The "art" in tumor transplantation is manifested in the ability to maintain these histologic characteristics over many transplant generations by "knowing," from gross appearance, which tissue is representative of the tumor and should be selected for transplantation. Histology, though necessary, is somewhat of a post facto confirmation of the selection made. The most careful technician can unwittingly convert a well-differentiated adenocarcinoma to an undifferentiated carcinoma, or even sarcoma, in a few passages. Where a transplantable tumor is being used for chemotherapy studies, it is also advisable to monitor its responsiveness to a known active compound. It is to be stressed, therefore, that transplantation-established syngeneic, as well as allogeneic and xenogeneic tumor systems are subject to change during serial transplantations, and characteristics such as histology, growth rates, chemotherapy responsiveness, and metastases need to be continually monitored. Cryopreserving a quantity of tissue in the early transplant generations of a syngeneic tumor provides a source for not only replacing lost tumor lines but also renewing long-transplanted lines. Alert to the need for a central repository and distribution center for well-characterized biological materials relevant to prostate cancer research, the National Prostatic Cancer Project has established such a tumor bank of animal and human tissues.

Table I indicates the three basic in vivo experimental systems that comprise the armamentarium of tumor models available for cancer research.

Autochthonous or nontransplanted tumors in both animals and man are of spontaneous (indicating etiology unknown) origin, or have been induced by hormones, viruses, chemical carcinogens, or combinations of these inducers. As an animal model of the human disease, each autochthonus tumor system requires the same stringent staging of tumors, with definition, monitoring, and randomization of the individual tumor-bearing animal for experimental use as does its human counterpart for effective management in phase II and III clinical trials.

The advent of the immunologically incompetent athymic nude mouse has permitted the "hybridization" of the human and animal systems. We have, as a result, transplantation-established human tumors, albeit in xenogeneic or allogeneic hosts. The DU 145 cell line of Dr. Mickey, the PC-3 cell line of Dr. Kaighn and the LNCaP cell line of Dr. Horoszewicz, established in serial transplantation in the athymic nude mouse, provide prostate cancer research with the potential for studying human tumor response under carefully controlled, defined, and reproducible in vivo conditions. Whether the human tumor xenograft predicts better for clinical response than its animal counterpart remains to be determined, however.

A compromise from the autochthonus tumor system is the first transplant generation animal tumor used in the F_1 hybrid. Here too, we have a human tumor/athymic nude mouse host counterpart. Development of the "subrenal capsule assay" [Bogden et al, 1978] has permitted the use of fresh surgical explants of human tumors to be used as first transplant generation xenografts in athymic nude or normal immunocompetent mice within a practicable time frame by evading the necessity of first establishing tumors in serial passage.

Table II summarizes the animal tumor models available for prostate cancer research. There are significant and basic differences between these animal tumor models. Though the Dunning and Noble tumors are transplantable syngeneic systems, the Dunning was of spontaneous origin, whereas the Noble tumors have been hormone induced. The Pollard tumors, though arising in the originally random-bred Wistar rat, are essentially transplantable syngeneic systems. The Lobund Wistar rat has been pen-bred in a closed colony for many years, resulting in a highly homogeneous genetic pool. The uniqueness of the Pollard tumors for the study of metastases has been pointed out. The A × C tumor, though not discussed here, is being used in prostate cancer research and represents the primary or autochthonus tumor model. It is poorly transplantable.

That rat prostatic tumor models represent a spectrum of hormone dependence and responsiveness, of metastasizing potential and histology, as is illustrated in Table III.

The androgen-dependent R3327-H tumor line metastasizes predictably when implanted in the normal prostate. The heterogeneity of the original Dunning tumor was shown by Dr. Lubaroff, who was able to develop four sublines having varying

TABLE I. Basic Animal and Human In Vivo Experimental Systems

Animal tumor systems	Human tumor systems

Non-transplanted
  Autochthonous (primary)
	Non-transplanted
	  Autochthonous (primary)

Transplantation established
  Syngeneic (inbred)
  Allogeneic (outbred)
	Transplantation established
	  Xenogeneic – the human tumor/
	  athymic nude mouse

First transplant generation
  Primary tumor in F_1 hybrid
	First transplant generation
	  Fresh surgical explants as xenografts
	  in the athymic nude or normal mouse

TABLE II. Rat Prostate Tumor Models

Prostate tumor models	Origin	Strain of origin or transplantability	Experimental systems
I. Dunning tumors	Spontaneous, in aged retired male breeder	Copenhagen 2331 inbred	Transplantable (syngeneic)
II. Noble tumors	Hormone induced	Nb inbred	Transplantable (syngeneic)
III. Pollard tumors	Spontaneous, in aged males	Lobund-Wistar (random-bred)	Transplantable (subline of origin)
IV. A × C tumors	Spontaneous, in aged virgin males	A × C inbred	Primary (autochthonous), poorly transplantable

degrees of hormone responsiveness. Metastasis to the bone has not, however, been demonstrated in this tumor system.

The Noble tumors also have definable hormonal characteristics. The steroid-dependent tumors metastasize with about a 35% frequency, whereas 55–60% of the autonomous tumors metastasize.

On the other hand, 100% of the Pollard tumors metastasize predictively from any site, PA-I and PA-III primarily via the lymphatics and PA-II hematogenously. All of the Pollard tumors are responsive to diethylstilbestrol.

That each tumor model also has its characteristic growth rate is shown in Table IV. The growth rates of the Pollard tumors in vivo can be ranked as PA-I > PA-III > PA-II. When thus compared (Table IV) it becomes evident that as transplantable systems the prostate tumor models exhibit a wide range of growth rates. In contrast to the autonomous tumors of Noble, for example, the Dunning R3327-H

TABLE III. Growth Characteristics of Rat Prostatic Tumor Models

Prostate tumor models	Hormonal status	Metastatic potential	Histology
Dunning tumors			
R3327-H	Androgen dependent	Metastasizing	Well-differentiated adenocarcinoma
R3327-A	Autonomous	–	Squamous cell carcinoma
R3327-At	Autonomous	–	Anaplastic carcinoma
Noble tumors			
2PR-128 2PR-129	Androgen dependent	Occasionally	Adenocarcinoma
52PR 114PR	Estrogen dependent	Occasionally	Adenocarcinoma
18PR 13PR 102PR	Autonomous	Metastasizing	Poorly differentiated carcinoma
Pollard tumors			
PA-I			Scirrhotic adenocarcinoma
PA-II	DES responsive	Metastasizing	Adenocarcinoma
PA-III			Scirrhotic adenocarcinoma
A × C tumors	Androgen responsive	None observed	Adenocarcinoma

TABLE IV. Growth Rates of Prostatic Tumor Models

Tumor model	Doubling time	Other
Dunning tumors		
R3327-H	20.9 days	80–100 days to reach 1-2 cm D
R3327-At	–	10–15 days to reach 1-2 cm D
Noble tumors		
Androgen dependent		
2PR-128	5.3 days	36 days to achieve 1 cm^3
2PR-129	7.5 days	51 days to achieve 1 cm^3
Estrogen dependent		
52PR	8.5 days	58 days to achieve 1 cm^3
114PR	7.3 days	50 days to achieve 1 cm^3
Autonomous		
13PR	4.3 days	29 days to achieve 1 cm^3
102PR	6.0 days	41 days to achieve 1 cm^3
18PR	4.6 days	31 days to achieve 1 cm^3
Pollard tumors		
PA-I	22 hours	
PA-II	–	in vitro culture
PA-III	18 hours	
A × C tumors	Spontaneously arising with a frequency of 70% in a population of 30–46-month-old virgin males	

tumor is slow growing. However, the growth of R3327-H exhibits a greater practicality for use as an experimental system in terms of the time frame required for study than the A X C tumors, which require 30 to 46 months to develop.

It should be stressed that, basically, animal models incorporate features of convenience for the experimentalist, a luxury not available to the clinician, and that animal model systems generally only represent, or model for, one facet of the disease. These modeling characteristics of experimental tumor systems are further illustrated in Table V, which summarizes the salient experimental features of the current animal prostate tumor models. It is important to note that a supplement to both the Dunning and Pollard tumor model systems has been the establishment of in vitro transplantable cell lines derived from each tumor system.

TABLE V. **Experimental Characteristics of Prostatic Tumor Models**

Tumor system	Characteristics
Dunning tumors	R3327-H tumor made up of androgen-dependent and autonomous cells. Tumor responds to androgens, castration, estrogens, and anti-androgens. A predictively relapsing model for evaluating ablation effects as well as single and combined therapies with hormonal and non-hormonal chemotherapeutic agents. Very slow growing, transplantable test system, Copenhagen or F_1 hybrid (Copenhagan X Fischer).
Noble tumors	Hormone-induced tumors with a variety of androgen, estrogen, and androgen + estrogen dependency. A model for study of reversion from hormone dependence to autonomy, and for evaluating ablation effects with and without nonhormonal chemotherapeutic agents. Relatively fast growing, easily transplantable test system, Nb strain.
Pollard tumors	Hormone independent, with predictable metastasizing patterns. Implanted into hind footpad. PA-I and III spread through draining chain of ipsilateral lymph nodes to the lungs in and on which they develop as distinct round focal tumors. PA-II spreads through lymphatic and hematogenous channels to many visceral organs. Livers and spleens much enlarged. A model for the study of organotropism and of agents modulating the rate and extent of spread of metastases. Relatively fast growing, easily transplantable in stock of origin, Lobund Wistar stock.
A X C tumors	Spontaneous adenocarcinomas of the ventral prostate gland associated with atypical hyperplasia in the aging A X C male rat. Provides a model for the study of the progression and pathogenesis of prostate neoplasia. Very slow growing, poorly transplantable, A X C strain.

This workshop has pointed out that investigators in prostate cancer research now have in their armamentarium of experimental models a spectrum of in vivo and in vitro test systems that have clinical relevance and that can serve to elucidate fundamental problems in tumor biology as well. Though the most artificial model has the potential to produce new information about the biology of cancer, if preclinical investigations are to generate guidelines for the realistic design of appropriate clinical studies, it is imperative that the experimentalist not be blinded to the limitation of his or her model systems. By the same token, the clinical oncologist must have a sufficient appreciation of model systems to know whether extrapolations can be made.

Drs. Coffey, Lubaroff, Drago, and Pollard should be congratulated for their studies directed to the further development and refinement of the various animal prostate tumor models discussed in this workshop. The number and types of questions that can be answered by clinical trials, controlled or otherwise, are limited by the resultant logistic and ethical problems. These limitations, however, are the very area in which animal experimentation offers significant advantages.

On the assumption that human tumors, albeit as xenografts in the athymic nude mouse host, are more representative of human tumor response than their animal counterparts, the Division of Cancer Treatment of the National Cancer Institute has incorporated into its preclinical test panel transplantable organ-specific tumors of human origin — eg, a breast tumor (MX-1), a lung tumor (LX-1), and colon tumors (CX-1 and CX-5). Based upon the current information on the in vivo and in vitro experimental systems presented by the various investigators at this workshop there is, it is hoped, a potential for the development and incorporation of at least one human prostatic tumor (PX-1?) into such a screening panel. From the standpoint of cost and practicality, however, transplantation-established human xenograft systems can most efficiently serve to further evaluate chemotherapeutic agents and treatment modalities first detected and defined in experimental animal tumor models.

REFERENCE

Bogden AE, Kelton DE, Cobb WR, Esber HJ: A rapid screening method for testing chemotherapeutic agents against human tumor xenografts. In Houchens DP, Ovejesa AA (eds): "Proceedings of the Symposium on the Use of Athymic Nude Mice in Cancer Research." New York: Gustav Fischer, Inc., 1978, pp 231-250.

Concepts in Prostatic Cancer Biology: Dunning R-3327 H, HI, and AT Tumors

John T. Isaacs, Robert M. Weissman, Donald S. Coffey, and William W. Scott

Human prostatic cancer is characterized by a wide spectrum of diversity in relation to pathology, state, and variability of differentiation, uniformity of growth rate, and differences in therapeutic responsiveness to hormonal, nonhormonal, and radiation treatment. Because of this variability, it is possible that more than one animal model may be required to correspond to these different states of the human disease. Based on this principle, the transplantable Dunning R-3327 rat prostatic adenocarcinomas have become an attractive animal model system since there are now several specific sublines each with distinct properties that mimic many of those found in various states of human prostatic cancer. At present, three forms of transplantable Dunning rat prostatic adenocarcinomas have been characterized in detail [1–4]: R-3327-H, a slow-growing, well-differentiated, hormone-sensitive tumor; R-3327-HI, a similar tumor that is slow growing, well-differentiated, and hormone-insensitive; and R-3327-AT, a rapidly growing anaplastic tumor, which is also hormone-insensitive. All of these transplantable prostatic tumors originated as sublines from the original Dunning R-3327, which was first described by W. F. Dunning in 1961 as a spontaneous tumor originating in the prostate of an aged, syngeneic Copenhagen rat [5]. The original tumor is hormone-sensitive and metabolizes testosterone to dihydrotestosterone [6].

In this chapter we summarize the biological concepts that have developed from the study of these three tumor sublines.

HORMONE SENSITIVITY

Many fundamental questions about prostatic cancer need to be resolved, and the answers will have impact on the rationale and development of new therapeutic modalities. For example, when prostatic cancer relapses from hormonal therapy, is this a reflection of the transformation of a hormone-sensitive cell to an insensitive

Models for Prostate Cancer, pages 311–323

form or, in contrast, is this the result of selecting the growth of hormone-insensitive clones existing from the time of tumor initiation in a multicellular tumor system? If transformation of cellular hormonal insensitivity occurs (Fig. 1, Model I or II), one would wish to study the prevention or reversal of this process. If, however, preexisting clones of hormonally insensitive cells are being permitted to continue their growth (Fig. 1, Model III), one would want to evaluate new nonhormonal chemotherapeutic agents affecting these types of cells. If this were possible, it would appear advisable to initiate this type of therapy simultaneously with hormonal therapy in the early phases of this disease.

The above models have been tested with the Dunning R-3327-H tumor, and it appears that Model III of Figure 1 can be supported by experimental evidence [2]. This evidence is illustrated in part with the following experiments.

The growth of the Dunning R-3327-H in various hormonally treated rats for 180 days is depicted in Figure 2, in which the silhouette of the tumor is compared to that of the rat sex accessory tissues. Although the tumor attains a larger size in the presence of androgens it has, nevertheless, been noted that some growth was observed in the castrate animals. When the growth of these tumors was monitored for a time and the log of the tumor volume was plotted against time a straight line was obtained [1]. These cell kinetic studies indicated clearly that a fraction (8–29%) of the original tumor cells inoculated were hormone-insensitive cells that were capable of growing in the absence of androgens. These hormone-insensitive cells doubled every 20 days in a manner similar to that of the hormone-sensitive cells (Table I). The data in Table I are derived from kinetic studies reported elsewhere [1] and indicate that hormone-insensitive cells were present as a subclone in the original R-3327-H tumor and that they grew out in the castrate.

Other experiments have indicated that when intact animals bearing an R-3327-H tumor for 120 days are castrated an involution and marked loss of tumor volume is observed. This is followed by a subsequent relapse as the smaller volume of hormone-insensitive cells continues to grow in the castrate animal [1]. The analysis of our data is best represented by Model III of Figure 1, which provides a schematic presentation of the development of the hormone-insensitive state following castration of male animals bearing the Dunning R-3327-H rat tumor.

If the selection of a clone of hormone-insensitive cells accounts for the development of relapse to hormone therapy in human prostatic cancer, then specific nonhormonal treatment for these types of cells should be initiated in the earliest phase of therapy. Furthermore, the ratio of hormone-sensitive to insensitive cells in the individual prostatic tumor would determine the response to hormonal therapy with estrogens and/or castration. Indeed, if any insensitive cells were present, one would not anticipate a permanent cure as the cells continue to grow and ultimately the patient succumbs. Documented cures of patients with advanced prostatic cancer treated with estrogen therapy or castration are rare. The

MODELS FOR DEVELOPMENT OF HORMONE INSENSITIVITY

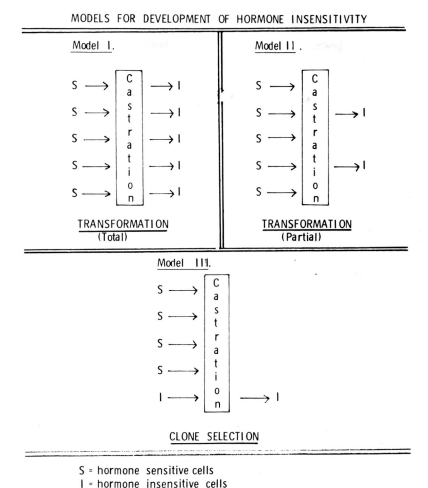

Model I.

Model II.

TRANSFORMATION
(Total)

TRANSFORMATION
(Partial)

Model III.

CLONE SELECTION

S = hormone sensitive cells
I = hormone insensitive cells

Fig. 1. Schematic of three models that may account for how a group of tumor cells can go from an androgen-sensitive (S) to an androgen-insensitive (I) state following castration.

same is true for the Dunning R-3327-H tumor; although the tumor involutes because of androgen deprivation, all animals finally die from the continued growth of the androgen-insensitive cells.

Even if cures are rare, is there any benefit from castration on survival time? This question has been debated for some time but the general feeling is yes. This can be tested with the Dunning R-3327-H animal tumor. Forty intact adult rats

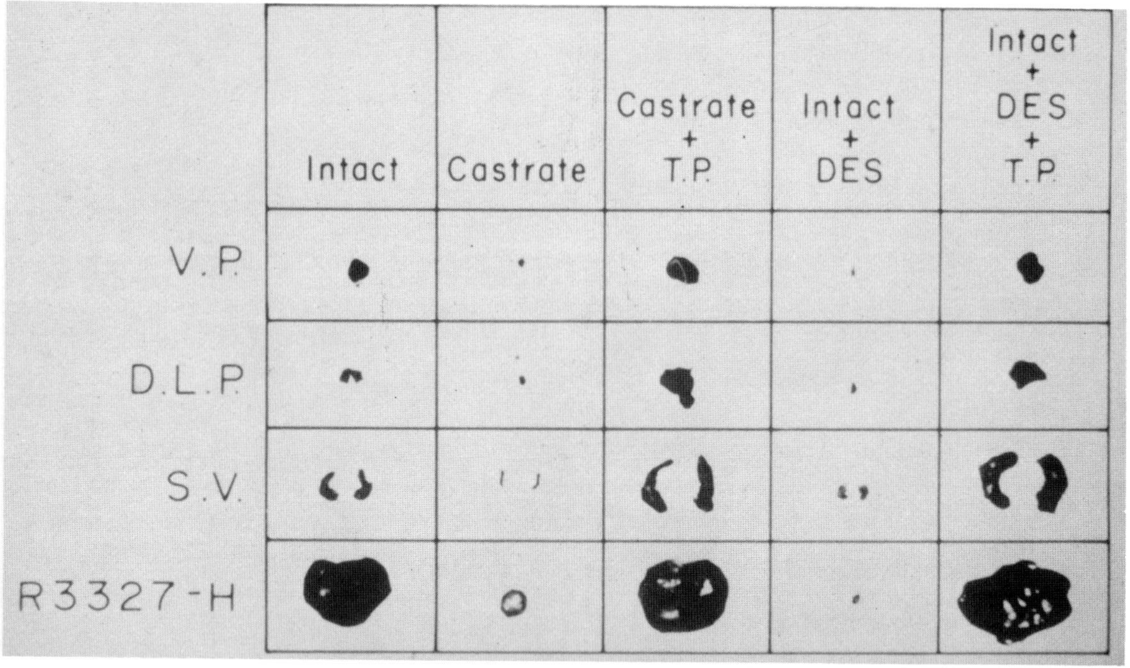

Fig. 2. Tissues removed from rats 180 days after subcutaneous injection of 1.5×10^6 viable Dunning tumor cells (R-3327-H). Animals were castrated at day 0 or treated daily for 180 days with 2 mg testosterone propionate or diethylstilbestrol at 100 μg/kg/day

TABLE I. 180-Day Growth of 1.5 × 10⁶ Cells of R-3327-H

	Total cell number		Fold increase in initial cell inoculum	% Inoculated cells growing	Cell doubling time (days)
Hormonal status	Relative	Absolute (10⁸)			
Intact	100	6.48 ± 2.7	432	93	20.9
Intact + testosterone propionate	99	6.40 ± 1.7	427	74	18.7
Intact + diethylstilbestrol	10	0.65 ± 0.21	43	8	20.2
Intact + flutamide	18	1.20 ± 0.32	80	16	20.3
Castrate	10	0.68 ± 0.16	45	29	24.8
Castrate + testosterone propionate	134	8.73 ± 3.0	582	83	19.8

were injected with 1.5×10^6 cells, and 120 days later when the tumor volume averaged 6.8 cubic centimeters, the animals were randomized to two groups, one left intact and the other group of 20 animals, castrated. The time of castrastion is indicated as day 0 in Figure 3, and the increase in survival time following castration is apparent. All animals in both intact and castrate groups subsequently died from tumor growth.

It would appear that hormone-insensitive cells may represent the culprit fraction that requires special therapeutic approaches. Means were therefore undertaken to develop such a subline to be termed the R-3327-HI and to use this line for therapeutic testing.

DEVELOPMENT OF THE HORMONE-INSENSITIVE LINES

The R-3327-H subline is routinely passaged in intact adult male rats in order to preserve the fraction (80%) of androgen-sensitive cells. In contrast, passage of this H subline in castrated male rats results in the selective loss of these androgen-sensitive cells with no effect on the proliferative growth of the androgen-insensitive cells. Therefore, by long-term passage of the H subline in castrated male rats, a new, slow-growing, well-differentiated, androgen-insensitive subline has been established and designated the R-3327-HI subline [4]. This HI subline contains both cytoplasmic receptor for DHT and 5α-reductase activity but does not respond to testosterone in terms of a stimulation of growth [4]. The R-3327-HI is therefore routinely passaged in castrate male rats.

A third tumor subline has spontaneously arisen from the R-3327-H tumor [1,

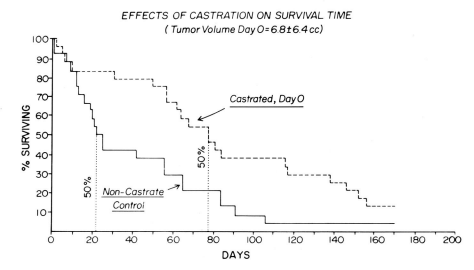

Fig. 3. Effect of castration on survival of animals with the Dunning R-3327-H tumor. Forty intact animals were inoculated with R-3327-H cells (1.5×10^6). After 120 days of growth the animals were randomized, and 20 were castrated and 20 were left intact. The time of castration after 120 days of initial growth is noted as day 0.

3, 4]. This subline is a rapidly growing, androgen-insensitive, anaplastic tumor termed the R-3327-AT. This anaplastic tumor does not contain receptor for DHT, nor does it possess 5α-reductase activity.

Using these three characterized R-3327 tumor sublines, a series of cellular parameters was examined to determine which of these indices could be used to predict the androgen sensitivity and the degree of differentiation of the prostatic adenocarcinomas.

Comparative Morphology of the R-3327 sublines (H, HI, and AT)

The morphology of the R-3327-H and HI tumors is very similar at the light microscopie level, with both of these sublines being composaed of glandular acini filled with PAS-positive secretions [3, 4]. The anaplastic AT tumor, in contrast, is composed of sheets of cells with no indication of secretory activity (Fig. 4). At the electron microscopic (EM) level, the H acinar cells have the characteristic appearance of epithelial cells. These cells possess both microvilli and desmosomes. The HI glandular cells have less prominent microvilli. Both the H and HI tumors contain cells that possess large filled vacuoles. The electron micrograph of the AT tumor reveals that there are few if any microvilli. Stains for collagen or reticular fibers fail to demonstrate any production of these components by the AT tumor. The AT tumor also does not contain cells that possess the large vacuoles.

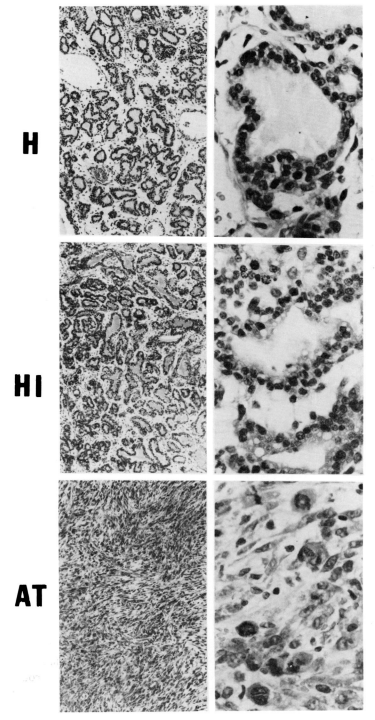

Fig. 4. Histology of the R-3327 sublines (top, H; middle, HI; bottom, AT).

It is clear that histological examination can only distinguish between the well-differentiated (H and HI) and anaplastic tumors (AT). This type of examination is totally unable to distinguish between the androgen-sensitive H and androgen-insensitive HI tumors.

Biochemical Methods to Identify the R-3327 (H, HI, and AT) Sublines

A comprehensive biochemical comparison of the three tumors was made [3, 4] to determine if it might be possible to distinguish hormone-sensitive from hormone-insensitive tumors. It was anticipated that these methods might be an alternate method to supplement the well-known steroid receptor methods being developed as prognostic indicators. Several parameters were compared, including morphology, testosterone metabolism, tissue protein profiles by sodium dodecyl sulfate (SDS) gel electrophoresis, stimulation of DNA synthesis, and finally the development of a relative enzymatic index (REI), which proved successful [4]. The general results are discussed in the paragraphs that follow. Additional details and methodology have been reported elsewhere [4].

The ability of the various tumor sublines to metabolize testosterone was not an effective discriminator. The well-differentiated androgen-insensitive HI tumor was able to metabolize testosterone as well as the H tumor. It would therefore appear that the 5α-reductase activity may not be a good index of androgen sensitivity in this model. The presence of secretory acid phosphatase also was not predictive of androgen sensitivity. The presence of the secretory acid phosphatase activity, however, does demonstrate again the prostatic origin of the Dunning tumors. The fact that the anaplastic tumor does not contain the secretory form of the enzyme indicates a degree of dedifferentiation resulting in the loss of this marker. Other methods are needed to establish the prostatic origin of this AT tumor. This is accomplished through the study of the tissue protein electrophoretic profiles, which clearly demonstrate that the AT tumor is uniquely related to the H and HI tumors.

The type of SDS-gel electrophoresis performed tends to reveal mainly structural components of tissue, since only these components are of sufficient quantity to be detected. Most enzymes are at too low a total protein concentration to be individually stained on gels. The fact that each tissue examined possessed a unique protein profile is thus not surprising when this is taken into consideration. Thus, even though the well-differentiated H and HI tumors have such different histology from the anaplastic AT tumor, their protein profiles are all virtually identical and different from other control tissues.

The ability of testosterone to stimulate selectively the DNA synthesis of the H tumor demonstrates once again the androgen sensitivity of this subline. This may represent the primary requirement for androgen in the growth cycle of the H tumor. The DNA synthesis of neither the HI nor the AT tumor was stimulated by exogenous testosterone. The lack of androgen receptor in the AT tumor could explain why this tumor does not respond to androgens. This rationale is, however, unsatisfactory for the explanation of the androgen insensitivity of HI tumor. This tumor possesses androgen receptor equal in amount and Kd with that of the normal androgen-sensitive dorsolateral prostate [7]. Since the rate of DNA synthesis has been shown to be related to prostatic growth rates [8], androgen stimulation of DNA synthesis may be a more sensitive predictor of androgen sensitivity than receptors per se. The fact that the HI tumor would be falsely classified as androgen sensitive on the basis of its androgen receptor content points to the requirement that receptor content must be correlated with some type of growth response in order to be predictive. Testosterone stimulation of DNA synthesis would thus appear to be an excellent alternative method to androgen receptors for discriminating androgen-sensitive and androgen-insensitive tumors. However, the limitations of this method to human tumors are obvious. It is conceivable that a biopsy specimen from a human prostatic tumor might be either maintained in organ culture or grown in a "nude" mouse and the effects of testosterone on DNA synthesis determined; however, this has not yet been accomplished.

The enzymatic profile appears to offer an alternative as a prognostic indicator. The relative enzymatic index (REI) has been tested with this model system and appears highly reliable in distinguishing the androgen sensitivity of these tumors.

DEVELOPMENT OF THE RELATIVE ENZYMATIC INDEX

In an earlier study it was observed that three enzymes — 3α-hydroxysteroid dehydrogenase (3αHSD), leucine amino peptidase (LAP), and lactic dehydrogenase (LHD) — increased, while another three enzymes — 5α-reductase (5αR), $7\alpha,6\alpha$-steroid hydroxylase ($7\alpha,6\alpha$HYD), and alkaline phosphatase (AlkP) — decreased in the R-3327 sublines that were androgen insensitive [3]. These enzymatic changes proved of value as discriminatory factors, particularly when combined into an arbitrary enzymatic index value [4]. Therefore normal dorsolateral prostates and R-3327-H, HI, and AT tumor tissues were obtained from ten different animals of each group, and these 30 tumor samples were assayed for the specific activities of the enzymes discussed earlier. These specific activities were then presented as relative values by normalizing each enzymatic activity separately, based on the mean activity for that enzyme in the dorsolateral prostate (mean activity of each enzyme in the dorsolateral prostate = 1). These average relative values were used to construct an arbitrary index termed the "relative enzymatic index" (REI) according to the formula:

$$\text{REI} = \frac{\text{Product of the relative activities of the three enzymes that increase}}{\text{Product of the relative activities of the three enzymes that decrease}} = \frac{(3\alpha\text{HSD})\,(\text{LAP})\,(\text{LDH})}{(5\alpha\text{R})\,(7\alpha,6\alpha\text{HYD})\,(\text{AlkP})}$$

The individual REI values for each individual sample of a tissue group (n = 10) was determined based on the actual relative enzymatic values that each separate sample possessed. These individual REI values are presented as a scattergram in Figure 5. Using the REI as a discriminatory factor, one can clearly separate the androgen-sensitive (R-3327-H) and androgen-insensitive (R-3327-HI) tumors. In making the proper classification of the 30 tumors from the REI values, we encountered no overlap of values between the tumors that would mistakenly produce misclassification [4].

In summary, in an attempt to develop new indices for predicting which prostatic cancers will respond to hormonal therapy, several possible approaches have been compared. These approaches have been tested for their abilities to discriminate between tumors of known androgen sensitivity using the well-characterized Dunning R-3327 rat prostate adenocarcinoma sublines as models. The overall findings are summarized in Table II.

It is important to note that the six enzymes used in the REI were chosen on a pragmatic basis related to the normal tissue of origin, in this case the normal adult rat dorsolateral prostate. By definition the low values approaching 1 would indicate relatedness in enzymatic profile to the androgen-stimulated (intact adult) rat dorsolateral prostate. It appears that the more closely related a tumor is to the

TABLE II. Parameters Studied to Discriminate Androgen Sensitivity of R-3227 Tumors

	Androgen-sensitive	Androgen-insensitive	
	Slow growth rate R-3327-H	Slow growth rate R-3327-HI	Fast growth rate R-3327-AT
Histology	Well-differentiated	Well-differentiated	Anaplastic
Steroid metabolism (5α-reductase activity)	Active	Active	Inactive
Protein electrophoretic profile	Similar	Similar	Similar
Acid phosphatase Secretory Lysosomal	Present Similar	Present Similar	Absent Similar
Androgen stimulation of DNA synthesis	Sensitive	Insensitive	Insensitive
Relative enzymatic index (range of 10 individual values)	Low — very similar to DL prostate (0.7–4)	Medium — distinct from DL prostate (26–110)	High — distinct from DL prostate (2,337–9,260)

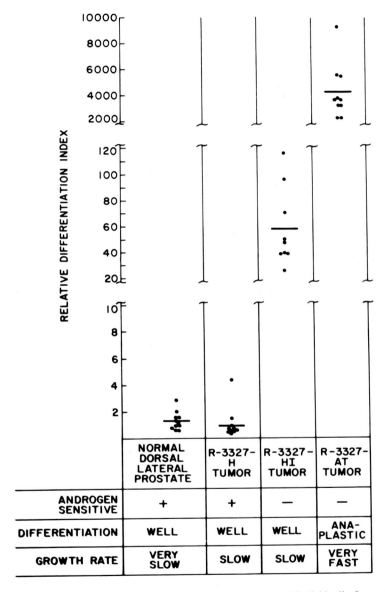

Fig. 5. Scattergram of the relative enzymatic indices determined individually for each sample tumor are compared to the normal dorsolateral prostate of the appropriate tissue groups. For details see text and References 3 and 4 (each group n = 10).

adult dorsolateral prostate, the higher is the probability that the tumor is androgen-sensitive. The relative enzymatic index also appears to discriminate the degree of differentiation of a tumor, The more closely related to the differentiated state of the tissue of origin, the more a tumor is, by definition, differentiated on a bio-chemical basis. Using the REI as a discriminator, then, the H tumor is well differentiated, the HI less differentiated, and the AT tumor anaplastic. It is important to note that differentiation is determined here by function as related through enzymatic profiles and not histology. In this case, however, the histology agrees completely with these interpretations.

One of the advantages of the REI is that this assay method could be scaled down and applied to needle biopsy samples, and multiple assays could be performed rapidly and with a high degree of reliability.

The present study did not consider the use of steroid-receptor assays, which might also prove useful in discriminating androgen-sensitive prostatic cancer; these studies are under way in several other laboratories [9]. It is conceivable that the REI and steroid-receptor assays might be used in concert to increase the discriminatory value of any prognostic indicators.

METASTASIS

One of the past limitations of the Dunning tumors has been the low rate of metastasis. More recently our laboratory has developed a new line, R-3327-AT-M, which has a very high rate of metastasis to the axillary lymph nodes and lungs. At present we are using the methods reported by Fidler [10] to develop new subclones that will metastasize to specific sites.

THERAPY

Hormonal and chemotherapy with Estracyt has been tested on the Dunning R-3327 tumors, and it indicates that this model may be applicable as a screen for drugs affecting prostatic cancer growth [1, 11, 12]. Adjuvant and immunotherapy have also been tested with the R-3327-AT tumor [13].

SUMMARY

The Dunning rat prostatic adenocarcinoma models (R-3327 series) are providing a valuable system for elucidating new principles of prostatic tumor biology. Each of the new lines provides a new tool for these studies, but each line must be carefully characterized and monitored.

ACKNOWLEDGMENTS

These investigations were supported by grant CA-15416, awarded by the National Prostatic Cancer Project of the National Cancer Institute, DHEW.

REFERENCES

1. Smolev JK, Heston WDW, Scott WW, Coffey DS: Characterization of the Dunning R-3327-H prostatic carcinoma: An appropriate animal model for prostatic cancer. Cancer Treat Rep 61:273–287, 1977.
2. Smolev JK, Coffey DS, Scott WW: Experimental models for the study of prostatic adenocarcinoma. J Urol 18:216–220, 1977.
3. Isaacs JT, Heston WDW, Weissman RM, Coffey DS: Animal model of hormone sensitive and insensitive prostatic adenocarcinomas: Dunning R-3327-H, R-3327-HI, and R-3327-AT. Cancer Res 38:4353–4359, 1978.
4. Isaacs JT, Isaacs WB, Coffey DS: Models for the development of non-receptor methods for distinguishing androgen sensitive and insensitive prostatic tumors. Cancer Res 36:2652–2659, 1979.
5. Dunning WF. Prostatic cancer in the rat. Natl Cancer Inst Monogr 12:351–369, 1963.
6. Voigt W, Feldman M, Dunning WF: 5α-Dihydrotestosterone-binding proteins and androgen sensitivity in prostatic cancers of Copenhagen rats. Cancer Res 35:1840–1846, 1975.
7. Heston WDW, Menon M, Tananis C, Walsh P: Androgen, estrogen, and progesterone receptors of the R-3327-H Copenhagen rat prostatic tumor. Cancer Lett 6:45–50, 1979.
8. Sufrin G, Coffey DS: A new model for studying the effect of drugs on prostatic growth. I. Antiandrogens and DNA synthesis. Invest Urol 11:45–54, 1973.
9. Menon M, Tananis CE, McLoughlin MG, Walsh PC: Androgen receptors in human prostatic tissue: A review. Cancer Treat Rep 61:265–271, 1977.
10. Fidler IJ: Tumor heterogeneity and the biology of cancer invasion and metastasis. Cancer Res 38:2651–2660, 1978.
11. Block NL, Camuzzi F, Donefrio J, Troner M, Claflin A, Stover B, Politano VA: Chemotherapy of the transplantable adenocarcinoma (R-3327) of the Copenhagen rat. Oncology 34:110–113, 1977.
12. Muntzing J, Kirdani RV, Saroff J, Murphy GP, Sandberg A: Inhibitory effects of Estracyt on R-3327 rat prostatic carcinoma. Urology 10:439–445, 1977.
13. Weissman RM, Coffey DS, Scott WW: Cell kinetic studies of prostatic cancer: Adjuvant therapy in animal models. Oncology 34:133–137, 1977.

Chemotherapeutic and Hormonal Considerations of the Nb Rat Prostatic Adenocarcinoma Model

Joseph R. Drago, MD, Laurence B. Goldman, MD, and
M. Eric Gershwin, MD

Carcinoma of the prostate is the most frequently occurring malignancy of the genitourinary tract. Sixty-two thousand cases were diagnosed in 1977, and 19,000 men died of this disease in the United States, alone [1]. Various approaches have been taken in the treatment of this malignancy and have included surgical removal of the local lesion through either a perineal or retropubic (abdominal) approach, radiotherapy, hormonal manipulation, cryosurgery, bilateral orchiectomy, surgical or medical adrenalectomy, hypophysectomy, and, most recently, chemotherapy. As in any condition where multiple modalities exist, there is controversy about which of the treatments is appropriate at the various stages of disease, from a small nidus of local carcinoma to extensive bony metastases.

Only recently has chemotherapy received attention, and it is now being explored with either single or multiple agents. Prior to 1973 only a handful of chemotherapeutic agents had been appropriately studied in a systematic fashion [2, 3]. There are obvious reasons for the lack of research. The variable nature of the disease, and the initial favorable response to hormonal manipulation are two reasons, perhaps, for the lack of appropriate chemotherapeutic trials earlier in the treatment of prostatic carcinoma. Traditionally, prostatic carcinoma patients were rarely included in phase II chemotherapeutic studies because of the difficulty in quantitating exact tumor extent or tumor response. Since phase II studies have traditionally been a springboard for more thorough evaluation, it is again apparent how chemotherapeutic application to treatment of prostatic cancer may have lagged behind chemotherapeutic treatment of other solid malignancies. How-

This investigation was supported by grant PHS-CA25032-01 awarded by the National Cancer Institute, DHEW (to J.R.D.) and by grant PHS-CA20816 awarded by the National Cancer Institute, DHEW (to M.E.G., who is the recipient of U.S. Public Health Service Research Career Development Award AI00193).

Models for Prostate Cancer, pages 325–363
© **1980 Alan R. Liss, Inc., 150 Fifth Ave., New York, NY 10011**

ever, several studies have recently been performed on hormone-resistant patients and include studies randomized by the National Prostatic Cancer Project, the ECOG, the Mayo Clinic, the NIC-VA Group, and the Western Cancer Study Group, to name but a few. Some single-agent chemotherapy has been shown to be effective in the treatment of prostatic carcinoma. Specific agents that have been shown to be efficacious include 5-fluorouracil, cyclophosphamide, estramustine, and streptozotocin, and these agents have produced objective response rates of 36%, 46%, 44%, and 32%, respectively, as compared to 19% for patients treated with hormonal manipulation, either castration or estrogen administration [4–7]. In another study, investigators have compared DTIC, procarbazine, and cyclophosphamide, obtaining response rates of 39%, 14%, and 21%, respectively [8]. Similarly, others have shown objective response rates of 5% and 25% for patients treated with single-agent 5-fluorouracil and Adriamycin [9, 10], whereas CCNU and 5-fluorouracil have shown 40% and 26% response rates [11, 12]. These investigations by Roswell Park researchers have also demonstrated a 33% objective response rate in patients with carcinoma of the prostate treated with cis-platinum [13]. Despite the generally encouraging chemotherapeutic objective response rates, difficulties arise in the relative activity of the various agents employed, since some studies include stabilization of disease in obtaining objective response rates. Other complications involved in using these agents include different patient populations with different performance states, different age of disease onset and different stage of disease at onset. Furthermore, a number of combination chemotherapeutic agents have been employed. Cyclophosphamide and 5-fluorouracil have yielded an objective response rate of 17% in 12 patients studied at the Mayo Clinic [14]. Objective response rates have been recorded, which include "stabilization," by the Roswell Park group, who have obtained objective response rates of 69% and 65% in combinations of Adriamycin plus cyclophosphamide and 5-fluorouracil plus cyclophosphamide, respectively [9]. With the multitude of chemotherapeutic agents available, several reports have been forthcoming evaluating the effects of various chemotherapeutic agents, singly or in combination, with varying degrees of objectivity or stabilization of disease (Table I).

As mentioned above, chemotherapy for disseminated prostatic cancer has been shown to increase survival and objective improvement of patients in selected instances [15–19]. Treatment for metastatic adenocarcinoma of the prostate has lagged behind treatment of other carcinomas. Only recently, since 1972 or 1973, has chemotherapy study in the treatment of patients with prostate carcinoma been undertaken in an effective manner. Chemotherapy with cyclophosphamide, vincristine, 5-fluorouracil, and methotrexate, as an adjunct for treatment of other solid malignancies, is well documented in the literature. A recent report has shown a 73% subjective and 24% objective response rate to a combination of 5-fluorouracil, melthan, methotrexate, vincristine, and prednisone in cases of advanced prostatic carcinoma [20]. Additionally, 16 patients have recently been treated

TABLE I. Chemotherapy Active in Human Prostate Cancer

Agent	Objective response and/or stabilization (%)[a]
5-Fluorouracil [5−7]	36
Cyclophosphamide [5, 7]	46
Estramustine [4]	44
Streptozotocin [4]	32
Standard hormonal therapy [5−7]	19
DTIC [8]	39
Procarbazine [8]	14
Cyclophosphamide [8]	21
5-Fluorouracil [9, 10]	5
Adriamycin [9, 10]	25
CCNU [11, 12]	40
5-Fluorouracil [11, 12]	26
Cis-platinum [13]	33
Cyclophosphamide and 5-fluorouracil [8, 14]	17
Adriamycin and cyclophosphamide [9]	69
5-Fluorouracil and cyclophosphamide [9]	65
Adriamycin and cis-platinum [15]	53
Adriamycin, cyclophosphamide, and cis-platinum [16]	75

[a]Patients in whom endocrine treatment failed.

with a similar regime consisting of cyclophosphamide, vincristine, 5-fluorouracil, and prednisone, with encouraging results. Six of 16 patients had objective responses, and 11 of 16 achieved subjective response rates [21]. In this report, cell tissue metastases were found to be more responsive than bony lesions. Of the 30 chemotherapeutic agents most active and effective in the treatment of other solid malignancies, only 5-fluorouracil and cyclophosphamide have been evaluated in more than 100 cases of prostatic cancer. However, data available from phase I evaluation show cause for some optimism with 5-fluorouracil, cyclophosphamide, and Adriamycin and lend support to the concept that appropriate single and/or combination chemotherapeutic agents for prostatic carcinoma must be sought. Yagoda has extensively, retrospectively reviewed drug therapy results at Memorial Hospital between 1959 and 1971 and found that, of the 601 patients who had metastatic prostate cancer, only 50% had cytotoxic chemotherapy. Despite the difficulties of such a retrospective analysis in evaluating objective responses, approximately 50% of the 88 patients so treated did have an objective response rate to nitrogen mustard, cyclophosphamide, and 5-fluorouracil [22]. Several controlled trial chemotherapeutic programs have been initiated, and the results have been previously described. Carter and Golden have ranked chemotherapeutic agents by activity in solid tumors and, in the most active group, active at least against two solid tumors [23], the Noble rat prostate adenocarcinoma has been evaluated with several of these agents (cyclophosphamide, Adriamycin, methotrexate, 5-fluorouracil, BCNU, and actinomycin-D). Additionally, agents active against one other solid tumor have also been evaluated, and the chemotherapeutic agents employed include vincristine, cis-platinum, and estramustine.

We have also applied this versatile rat prostatic adenocarcinoma model to study the various effects of chemotherapeutic agents on heterotransplanted Nb rat prostatic adenocarcinomas into congenitally athymic (nude) mice. The use of nude mice to rapidly identify numerous antitumor agents for clinical use is not a new one. Although our laboratory unit provided early evidence for the use of nude mice as biologic dosimeters for radiotherapeutic responsiveness [24], a number of other laboratories have seized upon the utility of human tumors in a graft nude mouse model to demonstrate the therapeutic agents clinically active, or inactive, retaining that level of anaplastic activity or inactivity when implanted in nude mice. Indeed, such approaches have demonstrated a well-documented clinical impression that the majority of solid tumor systems can be investigated in this manner. At present extensive work has been performed on human breast, endometrial, colon, and some human prostatic adenocarcinomas. The use of specific chemotherapeutic agents in nude mice has been reported and explored in this laboratory unit [25, 26]. Agents that have been studied, and for which the LD_{50} data are available (with 95% confidence levels) include BCNU, methotrexate, 5-fluorouracil, vincristine, Adriamycin, cyclophosphamide, actinomycin-D, vinblastine, and DTIC. The majority of these nonhormonal cytotoxic chemotherapeutic compounds have not been given adequate trials against human prostatic cancer. Indeed, a plethora of data exists for the 30 chemotherapeutic agents now in vogue for the treatment of other solid malignancies, and this situation is particularly noteworthy for prostatic adenocarcinoma.

Since the work of Huggins and Hodges, even prostatic carcinoma has been shown to be influenced by hormonal manipulation and to be primarily androgen dependent, at least initially. Thus, major therapeutic attempts have been directed at suppressing androgen stimulus to the prostate. The most common way of achieving this has been by bilateral orchiectomy, estrogen administration or other forms of hormonal manipulation — hypophysectomy and/or adrenalectomy. The use of the Noble rat prostatic adenocarcinoma model, with its androgen-dependent tumors, have been evaluated to assess the degree of efficacy of castration therapy on tumor size and tumor kinetics. Additionally, by using Silastic containing implants of either estrogen or testosterone, growth rates of these tumors could be altered (see chapter titled The Nb Rat Prostatic Adenocarcinoma Model System). Hormonal manipulation has been the mainstay of treatment of prostatic carcinoma over the last 30 years. This is based, in large part, upon the fact that some 70% of tumors respond to hormonal manipulation, at least initially, with both objective and subjective response rates. However, eventually these patients go on to relapse and their disease becomes refractory to hormonal manipulation. Additional hormonal studies have been carried out on such androgen-dependent tumors and include comparisons of castration therapy with various chemotherapies alone, including BCNU, 5-fluorouracil, cyclophosphamide, and Adriamycin. Similar studies have also been performed on heterotransplanted Nb rat tumors into congenitally athymic (nude) mice.

The use of radiation therapy for treatment of prostatic carcinoma has recently received widespread attention. Noteworthy are reports by Bagshaw, who used external radiotherapy treatment of prostatic carcinomas [27]. Additionally, interstitial radiation, as used by Whitmore and Carlton's group, has a place in treating patients with prostatic adenocarcinoma in some instances [28, 29]. Also well known are the effects of radiation therapy on local bony metastases and the efficacy of such treatment. It is with this in mind that radiotherapy of Nb rat tumors is considered. Determination of the effects of radiation therapy are correlated with tumor growth kinetics [24]. Quantitation of the dose necessary to arrest tumor growth is also described.

METHODS AND MATERIALS

Tumor Transplantation

As noted earlier, the major advantage of the Nb rat adenocarcinoma is the marked degree of tumor homogeneity. Thus, tumors can be transplanted into multiple recipients without attendant hazards of variable tumor transfer. Transplantation of tumors is performed in a manner similar to that described in the chapter on the Noble tumor (this volume). Briefly, an Nb rat prostatic tumor grows from a 2 mm^3 implant to a 1 cm^3 mass within four to eight weeks, depending on the specific tumor. The procedure for tumor transplantation into multiple recipients is as follows: After the tumor in the Nb rat host has reached a suitable size, the tumor is minced into 2 mm^3 fragments and transplanted directly under the skin in the area of the left flank of the Nb rat or nude mouse recipient. This procedure is performed under sterile conditions and takes approximately 15 seconds per transfer. The skin incision is made using a sterile scalpel, and the tumor is inserted with forceps into a subcutaneous tunnel. The wound is then closed with a single sterile surgical clip. It should be emphasized that all tumors transplanted for chemotherapeutic agents are derived directly from fresh tissue rather than from the frozen tissue bank. The tissue bank is maintained to permit storage and raising of larger volumes of tumor tissue needed for replicate copies. Thus, at a given time, attention can be focused intensely on individual tumors. The tumor nodule of 1.5 cm^3 is sufficient for implantation of 100 to 250 animals. Thus, it is possible to use transplantable tumors from the same transfer generation (ie, standardized replicate tissues). As emphasized, the reproducibility of this method of tissue transplantation is readily demonstrated by the similar growth pattern in multiple littermate recipients. Following tumor transplantation, animals are observed twice weekly, with specific tumor measurements begun when palpable masses are observed. The onset of tumor development varies with the individual tumor type. However, masses are usually observed at six to ten days following transplantation. The tumor masses are measured with the formula: tumor volume $(mm^3) = (width^2 \times length)/2$. Experiments treating both autonomous and hormone-dependent tumors with chemotherapy are as follows: Each group consists

TABLE II. Chemotherapy of Nb Rats

Androgen-dependent tumors	Adriamycin 1.25 mg/kg q week × 4
	Adriamycin 1.25 mg/kg q 10 days × 3
	Adriamycin 5 mg/kg q week × 4
	BCNU 2 mg/kg q 4 days × 3
	BCNU 2 mg/kg q 4 days × 3, 10-day rest, q 4 days × 2
	BCNU 2 mg/kg q week × 2
	BCNU 2 mg/kg q week × 3
	5-Fluorouracil 50 mg/kg q week × 4
	5-Fluorouracil 80 mg/kg q week × 4
	5-Fluorouracil 120 mg/kg q week × 4
	Methotrexate 25 mg/kg q week × 3
	Methotrexate 80 mg/kg q week × 4
	Methotrexate 100 mg/kg q week × 2
Autonomous tumors	Actinomycin-D 0.4 mg/kg q 4 days × 3
	Adriamycin 1.25 mg/kg q week × 4
	Adriamycin 2.5 mg/kg q week × 4
	Adriamycin 5 mg/kg q week × 4
	Alkeran 4 mg/kg q week × 2
	BCNU 2 mg/kg q 4 days × 3
	BCNU 10 mg/kg × 1
	Cis-platinum 1 mg/kg q week × 3
	Cis-platinum 10 mg/kg, 5 mg/kg × 1
	Cyclophosphamide 60 mg/kg q week × 3
	Cyclophosphamide 60 mg/kg q week × 4
	Cyclophosphamide 100 mg/kg q week × 4
	DTIC 5 mg/kg days 1 & 2, q 2 weeks × 2
	5-Fluorouracil 20 mg/kg q week × 3
	5-Fluorouracil 80 mg/kg q week × 3
	5-Fluorouracil 120 mg/kg q week × 3
	5-Fluorouracil 120 mg/kg q week × 4
	Ftorafur 30 mg/kg q week × 3
	Methotrexate 60 mg/kg q week × 4
	Methotrexate 80 mg/kg q week × 4
	Vincristine 0.2 mg/kg q 4 days × 3

TABLE III. Chemotherapy Heterotransplants: Nude Mice

Androgen-dependent tumors	Cyclophosphamide 100 mg/kg q week × 2
	5-Fluorouracil 80 mg/kg q week × 1
	5-Fluorouracil 80 mg/kg q week × 2
Autonomous tumors	Actinomycin-D 0.4 mg
	Adriamycin 2.5 mg/kg q week × 3
	Adriamycin 5 mg/kg q week × 4
	Adriamycin 5 mg/kg q week × 5
	BCNU 0.1 mg/kg q 4 days × 3
	Cyclophosphamide 100 mg/kg q week × 2
	Cyclophosphamide 100 mg/kg q week × 4
	5-Fluorouracil 80 mg/kg q week × 3
	5-Fluorouracil 80 mg/kg q week × 4
	5-Fluorouracil 120 mg/kg q week × 3
	Ftorafur 30 mg/kg q week × 3
	Methotrexate 60 mg/kg q week × 3
	Methotrexate 100 mg/kg q week × 3
	Methotrexate 100 mg/kg q week × 4

of eight to 12 animals with a standard saline control group. Chemotherapy is initiated after tumor volume is at least 60 mm^3. At this point, tumor viability and growth have been determined. The tumor take rate in Nb rat recipients is in the order of the magnitude of +95%, whereas in the nude mouse it is 90%. The chemotherapeutic agents employed include 5-fluorouracil, methotrexate, BCNU, melphalan (Alkeran), cis-platinum, Adriamycin, estramustine, actinomycin-D, cyclophosphamide, DTIC, and streptozotocin. Several agents have been employed at more than one dosage and have varying times of chemotherapeutic administration (Tables II and III). Evaluation of statistical significance has been carried out utilizing the Student t-test in all instances. Combination chemotherapy has not been employed to date. The length of the individual experiments varies, but all are continued a minimum of 30 days following the last chemotherapeutic administration. At the conclusion of the experiment, all animals are necropsied, and tumor samples as well as representative samples of pulmonary, liver, mediastinal, and other metastatic deposits are analyzed for histologic confirmation. Additionally, histologic evaluation is made of the liver, kidneys, bladder, and lungs for specific treatment groups.

Hormonal Studies

As noted earlier, Nb rat prostatic adenocarcinomas are derived by hormonal implantation of the Nb rats and have been characterized on the basis of being either androgen-dependent, autonomous, or estrogen-dependent. It is the purpose of this section to describe the methods and materials in evaluating the androgen-dependent tumors 2 Pr 128 and 2 Pr 129. The tumors are transplanted into groups of eight to 12 Nb rat or nude mouse recipients, as described previously. Tumor transplantation is carried out 48 hours prior to other experimental manipulation. The experimental groups include an intact saline control group, castration group, castration and implantation of 17-beta-estradiol Silastic implant, castration and implantation of a testosterone Silastic implant, castration alone, sham castration, as well as administration of various chemotherapeutic agents. Additional hormonal manipulation has been carried out on selected groups of androgen-dependent tumors and consists of removing testosterone Silastic implants as well as implanting estrogen Silastic implants for evaluation of this hormonal therapy late in the course of treatment, when the tumor burden is marked and the tumor volume is greater than 3 cm^3. Statistical significance is computed by the Student t-test (Tables IV and V). Figures 1 and 2 give a graphic representation of the results of

TABLE IV. Tumor Growth: Nb Rats*

	Number of tumors growing Number of tumors implanted
Autonomous tumors 18 Pr, 13 Pr 12, 102 Pr	
Normal males and normal females	343/351
Estrogenized males	72/74
Androgenized males	87/90
Estrogenized females	84/88
Androgenized females	76/79
Androgen-dependent tumors 2 Pr 128, 2 Pr 129	
Normal males	296/302
Estrogenized males	3/115[a]
Castrate males with testosterone implants	125/128
Normal females	2/78[a]
Androgenized females	135/139
Estrogen-dependent tumors 52 Pr, 114 Pr	
Normal females	48/52
Androgenized females	3/66[a]
Castrate females with estrogen implants	49/55
Normal males	3/46[a]
Estrogenized males	31/34

*Tumor volume $\geq$ 20% of control — ie, androgenized host control for androgen-dependent tumor study.
[a]$P < 0.01$ when compared to growth in these groups.
NOTE: For determination of hormonal influence and autonomy, groups of Nb rats with tumor in vivo were subjected to the following hormonal manipulations for the three main tumor types: Autonomous tumors were subjected to estrogenization and androgenization, androgen-dependent tumors were subjected to androgenization and estrogenization, and a similar procedure was carried out for the estrogen-dependent tumor-bearing Nb rats.

TABLE V. Tumor Growth: Classification for (Nude) Mice*

	Number of tumors growing / Number of tumors implanted
Autonomous tumors 18 Pr, 13 Pr 12, 102 Pr	
Normal males and females	99/100
Estrogenized males	67/70
Androgenized males	54/56
Estrogenized females	58/60
Androgenized females	69/70
Androgen-dependent tumors 2 Pr 128, 2 Pr 129	
Normal males	51/53
Estrogenized males	4/70[a]
Castrate males with testosterone implants	58/63
Normal females	3/58[a]
Androgenized females	41/45
Estrogen-dependent tumors 52 Pr, 114 Pr	
Normal females	43/45
Androgenized females	2/42[a]
Castrate females with estrogen implants	41/44
Normal males	3/39[a]
Estrogenized males	22/26

*Growth; tumor volume > 60 mm; statistical analysis by Student's t-test.
[a]$p < 0.01$ when compared to growth of tumors in these groups; ie, androgen-dependent tumor growth in androgenized hosts is significant when compared to tumor growth in estrogenized hosts.

the various hormonal manipulations employed. At the conclusion of the experiment, procedures for autopsy and histologic sections are followed as outlined in Methods and Materials.

Radiation Therapy

Tissue explants are irradiated prior to implantation into groups of 12 Nb rats and nude mice. Determination of the effects of radiation therapy are correlated with tumor growth kinetics. Quantitation of the dose necessary to arrest tumor growth has also been determined. Tumor nodules are removed from Nb rats bearing prostatic adenocarcinoma. Wedges of tumor, 2 mm^3, are prepared and placed in RPMI 1640 medium in a 100 mm Falcon plastic Petri dish. These dishes are irradiated from 0 to 1,500 rads at 162.7 rads/min using identical geometrical operational parameters and ambient temperature. Following radiation, the tissues are implanted into eight to 12 unmanipulated Nb rats. Tumor growth is followed for a period of ten weeks. The tumors used in this study included the autonomous tumors, 13 Pr 12 and 18 Pr, and the androgen-dependent tumor, 2 Pr 129.

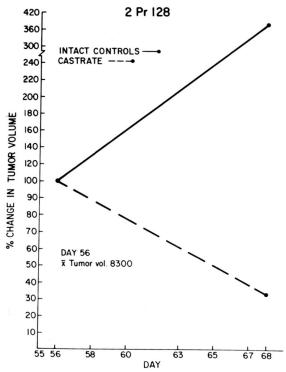

Fig. 1. Twenty animals were the subject of this experiment. All had the androgen-dependent tumor 2 Pr 128 growing to determine the effect of massive tumor volume in response to castration on the 56th day of tumor growth. One-half of the animals were castrated and the others were not. At this time, the mean tumor volume was 8,300 mm³ ± 1,287, and the animals were observed for the next 12 days. The intact controls increased tumor size to an average final volume of 31,700 mm³ ± 4,200, as opposed to the castrated group of which the final tumor volume was 5,500 mm³ ± 852.

Laboratory Results

Hematocrit and hemoglobin levels in Nb rats were evaluated in control groups without tumor, in saline-treated control groups with tumors in situ, and in the chemotherapeutic treatment groups. Additionally, standard laboratory evaluation of liver function tests, SGOT, SGPT, alkaline phosphatase, total bilirubin, BUN, total protein, albumin, LDH, and serum calcium levels were performed in the following groups: pretreatment controls that were to receive interperitoneal saline, controls without tumor, and the various chemotherapeutic groups. A range and a mean were determined for the control animals and compared to the various treatment groups and indicated as normal, decreased, or increased (Tables VI and VII).

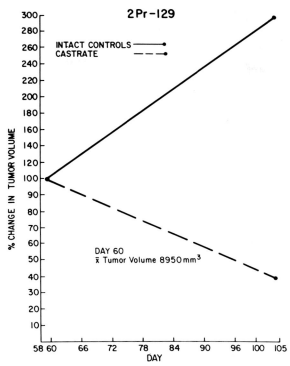

Fig. 2. The androgen-dependent tumor 2 Pr 129 was subject to the same experiment as outlined in Figure 1. The mean castrate groups' tumor volume at the conclusion of the experiment 55 days following initiation of therapy was 5,459 mm³ ± 985. The intact controls' mean tumor volume was 26,402 mm³ ± 3,750.

TABLE VI. Hematocrit and Hemoglobin: Chemotherapy

Group	Mean hematocrit (%)	Mean hemoglobin (gm %)
Saline control	43.5	13.1
Estramustine	43.0	15.0
Mephalan (Alkeran)	41.0	14.0
DTIC	43.5	13.0
Vincristine	41.0	13.6
BCNU	42.0	12.5
Cis-platinum	43.0	12.5
5-Fluorouracil, 80 mg	41.0	12.2
5-Fluorouracil, 120 mg	39.0	12.0
Methotrexate, 50 mg	38.0	12.0
Methotrexate, 150 mg	32.0	11.0
Adriamycin, 2.5 mg	41.0	12.5
Adriamycin, 5 mg	37.0	11.75
Cyclophosphamide, 80 mg	40.0	12.5
Testosterone implant	43.0	13.2
17-beta-estradiol implant	42.0	13.0

TABLE VII. Biochemistry*

Group	SGOT (units/liter)	SGPT (units/liter)	LDH (units/liter)	Alkaline phosphatase (units/liter)	Bilirubin (mg/dl)	BUN (mg/dl)	Calcium (mg/dl)	Albumin (gm/dl)	Total protein (gm/dl)
Control $\bar{X}$	193	75	860	383	0.1	21	9.1	3.2	5.7
Control range	111–306	28–220	575–1,436	175–1,000	0–0.4	12–32	3.8–12.8	1.7–3.7	3.4–7.6
Adriamycin	N	N	N	N	N	N	N	N	N
BCNU	N	N	↑	N	N	N	N	N	N
5-Fluorouracil	N	N	N	N	N	N	N	N	N
Cyclophosphamide	N	N	N	N	N	N	N	N	N
Actinomycin-D	N	N	N	N	N	N	N	N	N
Estrogen implant	N	N	N	N	N	N	N	N	N
Testosterone implant	N	N	N	↑	N	N	N	N	N
Saline (tumor in vivo)	N	N	↑	↑	N	N	N	N	N
Animals with metastases	N–↑	↑	↑	↑	N	N	N	N	N

N = normal; ↓ = decreased as compared to controls; ↑ = increased as compared to controls.

RESULTS

Nb Rat Hormone Considerations

2 pr 129. This androgen-dependent tumor was subjected to various therapeutic manipulations.

Experiment I. Sixty animals were the subject of this study to evaluate Adriamycin 1.25 mg/kg every week times four, 5-fluorouracil 50 mg/kg every week times four, and methotrexate 25 mg/kg and BCNU 2 mg/kg every week times three. None of these animals received testosterone supplementation. The mean tumor volume increases were as follows: saline control group 21,000 ± 4,500 mm^3; Adriamycin 694 ± 1,300 mm^3; methotrexate 186 ± 208 mm^3; BCNU 2,660 ± 2,600 mm^3; 5-fluorouracil 3,177 ± 3,558 mm^3; castration alone 5,726 ± 3,200 mm^3. All agents employed at these dosage schedules were statistically significant ($P < 0.01$). The castration group was $P < 0.0013$, and it is noted that all chemotherapeutic agents versus castration yielded statistically significant results ($P < 0.01$). In this experiment, methotrexate was the most efficacious. However, Adriamycin, BCNU, 5-fluorouracil, and castration were statistically significant. In the methotrexate group, 40% of the animals had complete tumor regression. In the Adriamycin group, one-third of the animals showed complete tumor regression. Additionally, in the 5-fluorouracil and BCNU groups, 15% of the animals had complete tumor regression. Metastatic disease was observed in 20% of the saline control animals as well as in 20% of the castrated animals. However, only 10% of the animals treated with Adriamycin, BCNU, and 5-fluorouracil had metastatic disease. Animals receiving methotrexate had no pulmonary or other metastatic disease (Table VIII and Fig. 3).

TABLE VIII. 2 Pr 129: Complete Regression and Metastasis at Necropsy

Group	Complete tumor regression (%)	Metastasis (%)
Saline	0	20
Castrate	0	20
5-Fluorouracil	15	10
BCNU	15	10
Adriamycin	33	10
Methotrexate	40	0

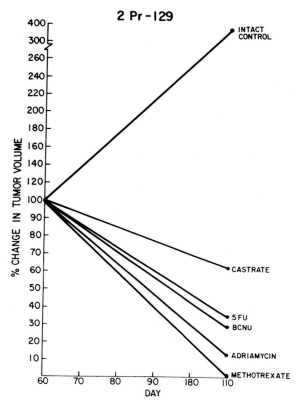

Fig. 3. Hormonal and chemotherapeutic manipulations on the 2 Pr 129 androgen-dependent tumors in intact controls, castrate animals, 5-fluorouracil-treated animals, BCNU-treated animals, Adriamycin-treated animals, and methotrexate-treated animals. Treatment was initiated on day 60 post-tumor implantation, at which time the mean tumor volume was 90 to 100 mm^3 ± 1,200 mm^3 and was observed to day 110.

Experiment II. The androgen-dependent tumor 2 pr 129 was subjected to the following chemotherapeutic agents, with chemotherapy initiated after a period of suitable tumor growth to a volume of at least 90 mm^3. Each group consisted of ten animals, which were treated as follows: intraperitoneal saline, Adriamycin 1.25 mg/kg every ten days times three, methotrexate 100 mg/kg every week times two, BCNU 2 mg/kg every week times two, and a castration group. The saline control animals had an average tumor growth of approximately 20,000 mm^3, whereas the Adriamycin-treated animals had tumor growth of approximately

TABLE IX. 2 Pr 129: Tumor Growth Comparison Treatment Groups
Versus Controls*

Group	% Tumor growth treatment groups versus controls
Saline controls	100.0
Castrate	35.0
Adriamycin 1.25 mg/kg every 10 days $\times$ 3	3.5
Methotrexate 100 mg/kg every week $\times$ 2	0.5
BCNU 2 mg/kg every week $\times$ 2	11.0

*All treatment modalities were effective, but chemotherapeutic agents had a more marked effect on tumor growth than did castration alone.

700 mm^3. Methotrexate-treated animals had an average tumor volume growth of 100 mm^3, and BCNU was associated with a tumor volume of 2,700 mm^3 at the conclusion of the experiment. Animals that were castrated at the time of initial chemotherapy had an average tumor growth of 7,100 mm^3. All results were statistically significant ($P < 0.005$). The chemotherapeutic agents employed were also significant when compared to the castrated group. The percentage of growth of the chemotherapeutic and castrated groups versus the saline groups showed the Adriamycin group to have an average tumor growth only 3.5% of that of the saline treatment group. Methotrexate had an average tumor growth of 0.5% of the control group, BCNU had 11% of the control group, and the castrated group had 35% of the control group (Table IX). Two animals treated with Adriamycin died. In both cases the cause of death was related to myocardial toxicity. Two animals treated with methotrexate also died after the second chemotherapeutic administration. The animals treated with BCNU and castration had no significant toxicity.

Experiment III. This experiment was designed to evaluate 5-fluorouracil versus saline controls. The dose of 5-fluorouracil used was 120 mg/kg every week times four. The chemotherapy was started when the tumor volume was at least 90 mm^3. Prior to that time, homogeneous tumor growth was demonstrated, as shown in Figure 4. This figure shows the homogeneous nature of tumor volume growth of the saline group throughout the experiment. Of 25 tumors treated with 5-fluorouracil at this dosage and schedule, homogeneous response was seen in 21 of these tumors, with abrupt cessation in tumor growth following the second chemotherapeutic administration (Fig. 5). Two tumors actually regressed completely by the mid-point of the chemotherapy. A third tumor was on its way to complete regression, which did occur approximately one month following the last chemotherapeutic administration (Fig. 6) ($P < 0.005$).

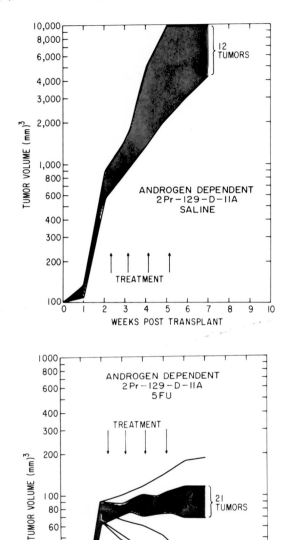

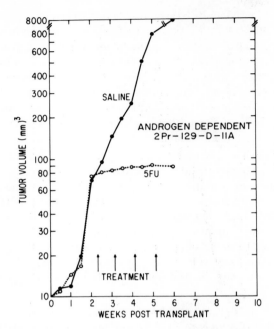

Fig. 6. Comparison of saline and 5-fluorouracil treatment on the androgen-dependent tumor 2 Pr 129.

Experiment IV. Nb rat females were subjected to the following manipulation: forty-eight hours prior to transplantation, 12 animals received testosterone Silastic implants, 12 animals were oophorectomized and implanted with 17-beta-estradiol implants, 11 animals were oophorectomized and implanted with testosterone implants, 11 animals were oophorectomized, and 11 animals received testosterone. This latter group was to receive chemotherapy consisting of BCNU at 2 mg/kg every week times two after the tumor had reached a volume of at least 90 mm^3. The design of this experiment was to enable our unit to ascertain the various growth parameters in animals with an androgenized milieu and an estrogenized

---

Fig. 4. Androgen-dependent tumor 2 Pr 129, subline D-11A, depicting the homogeneous tumor growth for the 12 tumors involved in the saline group.

Fig. 5. Effect of 5-fluorouracil treatment on androgen-dependent tumor 2 Pr 129, subline D-11A. Note two tumors completely regressed at six weeks during the 5-fluorouracil treatment, and a third tumor regressed at ten weeks. Also note homogeneous retardation of growth of the majority of the other tumors treated [21].

milieu as well as to evaluate BCNU chemotherapy. Oophorectomized animals that had received testosterone served as the controls. Their tumor volume increase was 13,000 mm^3. Animals that were oophorectomized alone had a tumor volume increase of 8,700 mm^3. Animals that had been oophorectomized and received estrogen implants had a tumor volume of only 1,475 mm^3, whereas females that had received testosterone implants showed a tumor volume of 8,500 mm^3. Thus, relatively androgenized females had significant tumor volume increase as opposed to estrogenized females. Females that had been implanted with testosterone were the control group for the females implanted with testosterone and subsequently treated with BCNU. There were statistically significant differences between these groups, in that the females treated with testosterone had a tumor volume increase of 8,500 mm^3 as opposed to the animals treated with testosterone implants and BCNU, which showed a tumor volume increase of only 700 mm^3 ($P < 0.001$). It was observed that animals that were androgenized either by testosterone implant alone or by oophorectomy plus testosterone had a significant increase in tumor volume, as opposed to animals that were actively estrogenized via oophorectomy plus estrogen. Also of interest is the fact that animals receiving testosterone then treated with chemotherapy showed that this BCNU chemotherapeutic trial was effective.

Experiment V. This protocol addressed the responsiveness of the androgen-dependent tumor Pr 129 to cytotoxic chemotherapy using BCNU, hormonal manipulation, and a combination of the two. Experimental groups were as follows:

   I. Sham incision — saline injections
  II. Sham incision — BCNU injections
 III. Orchiectomy with testosterone implant — saline injections
 IV. Orchiectomy with testosterone implant — BCNU injections
  V. Orchiectomy with testosterone implant — BCNU injections — removal of testosterone implant
 VI. Orchiectomy with testosterone implant — BCNU injections — removal of testosterone implant and placement of estrogen implant
VII. Orchiectomy with saline injections.

Seventy-two to 96 hours prior to the onset of cytotoxic chemotherapy, hormonal manipulation consisting of orchiectomy and subcutaneous placement of testosterone implants was performed.

BCNU 2 mg/kg was administered as an intraperitoneal injection. In all, five injections (10 mg/kg) were given during the experiment. The first three injections were administered every four days times three. This was followed by a ten-day "free" period, during which the second hormonal manipulations were performed at the mid-"free" point (day five). Cytotoxic chemotherapy was reinstituted on day 11, with the final two injections given every four days times two. Controls were treated with intraperitoneal saline at the time chemotherapy groups were administered the cytotoxic agents. Hormonal manipulation controls had scrotal incisions only. Five treatment cycles were administered to the seven groups. In the sham incision-saline injection group (I), the increase in tumor volume was 34,000 mm^3. Group III (orchiectomy, testosterone implant, and saline) had an increased tumor volume of 28,000 mm^3. No significance was observed between these groups (P < 0.15). However, the orchiectomy-saline group (VII) had a tumor increase of 14,600 mm^3. This was significant when compared to either group I or group III (P < 0.05). Group II (sham incision, BCNU injection) rats showed an average increase in tumor volume of 9,500 mm^3. This is compared to group IV (orchiectomy, testosterone implant, BCNU injection), which had an average tumor increase of 2,281 mm^3 (P < 0.02). Groups V (orchiectomy, testosterone implanted, BCNU injections, removal of testosterone implant) rats had an average tumor volume increase of 2,567 mm^3. Group VI (orchiectomy, testosterone implant, BCNU injection, removal of testosterone implant, addition of estrogen implant) rats showed an average tumor increase of 54 mm^3 at the termination of the experiment. Eighteen of 20 tumors in this group showed complete regression. In one of the remaining two tumors, significant retardation of growth occurred, and in only one tumor was there minimal progression (Figs. 7 and 8; Table X). One experimental animal died prior to the termination of the experiment. Metastases were noted in 16% of the rats at autopsy. Comparison of tumor growth demonstrates the significance of BCNU over saline controls. The efficacy of this agent was further increased by the removal of testosterone and the addition of estrogen. The combination of hormonal manipulation and cytotoxic chemotherapy was statistically more significant than the use of either modality by itself.

The addition of estrogen in combination with the removal of testosterone yielded greater tumor regression than the removal of testosterone alone. In fact, the removal of testosterone alone did not significantly alter tumor growth. This can be seen in both the saline and the BCNU-treated groups. The lack of response to the removal of testosterone may be due to the size of tumor burden at that time. Serum testosterone levels correlate well with final tumor volumes and attest to the hormonal dependency of Pr 129. These levels reveal that castrate animals had a reduction in serum testosterone to at least one-fifth the levels of normal intact males or males with testosterone implants.

Nb rat chemotherapy — 2 pr 128. In this experiment, all male rats were supplemented with 1 cm testosterone Silastic implants. The groups were as follows: a saline control group, an Adriamycin group, a 5-fluorouracil group, a methotrexate group, and a BCNU group. Adriamycin 5 mg/kg, 5-fluorouracil 80 mg/kg, and methotrexate 80 mg/kg were administered via the intraperitoneal route at weekly intervals times four. BCNU 2 mg/kg was administered every four days times three.

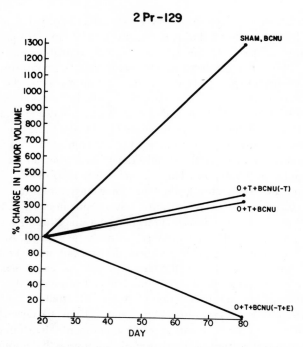

Fig. 7. Androgen-dependent tumor 2 Pr 129 subjected to BCNU chemotherapy as well as a combination of orchiectomy plus testosterone and orchiectomy plus testosterone with an exchange of a 17-beta-estradiol implant for the testosterone implant. Treatment in this experiment was initiated at day 21 and followed until day 80 of the experiment and is expressed as percentage changes in tumor volume at day 80 versus day 21.

In addition, one group was treated with a Silastic implant containing 17-beta-estradiol administered at the time of the first chemotherapeutic administration to the other groups. The saline control group had an average tumor volume of 98,000 mm^3; 5-fluorouracil had an average tumor volume of 18,000 mm^3; BCNU treatment yielded a tumor volume increase of 4,500 mm^3; Adriamycin yielded a tumor volume increase of 1,500 mm^3; methotrexate yielded a tumor volume increase of 122 mm^3. The 17-beta-estradiol implant resulted in tumor growth of only 330 mm^3 (Table XI). However, in the methotrexate-treated group, three animals died of chemotoxicity following the second chemotherapeutic administration. To ascertain the effect of hormonal milieu on activity of growing tumors in these testosterone-supplemented males, eight tumor-bearing animals had testosterone implants removed and replaced with estrogen implants. These animals

2 Pr –129

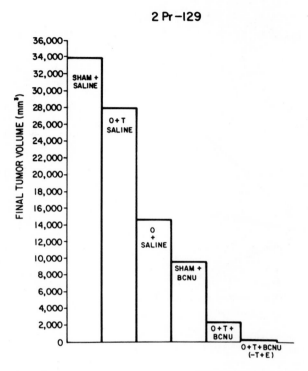

Fig. 8. Graphic representation of 2 Pr 129, the androgen-dependent tumor, and the effects of orchiectomy, testosterone, estrogen, and BCNU. This representation demonstrates the efficacy of combination chemotherapy and hormonal manipulation.

had tumor regression to a volume of 3,694 mm^3, as opposed to the animals that had the testosterone left in place during the same 12-day period, which had an increase in tumor size of 31,000 mm^3 (Fig. 9). Adriamycin-, 5-fluorouracil-, and BCNU-treated groups all showed statistical significance with $P < 0.0025$ as did the methotrexate with the same P value.

Nb rat chemotherapy — autonomous tumor 102 pr. Chemotherapy of the 102 pr autonomous tumor in syngeneic Nb rats consisted of 5-fluorouracil 80 mg/ kg and Ftorafur 30 mg/kg injected intraperitoneally at weekly intervals times three. This protocol was evaluated following prechemotherapy reduction of tumor growth to at least 90 mm^3. The saline control group received an injection of buf- fered saline in a 1 cc volume at the time chemotherapy was administered to the treatment groups. The saline control group had an average tumor increase of 2,100 mm^3, and the Ftorafur resulted in a 4,266 mm^3 increase in tumor volume

TABLE X. 2 Pr 129

	Group	Final tumor volume mm³	P value[a]
I	Sham incision saline	34,000	–
II	Sham incision BCNU	9,500	<0.01
III	Orchiectomy testosterone saline	28,000	<0.15 (NS)
IV	Orchiectomy testosterone BCNU	2,281	<0.005
V	Orchiectomy testosterone BCNU (testosterone removed)	2,567	<0.005
VI	Orchiectomy testosterone BCNU (testosterone removed and estrogen added)	54	<0.001
VII	Orchiectomy saline	14,648	<0.05

[a]Student's t-test.
NS = not significant.

TABLE XI. 2 Pr 128

Group[c]	Tumor volume (mm³)	% Tumor growth treatment groups vs controls	% Metastasis	% Complete tumor regression
Saline controls	98,000	100.00	25	0
Adriamycin 5 mg/kg q week × 4	1,500	1.50	16	17
5-Fluorouracil 80 mg/kg q week × 4	18,000	18.30	16	17
Methotrexate 80 mg/kg q week × 4	122	0.13	0	33
BCNU 2 mg/kg q 4 days × 3	4,500	4.60	16	17
Estradiol implant	330	0.34	16	33

*Except for the estradiol-implanted group, the experimental groups were supplemented with testosterone implants. Treatment was initiated when the tumor volume reached approximately 90 mm³.

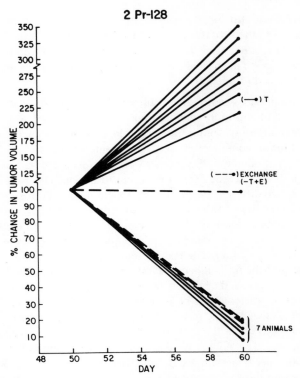

2 Pr-I28

Fig. 9. Individual tumor responses of androgen-dependent tumor 2 Pr 128 as determined by percentage changes in tumor volume from day 50 through day 60 in animals with testosterone implants as opposed to animals in which the testosterone implant was removed and a 17-beta-estradiol implant was placed. The "controls" were the animals in which the testosterone implant remained. At the initiation of the exchange (day 50 of the experiment) the tumor volume was 16,384 mm³ ± 2,576 mm³. Note the increase in doubling time of this tumor with supplemental testosterone being 4.2 days as opposed to the doubling time without supplementation with exogenous testosterone in the form of Silastic implant, which normally is 5.3 days.

at the completion of the experiment, as compared to the pre-treatment tumor volume. In the control animals there is a linear progression in tumor growth size throughout the course of the experiment, whereas in the chemotherapeutic treatment animals, there is a rapid fall-off of tumor volume following the second chemotherapeutic administration. However, at the completion of this experiment, there appeared to be a tendency toward regrowth and further progression in tumor volume. In this experiment, 5-fluorouracil-treated animals showed complete tumor regression in two of the 12 treated, whereas there were no complete tumor regression in the Ftorafur group. Significance of the 5-fluorouracil groups revealed $P <$ 0.008, as opposed to the Ftorafur group which had $P < 0.032$. Histologically, tumors treated with either agent resembled the primary donor tumor, except that there was some increase in stromal fibrosis. No significant toxicity in the dosages employed as observed (Table XII).

Nb rat chemotherapy — autonomous tumor 18 pr. This Nb rat autonomous tumor has been stable for more than 30 tumor transplant generations with no evidence of dedifferentiation. Tumor harvesting the implantation have already been described. At a tumor volume of 60 mm^3, the chemotherapy was initiated. Thirty days following chemotherapy, the animals were sacrificed and autopsied. Metastases were identified and sent for histologic confirmation. Three chemotherapeutic agents in two different experiments were employed. Testosterone was one of the modalities employed to reverify the autonomous nature of this tumor and was administered in the form of a Silastic implant. Adriamycin 5 mg/kg and methotrexate 60 mg/kg were used in the first experiment. They were administered at weekly intervals times four. The testosterone-containing implant was placed at the time of the first chemotherapeutic administration. Adriamycin 2.5 mg/kg, methotrexate 80 mg/kg, and cyclophosphamide 60 mg/kg were used in the second experiment and administered in 1 cc volumes every week times four. Controls for both experiments as well as the testosterone group received 1 cc intraperitoneal injections of sterile saline at the same time the treatment groups received cytotoxic chemotherapy. Ten animals were assigned to each group in the first experiment, and 12 rats per treatment group were used in the second experiment. The saline control group showed an average tumor increase in volume of 48,000 mm^3 in the first experiment and 56,000 mm^3 in the second. Adriamycin-treated groups had an average tumor increase of 11,725 mm^3 and 4,600 mm^3 at 5 mg/kg and 2.5 mg/kg dosages, respectively. The methotrexate treatment group showed an average tumor increase of 1,700 mm^3 at dosages of 60 mg/kg and 80 mg/kg, respectively. The cyclophosphamide-treated group revealed complete tumor regression in 66% of the animals treated and an average decrease of 51% in the remaining tumors. The testosterone-treated groups showed an average tumor increase of 44,000 mm^3, and this was not statistically significant compared to the controls ($P < 0.5$). Adriamycin therapy at 5 mg/kg and 2.5 mg/kg, and methotrexate therapy at 80 mg/kg and 60 mg/kg yielded retardation of tumor growth that was statistically significant ($P < 0.005$). Variations among chemotherapeutic agents may be dose related (Table XII). Noteworthy is the homogeneous tumor growth observed in all tumors prior to chemotherapy.

No deaths were observed in the saline control group or the Adriamycin group treated at 2.5 mg/kg. Mortality for the cyclophosphamide group was 15%. Mortality for the Adriamycin group at 5 mg/kg and the methotrexate group at 60 mg/kg was 37% and 10%, respectively. The mortality for the higher dose of methotrexate was 66%.

TABLE XII. Autonomous Tumors: 102 Pr, 18 Pr, Nb Rat Chemotherapy

Tumor		% Tumor growth treatment groups vs controls	% Metastasis	% Complete tumor regression
102 Pr	Saline	100.00	58	0
	5-Fluorouracil 80 mg/kg q week × 3	21.00	33	16
	Ftorafur 30 mg/kg q week × 3	42.00	33	0
18 Pr	Saline I	100.00	60	0
	Saline II	100.00	60	0
	Adriamycin 2.5 mg/kg q week × 4	8.00	0	16
	Adriamycin 5 mg/kg q week × 4	24.00	12	20
	Cyclophosphamide 60 mg/kg q week × 4	0.15	25	66
	Methotrexate 60 mg/kg q week × 4	4.00	25	25
	Methotrexate 80 mg/kg q week × 4	3.00	0	40
	Testosterone implant	92.00	60	0
18 Pr[a]	Saline	100.00	63	0
	Actinomycin-D 0.04 mg/kg q 4 days × 3	127.00	63	0
	BCNU 2 mg/kg q 4 days × 3	50.00	44	0
	Cyclophosphamide 60 mg/kg q week × 3	0.50	20	50
	5-Fluorouracil 20 mg/kg q week × 3	78.00	54	0
	5-Fluorouracil 80 mg/kg q week × 3	20.00	36	20

[a]Treatment initiated when tumor volume 900 mm^3 which is ten times the volume used for initiation of treatment in the other experiments.

Metastases were noted at autopsy in 60% of the saline control groups. No metastases were found in the Adriamycin group at 2.5 mg/kg or in the higher dose of methotrexate studied. Metastases were discovered in 25% of the animals treated with cyclophosphamide and were histologically similar to that of the donor tumor as well as the saline control tumors.

In this experiment, the autonomous Nb rat prostatic adenocarcinoma 18 Pr was subjected to chemotherapy when the tumor volume was large; approximately ten times the standard for initiation of chemotherapy was 90 mm^3, and in this experiment chemotherapy was initiated when the tumor volume was 900 mm^3. Animals were sacrificed 30 days following the last chemotherapeutic administration. Each treatment group received three intraperitoneal injections, and a saline control group received intraperitoneal injections at the same time. The cytotoxic agents employed were actinomycin-D, BCNU, cyclophosphamide, and 5-fluorouracil. Actinomycin-D and BCNU were administered every four days, and cyclophosphamide and 5-fluorouracil were administered weekly. The saline controls showed an average tumor volume increase of 40,000 mm^3. The actinomycin-D (0.04 mg/kg administered every four days times three) group showed a tumor volume increase of 51,000 mm^3. The 5-fluorouracil (20 mg/kg every week times three) group had an average tumor increase of 31,000 mm^3. BCNU (2 mg/kg administered every four days times three) had a tumor volume increase of 20,000 mm^3 compared to the cyclophosphamide group (60 mg/kg administered every week times three), which had an increase of only 200 mm^3. Actinomycin-D and 5-fluorouracil 20 mg/kg did not significantly alter tumor growth when compared to saline controls. Cyclophosphamide caused tumor regression in 66% of the animals treated, and the remaining animals showed marked retardation of tumor growth ($P < 0.002$). Growth retardation of the BCNU-treated groups was only slightly significant when compared to the saline controls at the termination of the experiment. However, this group did show significant tumor retardation during and immediately following chemotherapeutic administration. No deaths occurred in the saline, BCNU, or Actinomycin-D groups. However, the cyclophosphamide and 5-fluorouracil groups had a 9% mortality rate. Additionally, 5-fluorouracil was used in the dose of 80 mg/kg. At this dosage retardation of tumor growth was statistically significant when compared to the saline control groups ($P < 0.005$) (Table XII).

Nb rat chemotherapy — 13 pr 12. The initial chemotherapeutic agents evaluated were 5-fluorouracil 120 mg/kg, Adriamycin 1.25 mg/kg, cyclophosphamide 100 mg/kg, and methotrexate 80 mg/kg injected intraperitoneally every week times four. Additionally, a saline control group received 1 cc of normal saline injected intraperitoneally at weekly intervals times four at the same time as the chemotherapeutic agents were administered. The experiment was terminated 30 days following the last chemotherapeutic administration. Each group consisted of 12 animals. Of the agents employed, cyclophosphamide and methotrexate were statistically significant with $P < 0.04$ and 0.025, respectively. Adriamycin and 5-fluorouracil at the dosages employed were not statistically significant. Note is made of the fact that this is the only experiment involving Nb rats in which 5-fluorouracil 120 mg/kg was not significant. In other experiments using this tumor line this dosage has been significant. The explanation for this is not clear at this point. Chemotherapy was initiated at a time when the tumor volume in all animals was at least 90 mm^3. Again, it is noted that all tumors had homogeneous growth rates prior to initiation of chemotherapy. In this particular experiment chemotherapy was initiated 13 days after tumor implantation of the subcutaneous 2 mm^3

TABLE XIII. Autonomous Tumor: 13 Pr 12, Nb Rat Chemotherapy

Group	% Tumor growth treatment groups vs controls	% Metastasis	% Complete tumor regression
Saline controls	100	58	0
Adriamycin 1.25 mg/kg q week × 4	110	50	0
Cyclophosphamide 100 mg/kg q week × 4	23	16	50
5-Fluorouracil 120 mg/kg q week × 4	100	0	0
Methotrexate 80 mg/kg q week × 4	18	25	25
Saline controls	100	50	0
Alkeran 4 mg/kg q week × 2	21	0	25
BCNU 10 mg/kg × 1	8	16	8
Cis-platinum 1 mg/kg q week × 3	68	16	0
Cis-platinum 5 mg/kg × 1	24	0	0
Cis-platinum 10 mg/kg × 1	12	0	0
Cyclophosphamide 60 mg/kg q week × 3	14	24	42
DTIC 5 mg/kg days 1 & 2, 2 weeks × 2	27	0	8
5-Fluorouracil 120 mg/kg q week × 3	18	16	16
Vincristine 0.2 mg/kg q 4 days × 3	106	50	0

tumor wedge. At autopsy only two of the animals treated with cyclophosphamide had pulmonary metastases, and six animals showed complete tumor regression. Histologic evaluation of the tumor revealed central areas of necrosis with increased fibrosis and remnants of normal cellular architecture still present. Treatment with Adriamycin 1.25 mg/kg resulted in no deaths from chemotherapy. However, there was no tumor regression in this experiment. Pulmonary metastases were observed in one-half of the animals so treated with Adriamycin. The saline group had a pulmonary metastatic rate of 58%. In the methotrexate-treated group, 25% of the animals had pulmonary metastases, and none of the animals treated with 5-fluorouracil had metastatic disease (Table XIII).

In this experiment, 12 animals were assigned to each group to evaluate the response of autonomous tumor 13 Pr 12 and to demonstrate the efficacy of newer agents that traditionally have not been evaluated clinically for treatment of prostatic carcinoma. These include cis-platinum, mephalan, DTIC, BCNU, vincristine, cyclophosphamide, 5-fluorouracil, and Adriamycin. Cis-platinum was administered in three dosages of 10 mg/kg, 5 mg/kg, and 1 mg/kg. Mephalan was administered in 4 mg/kg dosages every week times two. DTIC was administered in 5 mg/kg dosages every day times two, then repeated in two weeks. Cyclophosphamide was administered at 60 mg/kg, 5-fluorouracil at 120 mg/kg, Adriamycin at 2.5 mg/kg, and vincristine at 0.2 mg/kg. Significant results were observed in the following treatment groups: 5-fluorouracil, mephalan, DTIC, cis-platinum 10 mg/kg and 5 mg/kg, BCNU, and Adriamycin ($P < 0.05$). Not significant were vincristine and cis-platinum 1 mg/kg and 10 mg/kg, which resulted in a 50% mortality rate. Animals receiving the other two dosages of cis-platinum did not die (Table XIII).

Radiation. Three Nb rat prostatic tumors have been subjected to in vitro radiation with dosages ranging from 0 to 1,500 rads. The tumors studied include 13 Pr 12, 18 Pr, and 2 Pr 129. The treatment was as follows: 2 mm^3 wedges of tumor tissue were placed in RPMI medium subjected to irradiation. Following irradiation, these wedges were implanted into groups of ten animals. The control group received no radiation to the tumor and had the standard tumor growth curve. Tumors that had received 1,500 rads had no growth throughout the experimental duration, which was ten weeks. It is apparent from Table XIV that tumors subjected to 250 rads were only slightly affected in terms of tumor volume. However, tumors receiving 500 and 1,000 rads had poor tumor growth rates as compared to the 0 radiation control group. The autonomous tumors were affected more than the androgen-dependent tumors. This was expected, as autonomous

TABLE XIV. Radiation Treatment

Rads	% Tumor volume $\left(\dfrac{\text{Treatment rads}}{\text{Control rads}}\right)$		
	13 Pr	18 Pr	2 Pr 129
0[a]	100	100	100
% Tumor present	100	100	100
250	71	67	85
% Tumor present	100	100	100
500	20	13	33
% Tumor present	80	90	100
1,000	3	0.3	25
% Tumor present	70	80	80
1,500	1	0.02	10
% Tumor present	20	20	40

[a]The 0 rad group for each tumor approximated the tumor volume observed in controls for other experiments. There was less than 5% variation for the respective tumors.

tumors are generally more anaplastic than the well-differentiated, gland-forming androgen-dependent tumors. The effect of radiation on this Nb rat prostatic adenocarcinoma has been demonstrated to be efficacious at 500 rads per 2 mm^3 wedge. We plan to perform radiotherapeutic kinetics on the other tumors outlined here as well as a trial of chemotherapy consisting of 5-fluorouracil, cyclophosphamide, and Adriamycin on irradiated tumors that have received 250 and 500 rads for determing the relative effect of chemotherapy and radiation on these tumors. Such a study could also ascertain whether chemotherapy will have an effect following radiation of these tumors. Histologically, the radiated tumors in the 0, 250, and 500 rad treatment groups resemble the primary tumor. However, tumors radiated with 1,000 rads that have eventually increased in size reveal a more marked fibrous stroma and some degree of anaplasia. When sacrificing the 1,500 rad-treated group, no prostatic tumor was identified.

Results with Athymic (Nude) Mice

Hormonal considerations of heterotransplanted Nb rat tumors into congenitally athymic (nude) mice. The autonomous tumors 13 Pr 12 and 18 Pr have been evaluated as follows: 2 mm^3 wedges were implanted in the left flank area in nude male and female recipients. The groups into which the tumors were implanted include normal males, normal females, males with 17-beta-estradiol implants, females with 17-beta-estradiol implants, castrate males with estradiol implants, castrate males with testosterone implants, castrate females with testosterone implants, and castrate females with 17-beta-estradiol implants. Tumor growth was achieved with a tumor volume of at least 100 mm^3 in 98% of all animals implanted. The autonomous tumor grew in all conditions whether estrogenized, androgenized, male, female, or castrated. Androgen-dependent tumors 2 Pr 128 and 2 Pr 129 were subjected to similar hormonal manipulation and treatment. The results revealed that androgenized animals, either female or male, subjected to the various hormonal manipulations had a tumor growth rate of $>$100 mm^3, as opposed to estrogenized animals in which tumors grew in 10% or less of the animals implanted. The statistical significance is shown with $P < 0.01$ in comparing androgenized versus estrogenized animals. Additionally, similar hormonal manipulation was carried out on the estrogen-dependent tumors, 14B and 52 pr 16. Estrogenized animals had significant tumor volume increase to 100 mm^3 in 98% of the animals, as opposed to animals that had been androgenized via either castration of the females with testosterone implants, normal males, or castrated males with testosterone implants (Table V).

Nude mouse chemotherapy — androgen-dependent tumor 2 pr 129. The initial choice of chemotherapeutic protocol in this unit was based on single-agent efficacy in treatment of human prostatic adenocarcinoma with 5-fluorouracil, and cyclophosphamide. Four groups were evaluated: saline control, 5-fluorouracil 80 mg/kg every week one time, 5-fluorouracil 80 mg/kg every week times two, and cyclophosphamide 100 mg/kg every week times two. Treatment was initiated after the tumor volumes were at least 90 mm^3 in size, and the experiment was terminated 30 days following the last chemotherapeutic administration. All groups revealed statistically significant results, with $P < 0.01$. The tumor volume change for the saline control group was 450 mm^3 ± 102, as opposed to the 5-fluorouracil treatment groups of -70 mm^3 ± 25 and -65 mm^3 ± 43 for the one-week and two-week cycles, respectively. The cyclophosphamide treatment group revealed complete tumor regression in 66% of the animals treated. The remaining four animals had a tumor volume that was only 50% of the prechemotherapy tumor volume.

Nude mouse chemotherapy — autonomous tumor 18 pr. Evaluation of Adriamycin 2.5 mg/kg every week times three and methotrexate at 60 mg/kg and 100 mg/kg every week times three was performed in groups of 14 animals. The saline control group of 18 animals had an average total tumor volume increase of 700 mm^3 over the course of the experiment. For all three chemotherapeutic groups the tumor volume decreased in comparison to the pretreatment levels. All agents employed had an effect that was statistically significant at $P < 0.05$. Four animals in the higher dose of the methotrexate group died of chemotherapeutic toxicity the day following the second chemotherapeutic administration. With the agents employed, the cessation of tumor growth was not apparent after the first chemotherapeutic administration. However, following the second administration in this three course, there was a noticeable regression of tumor volume. This was persistent even after the last chemotherapeutic administration had been given. Tumor regrowth did not occur during the course of this experiment, which lasted 30 days after the last chemotherapeutic administration.

Evaluation of cyclophosphamide and Adriamycin heterotransplanted into nude mice was done for the 18 pr prostate tumor. The treatment was initiated following tumor growth to a size of at least 60 mm^3. Cyclophosphamide was given at a dosage of 100 mg/kg intraperitoneally every week times two and Adriamycin at 5 mg/kg intraperitoneally every week times five. Fifteen animals were tumor transplant receipients for all groups, including the saline group. At this dosage schedule, both Adriamycin and cyclophosphamide were statistically significant, with $P < 0.01$. Cyclophosphamide resulted in complete tumor regression in seven of the animals, whereas the Adriamycin treatment group had no animals with complete tumor regression. Comparison of tumor size in the saline versus the Adriamycin and cyclophosphamide groups showed that the Adriamycin group had a tumor increase of 70% at the conclusion of the experiment, and the cyclophosphamide group had an average decrease in tumor size of -27%. The saline group tumor size increased 285% over the course of the experiment [25].

Chemotherapy of autonomous tumor 102 pr. This autonomous Nb rat prostatic adenocarcinoma was heterotransplanted into congenitally athymic (nude) mice in four groups: a saline control group, a 5-fluorouracil group at 80 mg/kg, a 5-fluorouracil group at 120 mg/kg, and a Ftorafur group at 30 mg/kg at a schedule of once-weekly intraperitoneal injections times three. The saline control group had an average tumor increase in volume of 7,000 mm^3 as opposed to the 5-fluorouracil groups, in which the tumor volume increase was 300 mm^3 and 700 mm^3 for the high and low dose, respectively. Ftorafur treatment was associated with a 2,800 mm^3 tumor increase. All agents employed were statistically significant with $P < 0.01$. However, only the higher dose of 5-fluorouracil was significant when compared to the Ftorafur. Note is made that, despite the statistical significance at the termination of the experiment, tumor volume for the lower 5-fluorouracil group and the Ftorafur group were increasing at the time of the conclusion of the experiment 35 days following the last chemotherapeutic administration. These agents have had a similar effect on Nb rat recipients, as has already been discussed.

Chemotherapy — autonomous tumor 13 pr 12. The autonomous Nb rat prostatic adenocarcinoma 13 Pr 12, heterotransplanted into nude mice, was subjected to four chemotherapeutic agents: 5-fluorouracil, cyclophosphamide, methotrexate, and Adriamycin. Treatment was carried out at weekly intervals times four. Statistical significance was observed in all agents at the dosage employed. Sixteen animals were treated with 5-fluorouracil at a dose of 80 mg/kg. Thirty animals were treated with cyclophosphamide at a dosage of 100 mg/kg. Adriamycin treatment was evaluated in 13 nude mouse recipients at a dose of 5 mg/kg. Methotrexate was utilized in treatment of 15 animals at a dose of 100 mg/kg. All results were statistically significant at $P < 0.001$. Chemotherapy was initiated on the twelfth post-transplant day at a time when the average tumor growth was 90 mm^3. The experiment was terminated 30 days following the last chemotherapeutic administration. The saline group had an average tumor volume increase of 550 mm^3 during this time, with a standard deviation of 156 mm^3. In both the cyclophosphamide and 5-fluorouracil groups, tumor volume actually shrunk or regressed from the pretreatment tumor volume. In the 5-fluorouracil-treated group four of the 16 animals showed complete tumor regression, whereas in the cyclophosphamide group, 21 animals had complete regression. The Adriamycin-treated group and the methotrexate-treated group did not have any animals with complete tumor regression. However, the tumor volume changed from the time of the initiation of chemotherapy to the termination of the experiment. In the Adriamycin group the change was 57 mm^3, and it was 22 mm^3 in the methotrexate group.

Chemotherapy — autonomous tumor 13 pr 12. The agents not usually employed to treat prostate cancer were evaluated in this experiment. These included BCNU and actinomycin-D. BCNU 1 mg/kg was administered intraperitoneally every four days times three in a volume of 0.1 cc into 13 animals. A similar volume of intraperitoneal saline was injected into the saline control group. Actinomycin-D 0.4 mg/kg was administered intraperitoneally every four days times three. All tumors were measured twice weekly. The average tumor volume increase in the saline control group was 440 mm^3 as opposed to the BCNU chemotherapy group. This group had a tumor volume increase of only 33 mm^3. The saline control group revealed a linear progression of tumor growth over the entire course of the experiment, whereas the BCNU group showed an abrupt cessation of tumor growth following the second administration of BCNU. Tumor regrowth was not demonstrated during the length of this experiment. Actinomycin-D at the dose schedule outlined above revealed a similar tumor growth to that observed in the saline control group. This was not statistically significant. Other experiments using the 13 Pr 12 tumor heterotransplanted into congenitally athymic (nude) mice revealed that BCNU at the dose of 2 mg/kg every four days times three resulted in only 21% tumor growth as compared to the control. Cyclophosphamide resulted in only 5% tumor growth as compared to the control at a dosage of 60 mg/kg every two weeks times two. Methotrexate at a dose of 150 mg/kg every week times four revealed only 5% tumor growth as compared to the control. At a 60 mg/kg dose, the chemotherapeutic group had a 27% growth rate as compared to the controls. Both of these were statistically significant with $P < 0.01$. However, Adriamycin administered at 1.25 mg/kg every week times three had a growth that was no different from the saline control group. Adriamycin at 2.5 and 5 mg/kg every week times three revealed tumor growth of 16% and 33%, respectively, of the tumor control growth ($P < 0.01$). Five-fluorouracil at 80 mg/kg and 50 mg/kg every week times four revealed a growth of only 7% of the saline control groups [32, 33].

DISCUSSION

The androgen-dependent tumor experiments demonstrated that these tumors increase significantly in volume in androgenized hosts as opposed to estrogenized hosts, and the addition of chemotherapy to androgenized animals does result in marked tumor volume decrease (Table IV). Furthermore, after estrogenization of animals bearing androgen-dependent tumors there is tumor regression, but it is often incomplete. With the administration of chemotherapeutic agents in addition to estrogen therapy, however, tumor retardation is more pronounced. This model may represent human prostatic adenocarcinoma that is no longer responsive to hormonal manipulation but that may benefit from the use of cytotoxic chemotherapeutic agents.

In the experiment involving Adriamycin 1.25 mg/kg, methotrexate 25 mg/kg, BCNU 2 mg/kg, 5-fluorouracil 50 mg/kg, and castration, the 2 Pr 129 tumor was shown to be hormonally responsive to castration. Additionally, these four chemotherapeutic agents have been efficacious and statistically significant (Table VIII; Fig. 3). Of the agents investigated, methotrexate and Adriamycin clearly have had the most effect. It is interesting to note that, despite the castrated group being significant when compared to chemotherapy, all cytotoxic therapeis resulted in a more marked effect on tumor growth in this androgen-dependent tumor, and each chemotherapy was significantly better than castration alone. Treatment of the androgen-dependent tumor 2 Pr 128 with 17-beta-estradiol resulted in marked tumor regression that paralleled the effect of chemotherapeutic agents employed in that experiment (Table XI).

Chemotherapy of disseminated metastatic prostate carcinoma has been hampered for several reasons that have been previously outlined. The Nb rat prostate animal model is hormonally dependent and histologically similar to human prostatic adenocarcinoma. It also metastasizes and has biochemical characteristics similar to human prostatic adenocarcinoma. In the experiment evaluating Adriamycin, BCNU, and methotrexate, those agents have been chosen because of their efficacy in treatment of other solid malignancies and occasional reports of success in treatment of human prostatic adenocarcinoma. These three chemotherapeutic agents had a marked effect on decreasing the rate of tumor growth and tumor progression. The effect of these agents versus castration was assessed and revealed that all modalities (Adriamycin, methotrexate, BCNU, 5-fluorouracil, as well as other agents herein) were statistically significant when compared to castration alone (Fig. 6, Table IX). Of the agents used, methotrexate resulted in the most toxicity. However, in the animals not suffering from chemotherapy toxicity, there were no pulmonary metastases. It has yet to be determined what dose of methotrexate will result in decreased tumor volume and decreased incidence of metastases, but it is compatible with a high level of survival in animals so treated.

Agents heretofore recognized as efficacious in the treatment of human prostatic adenocarcinoma (Table I) include 5-fluorouracil, cyclophosphamide, Adriamycin, estramustine, DTIC, streptozotocin, and an early experience with cisplatinum. Similarly, agents that have been employed in this animal model which caused complete tumor regression include Adriamycin, 5-fluorouracil, methotrexate, estradiol implantation, and BCNU. These agents have caused complete tumor regression in the androgen-dependent tumors in some animals treated (Table XI). BCNU and methotrexate traditionally have not been employed for the use in treatment of prostatic adenocarcinoma. However, in this model system, they are quite efficacious and cause complete tumor regression in tumor-bearing animals from 17% to over 30%. Additionally, both agents have a dramatic effect on tumor volume in the remaining animals which have not undergone complete tumor regression when compared to the controls. The efficacy of these agents is at least as good as that seen with the use of Adriamycin or 5-fluorouracil, which have been effective in the treatment of human prostatic adenocarcinoma. Reconsideration would be appropriate for evaluation of both methotrexate and BCNU in the clinical setting. The National Prostatic Cancer Project has already recommended methotrexate for the clinical setting. In this experimental model system only cyclophosphamide has given consistently better results in terms of complete tumor regression when compared to methotrexate or BCNU.

These Nb rat prostatic adenocarcinomas, the androgen-dependent tumors, provide a useful experimental approach for the evaluation of tumor-bearing animals to test the combination modality approach of either hormonal manipulation via orchiectomy or estrogenization with estradiol implantation and chemotherapy. This has been clearly illustrated in the experiments using BCNU, orchiectomy, testosterone implants, and estrogen implants. The most efficacious combination was orchiectomy followed by BCNU and estrogen administration (Table X). The added benefit of removing the androgen stimulus (testosterone implant) and placing a 17-beta-estradiol implant in animals that had already received chemotherapy consisting of BCNU is clearly depicted in Figure 7. If the testosterone implant was removed from previously orchiectomized and BCNU-treated animals, there was no difference between this group and the group in which treatment consisted of orchiectomy plus testosterone implant and BCNU without removal of the testosterone implant.

The versatility of this system is again pointed out in the experiments using the androgen-dependent tumor 2 Pr 128 (Fig. 9) in which the Silastic implants serve as an easy mechanism for reducing circulating androgen and adding estrogen. It is observed that all male animals with testosterone implants had continued tumor growth, whereas the animals in which the exchange took place showed a marked reduction of tumor volume over the same period. Future studies will be carried out using a similar scheme. However, prior to termination of the experiment, the animals that have been exchanged (testosterone implant removed and estrogen implant placed) will receive chemotherapy to determine if additional response can be obtained.

Nb rat chemotherapy — 18 pr. The cytotoxic agents used (cyclophosphamide, methotrexate, and Adriamycin) were statistically significant when compared to saline controls. Testosterone had no significant effect on tumor volume and again verifies the tumor's autonomous characteristics. Methotrexate and Adriamycin were evaluated at different dosage schedules with varying significance. These agents, which effective in retarding tumor growth and volume, also induced complete tumor regression in some animals studied (Table XII). The Adriamycin groups at different dosages were significant. However, there was a 37% mortality in the 5 mg/kg group, and there were no deaths in the 2.5 mg/kg group. Methotrexate 60 mg/kg was efficacious, with 10% mortality, as opposed to the 80 mg/kg group, with a 60% mortality.

Cyclophosphamide treatment yielded complete tumor regression repeatedly in the majority of the animals treated. In Experiment 1 of the 18 pr autonomous tumor most animals (eight of 12 treated) had complete tumor regression. In only three of the 12 animals treated with cyclophosphamide were pulmonary metastases observed. However, 60% of the animals in the saline group had pulmonary metastases. This is higher than the 15—25% metastatic rate seen in the saline control group of hormonally (androgen) dependent Nb rat tumors (Tables VIII and XI). At the higher dose of Adriamycin, a 37% mortality was observed. However, only 12% of the animals had metastases and, thus, the metastases alone could not be the sole cause of death in these animals. Attention must be given to the chemotherapy itself. Other experiments have indicated that at this dose of Adriamycin myocardiopathy exists with destruction of myocardial fibers. There is indeed an increased incidence of hepatic congestion and ascites. At autopsy both Adriamycin-treated groups showed evidence of cardiac toxicity, with the 5 mg/kg group having massive ascites and hepatomegaly in 100% of the animals. Hepatomegaly and ascites were not discovered in any of the experimental animals subjected to the other chemotherapeutic modalities employed. Cardiac toxicity in the rat following Adriamycin therapy is well documented and must be watched for when treating humans with Adriamycin [32, 33].

Cytotoxic chemotherapy for disseminated prostatic adenocarcinoma has been shown to increase patient survival in certain instances. Kane et al report a 24% objective and 72% subjective response rate to a combination of 5-fluorouracil, melphalan, methotrexate, vincristine, and prednisone [20]. Other encouraging reports of cytotoxic chemotherapy were mentioned at the beginning of this chapter. [As has been outlined in the Results, the use of single agent Adriamycin, methotrexate, and cyclophosphamide against the 18 Pr tumor in the experiment with 5-fluorouracil at 20 mg/kg, BCNU 2 mg/kg, cyclophosphamide 60 mg/kg, and Actinomycin-D 0.04 mg/kg, the results are examined.] The use of 5-fluorouracil 20 mg/kg was not significant as opposed to the use of 80 mg/kg against this autonomous tumor 18 Pr. The use of 5-fluorouracil was extremely significant at this latter dosage, and similar results have been obtained in the nude mouse system with this versatile animal model tumor. It is interesting to note that at the termination of this experiment, the BCNU group showed only slight statistical significance when compared to the saline controls. However, BCNU is extremely significant at the initiation of chemotherapy through three weeks post-treatment. BCNU appears to be effective in retarding tumor growth during ongoing chemotherapy at the dosage outlined above. These data suggest that longer pulsatile therapy using this agent may be efficacious. BCNU used at a similar dosage but pulsed throughout the experiment has resulted in statistically significant tumor retardation with no incidence of mortality.

Cyclophosphamide at 60 mg/kg yielded significant results, and complete tumor regression was observed in two-thirds of the animals treated. All tumors were affected by this cytotoxic agent, and no evidence of tumor regrowth was observed following chemotherapy.

Actinomycin-D 0.04 mg/kg did not significantly alter the tumor growth when compared to controls. No mortality was observed with this agent. Additional experimentation to determine whether increasing the dose or length of therapy may add to the efficacy of this agent may be needed. In one experiment, chemotherapy was initiated at a tumor volume of 900 mm^3, which is ten times the normal tumor load at which chemotherapy is initiated for the majority of the experimentations outlined in this chapter. The efficacy of the cytotoxic agents employed (cyclophosphamide, 5-fluorouracil, and BCNU), based upon the size of the primary tumor burden, has been determined. Despite this large tumor burden, cyclophosphamide 60 mg/kg and BCNU 2 mg/kg were efficacious (Table XII). However, actinomycin-D was not efficacious nor was 5-fluorouracil 20 mg/ kg. The 5-fluorouracil 80 mg/kg administered once a week times three was efficacious and statistically significant. As can be observed from the results, this model system can be used as a testing station to determine significance of chemotherapeutic agents that have been used with efficacy in clinical trials, as in the case of 5-fluorouracil and cyclophosphamide. In the case of actinomycin-D, which has not significantly altered tumor response, it is important to note that this agent has not been used clinically to treat carcinoma of the prostate. However, it is well known that it is efficacious in treatment of other solid malignancies. Perhaps this should be the work of future investigation. BCNU, on the other hand, is effective; however, a case can be made for either longer pulsatile therapy or administration at a higher dose. It is also known that this agent has not been subjected to much analysis in the treatment of human prostatic adenocarcinoma. These examples help illustrate this animal model system as useful and helpful in evaluating potentially lethal cytotoxic chemotherapeutic agents that have not been evaluated clinically to their fullest.

The autonomous Nb rat tumor, 18 Pr, subjected to Adriamycin, methotrexate, cyclophosphamide, 5-fluorouracil, and BCNU yielded statistically significant results ($P < 0.01$). These agents have also been employed and have been shown to be effective against the androgen-dependent tumors in a consistent pattern.

The use of the standard agents, Adriamycin, methotrexate, cyclophosphamide, and 5-fluorouracil as well as BCNU, vincristine, mephalan, DTIC, and cis-platinum, has been evaluated in treatment of the autonomous tumor 13 Pr 12. Cis-platinum was used in three different dose schedules and was significant in the two highest dosages employed, 10 mg/kg and 5 mg/kg, both administered once. However, the larger dose was associated with an unacceptable mortality rate. Only recently has the efficacy of cis-platinum for treatment of prostatic cancer been evaluated, as mentioned above. In the clinical situation, the use of cis-platinum in selected patients has given cause for some optimism. Of the other agents employed in treatment of this autonomous tumor, DTIC and alkeran warrant further investigation for clinical applicability. However, vincristine was not efficacious in treatment of this tumor model. Methotrexate and cyclophosphamide caused complete tumor regression in 25—50% of animals treated, a pattern similar to that observed in treatment of other Nb rat prostate tumors (Table XIII).

Preliminary radiation treatment of the 2 mm³ wedges of the 13 Pr 12, 18 Pr, and 2 Pr 129 tumors prior to tumor implantation has been carried out. These data are collected to aid in background information for future combination radiation and chemotherapeutic experiments. Briefly, efficacy in treatment of all tumor types was seen when 500 rads were delivered, and this dose also allowed for a high percentage of tumor takes of 80–100%. Doses greater than 500 rads resulted in poor tumor growth. We plan to use the 500 rad dose, evaluate it for ten weeks, then treat the animals with various chemotherapeutic agents to see if a further tumor reduction can be achieved. Even though this situation does not mimic the clinical setting in terms of local and systemic manifestations of radiation therapy, it will be used to determine if chemotherapeutic administration to irradiated tumor masses can yield complete tumor regression (Table XIV).

Heterotransplanted Nb rat prostatic adenocarcinomas into congenitally athymic (nude) mice have been evaluated. It can be stated that these heterotransplants maintain their hormonal dependency or autonomy when transplanted into athymic (nude) mice. Chemotherapeutic manipulation of heterotransplants thus far has shown qualitative similarities between tumor responses in nude mice to those seen in the direct treatment of tumor-bearing Nb rats. Agents that have been efficacious in the treatment of Nb rats have also been efficacious in treatment of nude mice. The major difference is the relative tumor volume, and this is probably related to the size of the animal; the nude mice are approximately one-tenth the volume of the Nb rats. It is beyond the scope of this chapter to discuss in detail all of the chemotherapeutic treatments of these heterotransplants. Suffice it to say that the chemotherapeutic agents that have been employed with success in treatment of human prostatic adenocarcinoma (Adriamycin, 5-fluorouracil, and cyclophosphamide) have also been efficacious in treatment of Nb rat prostatic adenocarcinomas and Nb rat heterotransplanted adenocarcinomas in the congenitally athymic (nude) mouse.

In summary, the Nb rat prostatic adenocarcinoma model is a versatile one that enables investigators to examine an androgen-dependent tumor model system as well as an autonomous tumor model system in which the origin has been induced by testosterone and esterone pellets in young rats. Hormonal manipulations such as castration, administration of estrogen, exchange of testosterone for 17-beta-estradiol implants, and combination hormonal manipulation with the various chemotherapeutic agents can be carried out with ease in this system. Additional parameters that make this system a good one include histologic stability, tumor growth kinetics stability, response to appropriate therapy, biochemical similarities to human prostatic adenocarcinoma, and a high tumor take rate. Finally, from the data generated from this project, it is hoped that better selection of chemotherapeutic agents can be made, based upon the response of the prostate adenocarcinomas in both Nb rats and heterotransplanted tumor in nude mice. It may be possible to treat the majority of patients with prostatic adenocarcinoma more effectively with a modality or a combination of modalities that has not been used to the fullest in the past. Additionally, evaluation of the endocrinology of these tumor-bearing animals may enable us to shed light on the hormonal milieu that may "contribute" to the etiology of this disease.

ACKNOWLEDGMENTS

The authors are grateful to David D. Eckels for his work on the statistical analysis, Boris Ruebner, MD, for his work on histochemical evaluations, and Mark Van de Water, Susan Shaw, and Herbert Ure for their technical support on this project.

REFERENCES

1. Cancer Statistics. CA 28:17–32, 1978.
2. Tejada F, Cohen MH: Initial chemotherapeutic trials in patients with inoperable or recurrent cancer of the prostate. Cancer Chemother Rep 59:243–249, 1975.
3. Murphy GP: Cancer of the prostate. Cancer 32:1089–1091, 1973.
4. Merrin C, Etra W, Wajsman S, Baumgartner M, Murphy G: Chemotherapy of advanced carcinoma of the prostate with 5-fluorouracil, cyclophosphamide and Adriamycin. J Urol 115:86–90, 1976.
5. Scott WW, Johnson DE, Schmidt JE, Gibbons RP, Prout GR, Joiner JR, Saroff J, Murphy GP: Chemotherapy of advanced prostatic carcinoma with cyclophosphamide or 5-fluorouracil: Results of first national randomized study. J Urol 114:909–111, 1975.
6. Scott WW, Gibbons RP, Johnson DE, Prout GR, Schmidt JD, Saroff J, Murphy GP: The continued evaluation of the effects of chemotherapy in patients with advanced carcinoma of the prostate. J Urol 116:211–213, 1976.
7. Scott WW, Gibbons RP, Johnson DE, Prout GR, Schmidt JD, Chu TM, Gaeta JR, Joiner J, Saroff J, Murphy GP: Comparison of 5-fluorouracil (NSC-19893) and cyclophosphamide (NSC-26271) in patients with advanced carcinoma of the prostate. Cancer Chemother Rep 59:195–201, 1975.
8. Eagan R, Hahn R, Myers R: Adriamycin (NSC-123127) versus 5-fluorouracil (NSC-19893) and cyclophosphamide (NSC-26271) in the treatment of metastatic prostate cancer. Cancer Treat Rep 60:115, 1976.
9. DeWys WD, Begg CB: Comparison of Adriamycin (Adria) and 5-fluorouracil (5-FU) in advanced prostatic cancer. ASCO Abstracts, March 1978.
10. DeWys WD: Comparison of Adriamycin (NSC-123127) and 5-fluorouracil (NSC-19893) in advanced prostatic cancer. Cancer Chemother Rep 59:215–217, 1975.
11. Tejada F, Eisenberger MA, Broder LA, et al: 5-Fluorouracil versus CCNU in the treatment of metastatic prostatic cancer. Cancer Treat Rep 61:1589, 1977.
12. Tejada F, Broder LE, Cohen MH, et al: Treatment of metastatic prostatic cancer with 5-fluorouracil (5-FU) versus 1-(2-chloroethyl)-3-cyclohexyl-1-nitrosourea (CCNU). Proc AACR ASCP. AACR Abstracts C-10:269, 1977.
13. Merrin C: PAACR-ASCO, 1977.
14. Eagan RT, Ulz DC, Myers RP, Furlow WL: Comparison of Adriamycin (NSC-123127) and the combination of 5-fluorouracil (NSC-19893) and cyclophosphamide (NSC-26271) in advanced prostatic cancer: A preliminary report. Cancer Chemother Rep 59:203–207, 1975.

15. Perloff M, Ohnuma T, Holland JR, et al: Adriamycin (Adm) and Diamminedichloro-platinum (DDP) in advanced prostatic carcinoma (PC). Proc AACR ASCO. AACR Abstracts C-265:333, 1977.
16. Strauss MJ, Parmelee J, Olsson C, et al: Cytoxan, Adriamycin and methotrexate (CAM) therapy of stage D prostate cancer. PAACR-ASCO 19:314, 1978.
17. Lerner JH, Malloy TR: Hydroxyurea in stage D carcinoma of prostate. Urology 10:35–38, 1977.
18. Murphy GP, Gibbons R, Johnson DE, Loening SA, Prout GR, Schmidt JD, Bross DS, Chu TM, Gaeta JR, Saroff J, Scott WW: A comparison of estramustine phosphate and streptozotocin in patients with advanced prostatic carcinoma who have had extensive irradiation. J Urol 118:288–291, 1977.
19. Blokhina NG, Vozny EK, Garin AM: Results of treatment of malignant tumors with Ftorafur. Cancer 30:390–392, 1972.
20. Kane RD, Stocks LH, Paulson DF: Multiple drug chemotherapy regimen for patients with hormonally-unresponsive carcinoma of the prostate: A preliminary report. J Urol 117:467–471, 1977.
21. Buell BV, Saiers JH, Saiki JH, Gergreen TW: Chemotherapy trial with comp-F regimen in advanced adenocarcinoma of the prostate. Urology 11:247–250, 1978.
22. Yagoda A: Nonhormonal cytotoxic agents in the treatment of prostatic adenocarcinoma. Cancer 32:1131–1140, 1973.
23. Carter SK, Goldin A: Experimental models and their clinical correlations. In USA-USSR Monograph, methods of development of new anticancer drugs. National Cancer Institute: Washington, DC, pp 63–75, 1977.
24. Ikeda RM, Gershwin ME, Shifrine M, Kawakami T: The kinetics and radiobiology of a heterotransplanted human endometrial carcinoma to nude mice. Cancer Treat Rep (in press).
25. Drago JR, Maurer RE, Gershwin ME, Eckels DD, Palmer JM: The effect of 5-fluorouracil and Adriamycin on heterotransplantation of Noble rat prostatic tumors in congenitally athymic (nude) mice. Cancer (in press).
26. Drago JR, Maurer RE, Gershwin ME, Eckels DD, Goldman LB: Chemotherapy of Nb rat adenocarcinoma of the prostate heterotransplanted into congenitally athymic (nude) mice: Report of 5-fluorouracil and cyclophosphamide. J Surg Res (in press).
27. Bagshaw MA, Pistenma DA, Ray GR, Freiha FS, Kempson RL: Evaluation of extended-field radiotherapy for prostatic neoplasm: 1976 progress report. Cancer Treat Rep 61:297–306, 1977.
28. Whitmore WF Jr: Retropubic implantation of I-125 in treatment of prostatic cancer. In "Prostatic Disease." New York: Alan R. Liss, Inc., 1976, pp 223–233.
29. Carlton CE Jr: Radioactive isotope implantation for cancer of the prostate. In Skinner D, deKernion G (eds): "Genitourinary Cancer." Philadelphia: W. B. Saunders Co., 1978, pp 380–387.
30. Drago JR, Goldman LB, Gershwin ME: Heterotransplanted Nb rat prostatic adeno-carcinoma into congenitally athymic nude mice: Chemotherapy of autonomous tumors pr 90 and 13 pr 12 with methotrexate, Adriamycin and cyclophosphamide. Cancer (in press).

Immunological Studies of Prostate Adenocarcinoma in an Animal Model

Alice J. Claflin, PhD, E. Churchill McKinney, PhD, and Mary A. Fletcher, PhD

A variety of deficiencies involving the immune system have been associated with prostate carcinoma in man. A depression in cellular immune reactions as determined by in vivo and in vitro testing has been observed. Impaired delayed hypersensitive skin responses and depressed inflammatory reactions that correlate with metastatic disease have been reported [1–3]. Studies of lymphocyte transformation in response to mitogens as a reflection of cell-mediated immunity have also shown diminished reactivity, although there are conflicting results concerning correlation with stage of disease. Some investigators have observed a marked depression in responsiveness of lymphocytes from patients with advanced metastatic disease to phytohemagglutinin (PHA) [4, 5]. Those patients with localized disease showed normal reactivity. Other investigators found no difference in response to PHA among patients with stage B, C, or D prostate cancer [6]. Still others found a significant reduction in PHA responsiveness in prostate cancer patients irrespective of the stage of disease [7]. Other host defense mechanisms are also impaired in these patients. Monocyte chemotactic responses were reported to be depressed, especially in patients with metastatic disease [2]. It has been shown that serum from prostate cancer patients can inhibit the migration of allogeneic leukocytes [8]. In addition, elevated $C'3$ and IgA levels have been noted [9, 10].

The evidence for an antigen specific for prostate tumors in humans is conflicting [11–14]. While species-specific and organ-specific antigens appear to be present, there is no good evidence for a tumor-specific antigen.

Animal models of human disease permit investigations that otherwise could not be carried out. With an animal model, the study of the mechanisms of disease and the role of factors involved in or controlling the disease can be studied. Generally in animal models there is often an increase in immune response to tumor antigens in early stages of the disease, followed by immunological depression or anergy in the terminal stages. These immunologic variations are influenced by therapeutic intervention such as surgery and chemotherapy. It must also be remembered that in aged animals, as in man, there is immunologic senescence [15].

Models for Prostate Cancer, pages 365–377

We have been studying the role of the immune system with the transplantable Dunning R3327 prostate adenocarcinoma. We are purifying the membrane glycoproteins in an attempt to determine the presence of an antigen specific for the tumor. The presence of a tumor-specific antigen will make it possible to assess the specific role of the immune system in tumor development, progression, and outcome.

MATERIALS AND METHODS

Transplantation of Tumors

Tumors were selected for transplant and dispersed with enzymes as previously described [16]. For the immunological studies, two groups of rats were used. One group consisted of rats one to two years of age; the other was made up of animals two years or older.

Humoral immune assays. Sheep erythrocytes (Srbc) were obtained from Cordis Laboratories, Miami, Florida. Animals were immunized by intraperitoneal injection of the antigen [16]. Four days after antigen administration, the spleens were removed, homogenized in a glass tissue grinder, washed, and tested for the presence of antibody-producing cells (pfc) [17, 18].

Preparation of peripheral blood lymphocytes. Rats were anesthetized and bled by retro-orbital sinus puncture into a heparinized tube. The rats were bled two weeks after tumor transplantation and at weekly intervals for five weeks. The whole blood was diluted with two volumes of phosphate-buffered saline (PBS). The blood was layered over the lymphocyte separation medium (Litton Bionetics) in a 4:3 proportion, and the gradient was centrifuged at 400g for 20 minutes at room temperature. Mononuclear cells were recovered from the interface and washed at least twice in Hanks BSS before testing.

Mitogens. Concanavalin A (Con A) was obtained from Calbiochem, phytohemagglutinin (PHA) from Difco Laboratories, and wheat germ agglutinin (WGA) from Sigma.

Blastogenic response to mitogens. Microcultures (200 μl) consisted of 10^5 lymphocytes in Eagle Hank's medium with 10% heat inactivated fetal calf serum and the appropriate amount of mitogen [16, 19]. The cultures were incubated for three days in 5% CO_2 in air at $37°C$. ^{3}H-thymidine was added to cultures 18 hours prior to culture termination, carried out by using a multiple-cell culture harvester (Flow Laboratories, Inc.). Incorporated radioactivity was determined by counting in a Packard liquid scintillation counter. Stimulation index was calculated as cpm (test)/cpm (background).

Membrane receptors. IgG on the peripheral blood lymphocytes was determined using fluorescein isothiocyanate (FITC) conjugated anti-rat IgG [20]. Lymphocytes for immunofluorescent studies were washed in 0.03 M NaN_3 in Hank's BSS. The cell pellet was resuspended in 50 μl of the buffer, and the conjugates were added to the cell suspension, incubated for one hour at 4°C, and washed twice. The cell suspension was mounted on a slide and examined at 1,000 × magnification with a Leitz fluorescent microscope. The complement receptor C_3b was determined using yeast incubated in fresh rat serum [21].

Cytotoxic assays. PHA-induced lymphocyte-mediated cytotoxicity and antibody-dependent cellular cytotoxicity (ADCC) were carried out with 1.25 × 10^6 peripheral lymphocytes cultured with either 25.0 μg of PHA or 10^{-4} to 10^{-6} M antibody plus $Na_2{}^{51}CrO_4$-labeled chicken erythrocytes (Crbc) as the target cell [22, 23]. The cells were cultured for 18–20 hours at 37°C in 5% CO_2 in air. The cultures were centrifuged, and the cell pellet and supernatant were counted separately. The percent cytotoxicity was calculated as shown:

$$\% \text{ release} = \frac{\text{cpm supernatant}}{\text{cpm supernatant } + \text{ pellet}} \times 100$$

$$\% \text{ cytotoxicity} = \% \text{ release (test)} - \% \text{ release (control)}$$

Tumor homogenates. Tumors were removed, washed well in PBS, minced, and homogenized in a Kontes glass tissue grinder. The homogenate was centrifuged at 100g and the supernatant removed. The protein concentration was determined on the supernatant by A_{280} nm reading in a Beckman DU spectrophotometer.

Membrane isolation. Cell membranes from the H and G sublines of the R3327 tumor were prepared by homogenization, differential centrifugation, and sucrose step-gradient ultracentrifugation as previously described [24]. Aliquots of each fraction were removed for determination of protein, sialic acid, and enzyme activity. Total protein was measured and sialic acids were determined by the thiobarbituric acid method [25, 26]. Before assay the samples were hydrolysed in 0.1 M H_2SO_4 at 80°C for one hour, and the released sialic acid was purified by chromatography on Dowex 1 × 8 formate form [27]. The 5′ nucleotidase activity, a plasma membrane marker, was assayed as described by Aronson [28].

Iodination of lectins. Con A and WGA were iodinated by the chloramine T method in the presence of inhibitor sugar [29]. After separation of the free iodine and sugar from the ^{125}I-lectins by gel filtration, affinity chromatography was used to achieve a product with high specific activity.

Fractionation of membranes. Membranes were fractionated by electrophoresis on sodium dodecylsulfate (SDS) gels, and the localization of the bands was carried out as shown in Figure 1, or by staining with periodic acid Schiff (PAS) or Coomassie blue (CB).

RESULTS

Dispersion of tumor tissue routinely results in the recovery of $0.5-1 \times 10^8$ cells per gram of tissue. Palpable G tumors are present in about three weeks if 2×10^7 dispersed cells are injected subcutaneously in male rats. The same number of H tumor cells results in palpable tumor in 8–12 weeks.

The numbers of antibody-producing cells present in the spleens of G tumor-bearing animals of both age groups were determined on the fourth day of the primary immune response. We have previously shown that this is the time of maximum antigenic stimulation with the immunization schedule followed [16]. The spleens of the tumor-bearing rats of both age groups displayed splenomegaly, with approximately two times the numbers of leukocytes compared to the controls. The numbers of antibody-producing cells differed in the controls. There were no differences between the two age groups of tumor-bearing animals (Table I). Lymphocyte blastogenic response to mitogens Con A and PHA resulted in little difference noted between tumor-bearing animals of the different

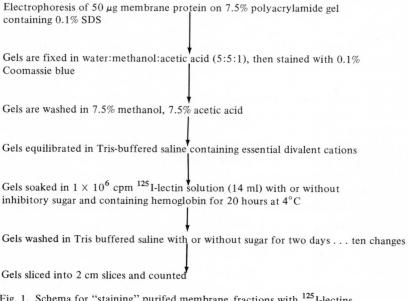

Fig. 1. Schema for "staining" purifed membrane fractions with ^{125}I-lectins.

TABLE I. Primary Immune Response to Sheep Erythrocytes*

	pfc/spleens ($\times 10^5$)	wbc spleen ($\times 10^8$)
Non-tumor-bearing		
< 2 years	1.97 (0.57)	2.87 (0.17)
> 2 years	0.34 (0.08)	2.62 (0.53)
Tumor-bearing		
< 2 years	1.77 (0.75)	5.64 (1.50)
> 2 years	2.3 (1.10)	4.6 (0.50)

*Mean (1 SD) using five animals/group.

age groups. The blastogenic response of those non-tumor-bearing rats over two years of age was consistently lower than in the younger animals. The age effect was evident, but there was little evidence of a tumor effect on this in vitro immunological assay. Two B lymphocyte markers were analyzed during a seven-week period following tumor implantation: surface immunoglobulin (SIg) and complement receptors (CR). No significant changes in the proportion of SIg or CR bearing peripheral blood lymphocytes were observed during this period.

Antibody-dependent cell-mediated cytotoxic (ADCC) capability was assayed over a seven-week period following tumor implantation in both one- to two-year-old and aged rats. The results of this study indicated that neither G tumor growth nor advanced age causes significant changes in the responsiveness of these animals. The reactivity of Fc receptor-bearing lymphocytes responsible for ADCC would appear to be unaffected by the prostate adenocarcinoma [23].

PHA-induced cytotoxicity was studied in a manner analogous to ADCC. Again, no age- or tumor-related alterations in reactivity were observed. This is in contrast to the PHA-induced blastogenic response. The cells responsible for the cytotoxic and blastogenic response to PHA have been shown to be distinct from one another [30]. Thus, it may be inferred that the lymphocyte population that incorporates ^{3}H-thymidine in response to PHA is more susceptible to age changes than the cytotoxic cell responsive to PHA.

Fresh and cryopreserved lymphocytes from non-tumor-bearing rats were tested with varying concentrations of homogenized tumor from either the G or the H subline. In no instance was there a response as determined by the incorporation of ^{3}H-thymidine. Fresh and cryopreserved lymphocytes from H tumor-bearing rats responded to the H tumor homogenate with a 2- to 5.6-fold increase in ^{3}H-thymidine incorporation compared to background (Table II).

Highly purified membrane fractions were isolated from both the H and the G tumors, as evidenced by a 6—10-fold increase in membrane-associated 5' nucleotidase and sialic acid and by negligible contamination with lysosomal enzyme

TABLE II. Blastogenic Response to Homogenized H Tumor

Lymphocytes		cpm ^{3}H-thymidine (SD)		Stimulation index
		Background	Homogenate	
Tumor-bearing animals	1)	110 (20)	400 (225)	3.7
	2)	236 (111)	1,314 (290)	5.6
Non-tumor-bearing animals	1)	269 (156)	257 (162)	1
	2)	1,793 (874)	1,253 (72)	1

(N-acetylglucosaminidase) or by DNA. Our experiments with ^{125}I-labeled Con A indicate that the G membrane fraction has four major Con A binding glycoproteins with apparent molecular weights of $>$ 150,000, 110,000, 86,000, and 61,000 (Fig. 2A). The binding pattern of this membrane fraction with ^{125}I-WGA was similar except for the absence of the 61,000 mol wt band (Fig. 2B). In contrast, the H tumor membrane fraction had a glocoprotein, band 2, of 105,000–109,000 apparent molecular weight, which bound nearly twice as much ^{125}I-Con A and WGA as did the band 2 of the G tumor preparation (Fig. 3). The gels of both H and G tumors stained with PAS are similar, except for some differences in minor bands. A major PAS-staining glycoprotein is present in both tumor sublines and has a molecular weight of approximately 95,000–100,000 (Figs. 4A and 5A). This glycoprotein is apparently not reactive with either Con A or WGA. For comparison, the Coomassie blue staining (CB) pattern for both of these membrane preparations is shown in Figures 4B and 5B.

DISCUSSION

The G subline of the Dunning R3327 tumor is a poorly differentiated, rapidly growing carcinoma. The animals bearing these tumors, when tested by a variety of immunological assays, show few differences between tumor-bearing and non-tumor-bearing rats. The aged non-tumor-bearing animals show some immunological senescence in that the number of antibody-producing cells, the amount of circulating antibody, and the magnitude of blastogenic responses to mitogens are depressed. This effect in the aged control animals is not evident in the aged tumor-bearing animals. The pfcs and blastogenic responses of the aged tumor-bearing rats are not different from the younger animals and are increased compared to aged controls. This observation appears to be a tumor effect. All of the tumor-bearing rats at the time of sacrifice show pronounced splenomegaly compared to the controls.

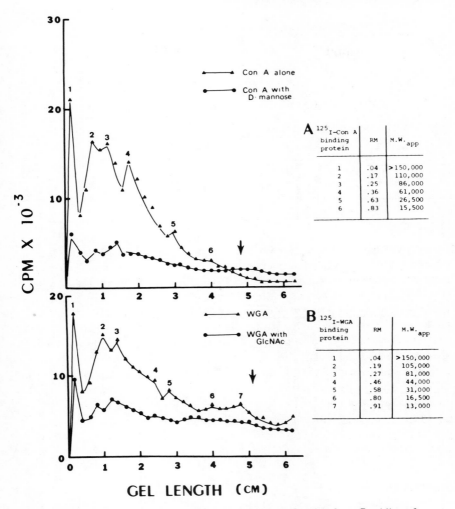

A

^{125}I-Con A binding protein	RM	M.W.$_{app}$
1	.04	>150,000
2	.17	110,000
3	.25	86,000
4	.36	61,000
5	.63	26,500
6	.83	15,500

B

^{125}I-WGA binding protein	RM	M.W.$_{app}$
1	.04	>150,000
2	.19	105,000
3	.27	81,000
4	.46	44,000
5	.58	31,000
6	.80	16,500
7	.91	13,000

Fig. 2. Electropherograms of 50 μg of purified membrane fraction from G subline of R3327 rat prostate tumor on 7.5% polyacrylamide gels containing 0.1% sodium dodecyl sulfate, 0.01 M phosphate, pH 7.0. Gels were fixed and washed extensively with 0.15 M NaCl, 0.1% NaN$_3$, 0.1 M Tris-HCl, pH 7.5 (for Con A, 0.5 mM MnCl$_2$ and CaCl$_2$ were added). The gels were then soaked in solutions containing ^{125}I-lectins with or without inhibitory monosaccharides, washed free of unbound radiolabeled lectins with Tris buffer (pH 7.5), and sliced into 2 mm segments and radioactivity determined. Arrows mark the point of dye (bromphenol blue) migration. A. Gels were "stained" with ^{125}I-Con A. B. Gels were "stained" with ^{125}I-wheat germ agglutinin. In both figures, the points represent an average of two gels. The apparent molecular weights were calculated by comparison of the relative mobility (RM) of each peak to RM of standard molecular weight marker proteins (N-acetyglucosamine-[GlcNAc]).

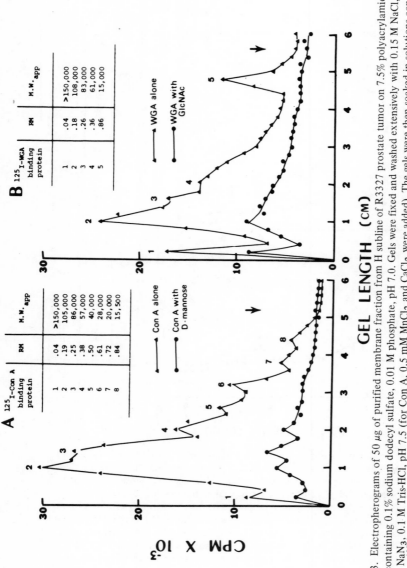

Fig. 3. Electropherograms of 50 μg of purified membrane fraction from H subline of R3327 prostate tumor on 7.5% polyacrylamide gels containing 0.1% sodium dodecyl sulfate, 0.01 M phosphate, pH 7.0. Gels were fixed and washed extensively with 0.15 M NaCl, 0.1% NaN₃, 0.1 M Tris-HCl, pH 7.5 (for Con A, 0.5 mM MnCl₂ and CaCl₂ were added). The gels were then soaked in solutions containing ¹²⁵I-lectins with or without inhibitory monosaccharides, washed free of unbound radiolabeled lectins with Tris buffer (pH 7.5) and sliced into 2 mm segments and radioactivity determined. Arrows mark the point of dye (bromphenol blue) migration. A. Gels were "stained" with ¹²⁵I-Con A. B. Gels were "stained" with ¹²⁵I-wheat germ agglutinin. In both figures the points represent an average of two gels. The apparent molecular weights were calculated by comparison of the relative mobility (RM) of each peak to RM of standard molecular weight marker proteins.

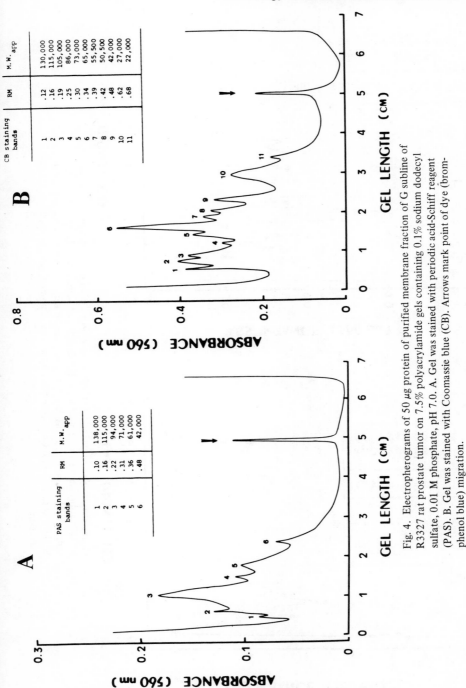

Fig. 4. Electropherograms of 50 μg protein of purified membrane fraction of G subline of R3327 rat prostate tumor on 7.5% polyacrylamide gels containing 0.1% sodium dodecyl sulfate, 0.01 M phosphate, pH 7.0. A. Gel was stained with periodic acid-Schiff reagent (PAS). B. Gel was stained with Coomassie blue (CB). Arrows mark point of dye (brom-phenol blue) migration.

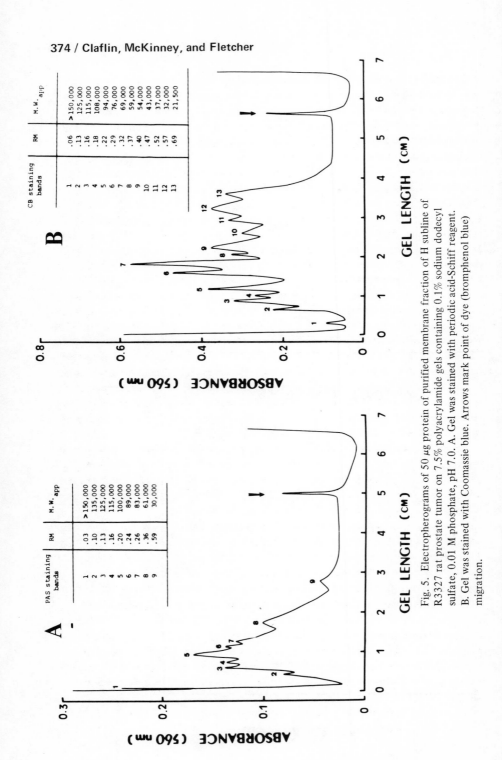

Fig. 5. Electropherograms of 50 μg protein of purified membrane fraction of H subline of R3327 rat prostate tumor on 7.5% polyacrylamide gels containing 0.1% sodium dodecyl sulfate, 0.01 M phosphate, pH 7.0. A. Gel was stained with periodic acid-Schiff reagent. B. Gel was stained with Coomassie blue. Arrows mark point of dye (bromphenol blue) migration.

Lymphocyte subpopulations characterized by various membrane markers have been shown to change in proportion to one another and in actual numbers during malignancy [31]. The B lymphocyte markers determined in spleen and peripheral blood lymphocytes in these animals did not change appreciably with tumor growth or with age of the animal. The cytotoxicity assays, ADCC- and PHA-induced, did not reflect any effect of tumor progression or advanced age. Rats bearing G tumors have had their tumor masses surgically removed, and a number of these animals did not develop tumors after an extended period. When these animals were reinjected with tumor cells, all developed palpable tumors in a predictable time. The second tumors did not differ histologically from the original tumor. At this time, there is no indication that the G tumor is immunogenic. The immunological testing that has been carried out supports this, as does the regrowth of the tumor in animals that were reinoculated following surgical removal of the tumor. The G and H sublines of the Dunning R3327 tumor represent the extremes in growth potential differentiation and ultimate size of this transplantable prostate adenocarcinoma. There is some evidence that the H tumor-bearing rats respond differently than the G tumor-bearing rats [32]. We have shown here that there is a minimal blastogenic response of the H tumor-bearing animals to the tumor. This response has not been observed in G tumor-bearing rats to G or H tumor homogenates. Further, rats bearing H tumors have had their tumor masses surgically removed and survived for 12 weeks without detectable regrowth of the tumor. These animals have been injected with tumor cells a second time, and at the time of this report (six weeks post-injection) do not have palpable tumors.

The initial investigation of the surface glycoproteins has been carried out on tumors of both the G and H sublines. The membranes were fractionated by SDS polyacrylamide gel electrophoresis. The proteins and glycoproteins which banded at various positions in the gels were located by staining reactions and by reactivity with two radiolabeled lectins, ^{125}I-Con A and ^{125}I-WGA.

Protein lectins with specific affinities for sugar molecules are widely distributed in nature, and interest has centered on their reactions with tumor cells. The number of carbohydrate receptors as defined by these lectins may appear to increase, appear de novo, become serologically available, or become redistributed during malignant transformation. Surface glycoprotein differences have been reported in several tumor systems by the use of lectins with well-characterized carbohydrate specificities [33, 34]. ^{125}I-Con A and ^{125}I-WGA in conjunction with staining techniques have shown quantitative and qualitative differences in the surface proteins of these two sublines. The PAS stains on gels of G and H tumor membrane preparations show some differences in minor bands. The H tumor, however, has a glycoprotein band with an apparent molecular weight of 105,000–109,000, which binds nearly twice as much ^{125}I-Con A and ^{125}I-WGA as the glycoprotein of similar molecular weight in the G tumor. These differences must be localized for further comparative studies in order to define the biochemical and immunological characteristics of the G and H sublines of the Dunning R3327 tumor.

In conclusion, it has been demonstrated that rats bearing the G subline of the Dunning R3327 tumor show some effect of the tumor implanted in aged rats. This effect is not apparent using younger animals. The G tumor, a poorly differentiated carcinoma, does not appear to be immunogenic. The H subline, a well-differentiated adenocarcinoma, has been shown to have an increased quantity of a Con A and WGA binding glycoprotein. Immunologically, the rats bearing H tumors respond to H tumor homogenate, in contrast to G tumor-bearing rats. This animal model, with the sublines of the R3327 tumor, permits comparative immunological and biochemical studies of the extremes of differentiation in prostatic adenocarcinoma.

ACKNOWLEDGMENTS

This investigation was supported by 5R26 CA 21696-02 awarded by NCI National Prostatic Cancer Project, DHEW.

REFERENCES

1. Huus JC, Kursh ED, Poor P, Persky L: Delayed cutaneous hypersensitivity in patients with prostatic adenocarcinoma. J Urol 114:86–87, 1975.
2. Brosman S, Hausman M, Shacks S: Immunologic alterations in patients with prostatic carcinoma. J Urol 113:841–845, 1975.
3. Decenzo JM, Allison R, Leadbetter GW Jr: Skin testing in genitourinary carcinoma: 2-year followup. J Urol 114:271–273, 1975.
4. Robinson MRG, Nakhla LS, Whitaker RH: Lymphocyte transormation in carcinoma of the prostate. Br J Urol 43:480–486, 1971.
5. Robinson MRG, Nakhla LS, Whitaker RH: A new concept in the management of carcinoma of the prostate. Br J Urol 43:728–732, 1971.
6. McLaughlin AP III, Brooks JD: A plasma factor inhibiting lymphocyte reactivity in urologic cancer patients. J Urol 112:366–372, 1974.
7. Catalona WJ, Tarpley JL, Chretien PB, Castle JR: Lymphocyte stimulation and urologic cancer patients. J Urol 112:373–377, 1974.
8. Ablin RJ, Bruno GR, Guinan PD, Bush IM: Migration-inhibitory effect of serum from patients with prostatic cancer. Oncology 30:423–428, 1974.
9. Ablin RJ, Gonder WJ, Soanes WH: Levels of immunoglobulins in the serum of patients with carcinoma of the prostate. Neoplasma 19:57–60, 1972.
10. Ablin RJ, Gonder WJ, Soanes WH: Levels of C'3 in the serum of patients with benign and malignant diseases of the prostate. Neoplasma 19:61–63, 1972.
11. Flocks RH, Urich VC, Patle C, Bagley BJ: Studies of the antigenic properties of prostate tissue. J Urol 84:134–143, 1960.
12. Ablin RJ: Immunologic studies of normal, benign and malignant human prostatic tissue. Cancer 29:1570–1574, 1972.
13. Brannen GE, Gomolka DM, Coffey DS: Specificity of cell membrane antigens in prostatic cancer. Cancer Chemother Rep 59:127–138, 1975.

14. Drucker JR, Moncure CW, Johnson CL, Smith MJV, Koontz WW Jr: Immunologic staging of prostatic carcinoma: Three years' experience. J Urol 119:94–98, 1978.

15. Bilder GE: Studies on immune competence in the rat: Changes with age, sex and strain. J Gerontol 30:641–646, 1975.

16. Claflin AJ, McKinney EC, Fletcher MA: The Dunning R3327 prostate adenocarcinoma in the Fischer-Copenhagen F_1 rat: A useful model for immunologic studies. Oncology 34:105–109, 1977.

17. Cunningham AJ, Szenberg A: Further improvements in the plaque technique for detecting single antibody-forming cells. Immunology 14:599–600, 1968.

18. Claflin AJ, Smithies O, Meyer RK: Antibody responses in bursa-deficient chickens. J Immunol 97:696–699, 1966.

19. Heber-Katz E, Click RE: Immune responses in vitro. V. Role of mercaptoethanol in the mixed-leucocyte reaction. Cell Immunol 5:410–418, 1972.

20. Rabellino E, Colon S, Grey HM, Uhanue ER: Immunoglobulin on the surface of lymphocytes. I. Distribution and quantitation. J Exp Med 133:156–157, 1971.

21. Mendes NF, Miki SS, Peixinho ZF: Combined detection of human T and B lymphocytes by rosette formation with sheep erythrocytes and zymosan-C^3 complexes. J Immunol 113:531–536, 1974.

22. Perlmann P, Perlmann H: ^{51}Cr-release from chicken erythrocytes: An assay system for measuring cytotoxic activity of non-specifically activated lymphocytes in vitro. In Bloom B, Glade PR (eds): "In Vitro Methods in Cell Mediated Immunity." New York: Academic Press, 1971.

23. Perlmann P, Perlmann H, Wigzell H: Lymphocyte-mediated cytotoxicity in vitro. Induction and inhibition by humoral antibody and nature of effector cells. Transplant Rev 13:91–114, 1972.

24. Fletcher MA, Lo TM, Graves WR, Robles AM: Isolation of plasma membrane glycoprotein from bovine thymocytes. Biochim Biophys Acta 465:341–352, 1977.

25. Lowry PH, Rosenbrough NJ, Farr AL, Randall RJ: Protein measurement with the Folin phenol reagent. J Biol Chem 193:265–275, 1951.

26. Aminoff D: Methods for the quantitative estimation of N-acetylneuraminic acid and their application to hydrolysates of sialomucoids. Biochem J 181:384–392, 1961.

27. Spiro RG: Analysis of sugar found in glycoproteins. In Neufeld EF, Ginsburg V (eds): "Methods in Enzymology." New York: Academic Press, 1961.

28. Aronson NM, Fouster DM: Isolation of rat liver plasma membrane fragments in isotonic sucrose. In Fleischer S, Packer L (eds): "Methods in Enzymology." New York: Academic Press, 1974.

29. Greenwood FC, Hunter WM, Glover JS: The preparation of ^{131}I-labeled human growth hormone of high specific radioactivity. Biochem J 89:114–123, 1963.

30. Dawkins RL, Zilko PJ: Separation of cell involved in phytohaemagglutin-induced mitogenesis and cytotoxicity. Nature 254:144–145, 1975.

31. Dorizzi M, Ortiz-Muniz G, Lopez DM, Sigel MM, Epstein RS: Increase in the proportion of cells with the C'3 receptor in Balb-C mice bearing mammary tumors. Int J Cancer 16:1015–1021, 1975.

32. Lopez DM, Voigt W: Adenocarcinoma R3327 of the Copenhagen rat as a suitable model for immunological studies of prostate cancer. Cancer Res 35:2057–2061, 1977.

33. Nicolson GL, Blaustein J, Etzler ME: Characterization of two plant lectins from Ricinus communis and their quantitative interaction with a murine lymphoma. Biochemistry 13:196–204, 1974.

34. Sharon N, Lis H: Lectins: Cell-agglutinating and sugar-specific proteins. Science 177:949–959, 1972.

Requirements for an Idealized Animal Model of Prostatic Cancer

Donald S. Coffey and John T. Isaacs

IS IT APPROPRIATE TO SEEK AN ANIMAL MODEL TO AID IN THE STUDY OF HUMAN PROSTATIC CANCER?

In attempting to study animal tumors as models for the corresponding human disease the appropriateness of the nature and merits of these models must first be established. Investigators will often be reminded that one cannot extrapolate results from experimental animals to the human [1]. We should be advised that many of these models are in species far removed from the human in evolutionary developments and that marked differences are often apparent at the anatomic and physiologic levels. Although caution is always in order, it is important to recognize that a great portion of our recent progress in biological and medical science has been obtained through animal studies. In fact, *most of our basic knowledge of human biochemistry, physiology, endocrinology, and pharmacology has been derived from initial studies in subhuman animal models.* Indeed, most of these discoveries were first made in mice, rats, guinea pigs, and dogs. Let us examine the support for the previous statements as they relate to our knowledge of the human prostate gland and list some important insights obtained from animal studies.

The following well-accepted concepts were first observed in studies with lower animals:

Hormonal Response of the Prostate

Castration produces involution of the prostate size and growth; estrogen therapy or hypophysectomy produces a similar glandular involution. This atrophy can be reversed by treatment with exogenous androgens.

Models for Prostate Cancer, pages 379–391

Endocrine Pharmacology

The classification of any chemical substance as an androgen, estrogen, anti-androgen, or antiestrogen is determined and defined through bioassays in rodents. The pharmacological potency of these compounds is compared to the units of activity in these animal bioassays. At present there are no compounds identified as androgens, estrogens, antiandrogens, or antiestrogens in animal bioassays that do not have similar pharmacological properties when tested in well-documented human trials. Although dose responses of many drugs appear different in man and animals, many of these apparent differences can be normalized when the route of administration is similar and the dose is equalized on a square meter body area basis. In addition, the mechanism of action of most drugs has been determined first in lower animals; metabolic rates may differ, but it is rare for a drug to have a different mechanism of action in man.

Endocrine Physiology

Knowledge of the basic physiology and endocrinology of the entire male reproductive system has resulted from animal studies that have been later confirmed in human investigations. These generalized properties include the mechanism of the hypothalamic-pituitary-gonadal axis; the biochemical pathway for the synthesis of testosterone by the Leydig cells; testosterone transport and binding to serum proteins; and steroid uptake and retention in the prostate gland. It should not be concluded that all species are identical; however, the similarities are more common than the differences.

Endocrine Biochemistry

The well-established mechanisms in the prostate for the enzymatic biotransformation of testosterone to dihydrotestosterone (DHT) through the action of membrane-bound 5α-reductase and the subsequent binding of DHT to steroid receptor proteins was first established in animal studies. The identification of DHT, 5α-reductase, and steroid receptors in the human prostate is now a well-accepted extrapolation from animal to human.

Prostatic Pathology

Although there may be some agreement on the merits of deriving useful information from animal studies that can be related to normal human physiology, can one also justify the study of pathological changes in the prostate in animal models and derive useful information that may be related to the human? This is, of course, a far more difficult and cautious endeavor. We also are reminded that no two human cancers are identical. Therefore, comparing two humans with the same disease may not be justified; however, enough generalizations have been developed through such comparisons to justify the discipline of oncology. Indeed, useful correlations have been derived for each general type of human cancer, once it is properly classified. The same may be the case for animal models of prostatic cancer. Thus each may provide distinct advantages for developing basic principles of prostatic cancer that may be more or less appropriate to one or more of the many types of human prostatic cancer. It is recognized that there are many types of human prostatic cancer, and there are also many corresponding types of animal prostatic cancers. The wisdom may come from the proper matching of appropriate types between species in developing useful concepts.

Does any prostatic cancer in animals produce a similar pathological situation as the human disease? Good pathological correlations are observed in spontaneous (not transplanted) prostatic adenocarcinoma between dog and man. In 1968, Leav and Ling reported a pathology study of 392 dogs greater than six years in age [2]. They observed metastatic prostatic adenocarcinoma in 20 of these animals, and the pathology of the disease was very similar to that of the human disease. These included morphological similarities, increased frequency in older animals, skeletal metastases, route of metastases, presence of acid phosphatase, and lipid particles in neoplastic cells. Differences from the human disease were also noted, such as the absence of a high incidence of latent prostatic adenocarcinoma in the dog.

Therapy of Prostatic Cancer

In oncology many important therapeutic concepts have been derived from studies using animal models of cancer. Among these accomplishments are the development and application of principles of tumor growth and cell kinetics, the testing of new concepts in combination and adjuvant therapy, and the preliminary screening of new cancer chemotherapeutic agents. In addition, these animal tumor models have been of value in elucidating basic principles of radiotherapy and immunotherapy.

The ultimate evaluation of any therapeutic modality will require careful randomized and controlled clinical studies; however, to define all therapeutic parameters and principles only in human studies would be prohibitively expensive, time consuming, and would in many cases involve ethical limitations. Waiting for clinical studies to resolve basic therapeutic questions has often been slow and frustrating because of the inherent difficulty of the task. Even after extensive clinical experience with estrogen therapy for human prostatic cancer, which has been employed for over 30 years, it has only recently become evident that no real estrogen dose-response data for benefit and risk were available to guide the clinician. In addition, the timing and beneficial effects of castration in the different disease states of prostatic cancer have not been resolved in a very compelling manner. In spite of these uncertainties it is still difficult – perhaps rightfully so – to have new and untreated early stage patients entered on experimental protocols using rather toxic cancer chemotherapeutic drugs with unknown but hoped for benefits in the control of human prostatic cancer. And yet this choice may be necessary if any real progress is to be made against this common and stubborn form of cancer. In these matters it would be most helpful in making these difficult clinical decisions if we had experimental evidence that a proposed regimen showed promise in a well controlled and appropriate animal model. Emphasis should be placed on controls, because many important factors that can be controlled properly in the laboratory are difficult or almost impossible to control adequately in similar clinical studies. These factors include 1) uniformity of genetic strain and age of host; 2) controlled onset of tumor growth; 3) uniformity of tumor type; 4) precise knowledge of tumor load and growth rates; 5) regulation of dietary elements and physical stress; 6) total compliance to drug intake and timing; 7) complete follow-up; 8) uniform control over the onset and termination of the study and subject with all subjects available for autopsy; 9) large numbers in each study group, all monitored at the same time; 10) one physician or observer making all evaluations. Other important variables could be listed that can best be controlled in the laboratory, and the fact that many of these variables are not or cannot be regulated within a clinical setting further emphasizes some of the difficulties that we must face in a realistic manner in resolving differences in human studies. Pioneering efforts are under way by the National Prostatic Cancer Project to provide the best rational basis for establishing clinical criteria for the evaluation of cancer chemotherapeutic drugs in a national cooperative study. Furthermore, effort is being expended to evaluate animal models for prostatic cancer and to characterize their properties and determine if these models can be helpful in providing new leads in the control of prostatic cancer. It may be important to emphasize that all established treatments of human prostatic cancer can also be shown to be effective in animal models of this disease. For example, castration and estrogen therapy of the Dunning rat prostatic cancer produces some involution of the disease, but there is subsequent relapse to a hormonal insensitive state and ultimate death from the disease [3].

It is obvious that animal models alone are not sufficient within themselves to assess the full clinical importance of a therapeutic approach; however, animal models do provide a unique opportunity to develop new concepts that are most difficult to obtain through available clinical studies and within reasonable cost, time, and ethical restraints. Appropriate animal studies with well-characterized tumors in controlled experiments and careful clinical trials must both work in concert to assist the search for new and more effective management of prostatic cancer.

Conclusion

In summary to answer the original question of whether it is important to develop animal models for prostatic cancer, I believe the answer is yes. Our physiology and biochemistry textbooks attest to the general statement that, more often than not, one can extrapolate useful information from animal studies. Certainly not all information derived from animal studies has been found to be applicable to humans; however, these are exceptions that catch our attention, but these few limitations should in no way detract from the major contributions that have been derived from animal studies. Caution is always in order, and scientific proof of similarity will always be required; however, we must not paralyze our efforts with outdated cliches stating that animal experimentation has little relevance to the study of the human disease.

Selecting a *single* animal model for prostatic cancer may not be realistic, because the human cancer counterpart is itself a variable and multifaceted disease. Each type of human tumor is often characterized by a wide spectrum of diversity in relation to pathology, state and variability of cellular differentiation, growth rate, and differences in therapeutic responsiveness to hormonal, nonhormonal, and radiation treatment. Indeed, many of these variations can sometimes be observed in one patient and may be due to the heterogeneity of the individual tumor. Because of this variability of human prostatic cancer, it is possible that more than one animal model may be required to correspond to these different states of human cancer. Even through we are aware of these variations within human and animal prostatic cancer, we can refer to the typical clinical picture and strive toward an animal model with similar properties and response. Some generalized properties of human prostatic cancer are summarized in Table I. (For more specific details of these properties refer to the recent review of Catalona and Scott [4]).

TABLE I. Generalized Properties of Human Prostate Cancer

Unknown etiology. Hormonal events suggested but not established.
Increased spontaneous incidence with age.
High incidence of latent cancer.
Localized to specific regions (lobes?) of prostate.
Adenocarcinoma.
Variable degrees of differentiation, sometimes within same tumor.
Suggested tumor cell heterogeneity.
Variable elevation in serum acid phosphatase.
Slow tumor growth rate; tumor doubling time probably > 30 days.
General pattern of metastasis to specific lymph nodes, bone, liver.
Amount of metastases and pattern can be variable.
Variable response to androgen deprivation (castration and/or estrogen therapy).
Subsequent relapse to hormonal therapy with time. No significant increase in cure rate; marginal to modest increase in survival time.
Low therapeutic response of hormonal relapsed tumors to chemotherapy with common cytotoxic agents (Cytoxan, 5-FU, Estracyt, hydroxyurea, DTIC) in controlled trials by the NPCP. Less than 15% of treated tumors produce > 50% reduction in tumor or partial regression following three-month therapy.
Low to modest sensitivity to radiation.
Tumor-associated antigen has been reported.

THE ANIMAL MODEL

The generalized properties of the animal model are listed in Table II and are derived from the human counterpart described in Table I, with the addition of practical experimental requirements to permit adequate study. The specific aspects of these requirements for the model are discussed in additional detail in the paragraphs that follow.

Species and Origin

The etiology of human prostatic cancer is still unknown, and while external factors such as carcinogens and viruses are possible causative factors, they have nevertheless failed to be proven as direct etiological agents. Efforts must continue to resolve the roles of these potentially important factors, but they remain very speculative. The only firm evidence is that prostatic cancer develops spontaneously in aged males who were not castrated prepubertally; therefore, this should be a prime prerequisite for the animal model. The dog develops spontan-

---

TABLE II. Generalized Properties of Animal Models of Prostatic Cancer

Spontaneous in origin.
Developed in aged animals.
Proven origin from prostatic tissue.
Adenocarcinoma.
Slow-growing tumor.
Histologic similarity to human prostatic cancer, with diversity in form.
Biochemical profile similar to normal prostate and human prostatic cancer.
Malignant and metastatic patterns to bone and lymph nodes.
Elevated serum prostatic acid phosphatase levels.
Hormone sensitive; requires presence of androgen for maximal growth or maintenance.
Capable of responding to castration and estrogen therapy followed by subsequent relapse to hormone insensitive state. Not cured by androgen deprivation.
Immunological parameters:
    1) Developed in syngeneic animals.
    2) Transplantable or easily induced.
    3) Contains tumor-specific antigens.
Large numbers of animals are available for statistical considerations.
Similar therapeutic response to human prostatic cancer; correlates with past clinical experience with
    1) Hormonal therapy
    2) Nonhormonal therapy
    3) Radiation sensitivity
Wide diversity of tumor types (differentiation, hormonal response, etc) corresponding to human tumor variability.
Accurately predicts response to future modalities of human therapy.

TABLE III. Spontaneous Prostatic Adenocarcinomas in Animals

Species	Year	Investigator	Tumor
Rat	1961	W.F. Dunning	From dorsal prostate of aged (22 months) Copenhagen rat, syngeneic; androgen dependent; transplantable
	1973	M. Pollard P.H. Luckert	Aged, germ-free Lobund Wistar; ?lobe, prostate; hormone sensitive; transplantable
	1975	S.A. Shain B. McCullough A. Segaloff	Aged A × C rats; ventral prostate; no metastases; not transplanted
Hamster	1960	J.G. Fortner J.W. Funkhauser M.R. Cullen	Aged Syrian golden hamster; transplantable; tumor has been lost
Dog	1968	I. Leav G.V. Ling	Aged (> 8 yr) mongrels; metastases; no occult tumor
Mastomy	1965	K.C. Snell H.L. Stewart	Aged female African rodent prostate
	1970	J. Holland	
Monkey	1940	E.T. Engle A.P. Stout	Aged Macaca mulatta

eous prostatic cancer with age [2], and a few old rats have likewise produced prostatic adenocarcinomas that can be propagated by transplantation. The most popular include the rat prostatic adenocarcinoma of Dunning R-3327 [5], the Pollard tumors [6–8], and the A × C tumors [9, 10]. (For a more complete list see Table III.) Detailed reviews of animal models have been presented recently [11, 12], and these reviews should be consulted for a broader discussion of available models that also include carcinogen-induced tumors.

Older primates have not been adequately studied in large numbers to determine the true spontaneous incidence of either prostatic cancer or spontaneous benign prostatic hyperplasia. This is due in part to the great expense of maintaining large numbers of aged primates and to the difficulty in permitting them to age sufficiently in captivity to develop these diseases. It is also very difficult to capture large numbers of older males for study. Because of evolutionary considerations, the ideal animal model for prostatic cancer might be the higher primates, and it is anticipated that increasing interest in animal models of abnormal prostatic growth will soon involve these important species.

Organ

In animal models it is essential to establish the organ of tumor origin. In the human, prostatic cancer primarily develops in the outer regions of the prostate. The dog and human have no clearly defined prostatic lobes, and it is difficult to draw clear analogies to homologous lobes in rats and other species, although it is obvious that the histology of the dorsal lobe of the rat is more similar to the overall normal human prostate than is the larger ventral lobe, which is almost devoid of stromal elements. Although the dog and human have no clearly defined anatomical lobes, they may nevertheless have different functional zones or areas of different embryological origins. This has not been established but is the basis of several active studies. It is important to know why prostatic cancer in humans is primarily limited to specific areas of the prostate and why the aged prostates of other species are devoid of these tumors.

Histology

Many carcinogen-induced animal prostatic tumors are squamous carcinomas and therefore are not similar to the human prostatic adenocarcinomas. In contrast, the spontaneous canine and rat tumors, both Dunning R-3327 and Pollard, are adenocarcinomas. 'Therefore, the epithelial nature of the animal tumor must be substantiated by appropriate histochemical similarities to the prostate epithelium. The presence of microvilli and secretory granules helps to establish the epithelial nature. Nuclear analysis should indicate the pleiomorphic nature of a cancer nucleus, and karyotyping is required for species identity and continued identification of the transplanted cells.

Biochemical Studies

Several biochemical markers have been used in concert to identify cells of prostatic origin, and although no single test is completely definitive, when taken together they do provide an overall biochemical profile of the tumor and prostate. In addition, many markers are decreased or lost as cells become malignant or dedifferentiated to a more anaplastic nature. In all cases, the monitoring of the biochemical profile usually provides an identity of the state of the tumor. There are many biochemical factors associated with prostatic tissue, and some of the more important of them follow:

Enzymes and isozyme patterns
    Acid and alkaline phosphatase
    Leucine aminopeptidase
    β-glucuronidase
    Arginase, lactic dehydrogenase
    Fibrinolysin
    5α-reductase
    3α and 3β-hydroxy steroid dehydrogenases
    3β-hydroxy steroid 6α and 7α-steroid hydroxylase

Small molecules
   High ratio of dihydrotestosterone to testosterone
   Pattern of steroid conjugates
   Zinc, cadmium
   Spermine and spermidine
   Citric acid

Receptors, cytoplasmic and nuclear
   Dihydrotestosterone (DHT)
   17 β-estradiol
   Nuclear uptake of DHT

Tissue-specific and secretory proteins
   Electrophoretic profiles
   Tissue- and tumor-specific antigens

Elevated serum acid phosphatase levels have provided one of the useful biomarkers of metastatic human prostatic cancer. This is due primarily to the extreme high tissue levels of acid phosphatase that under normal conditions enter the secretions of the pro- state; however, from metastatic prostatic adenocarcinoma cells the enzyme enters directly into the general circulation, raising the serum levels and providing an enzyma- tic marker. The prostatic tissue levels of acid phosphatase are the highest in humans and decrease in other species. For example. the level per unit of tissue in the mouse prostate is only 1/6,000 of that of the human prostate. Relative prostatic tissue le- vels of acid phosphatase activity are as follows: man, 1,200; baboon, 1,100; Rhesus monkey, 130; dog, 60; rat, 1.0; and mouse, 0.20. Therefore the extent of elevation of the serum levels of prostatic acid phosphatse in animal tumor models would be dependent on five factors: 1) the levels of acid phosphatase in the animal prostate from which the tumor was derived; 2) the state of maintained differentiation of the tumor; 3) the location of the tumor implant and metastasis; 4) the overall tumor load in the animal; and 5) the specificity of the assay and the stability of the en- zyme in serum. Therefore, all animal tumor models may not exhibit the eleva- tion in serum prostatic acid phosphatase.

Metastatic Pattern

Factors controlling the extent and route of metastasis of human tumors are still poorly understood. Human prostatic cancer invades locally and metastasizes primarily to the lymph drainage and bone. Spontaneous tumors in the prostates of animals such as the dog follow similar patterns of metastasis and also produce elevated serum acid phosphatase values [2]. Many other animal tumors such as the Dunning R-3327 and Pollard tumors are transplanted subcutaneously and would, by necessity, follow different routes of metastasis from that of spontaneous prostatic tumor, although the end result may be nearly the same. Site of injection of the tumors (subcutaneous, intraperitoneal, intraprostatic), number of cells and state (free cell suspension or small tumor tissue implants), hormonal treament, and drug therapy can have marked effects on metastasis [8]. Metastatic cells may also represent a selection of a subclone or population of cells "preprogrammed" to home to specific metastatic sites [13].

Hormonal Response

The tumor should be hormonally sensitive, requiring the presence of androgens for full growth, and it should demonstrate growth inhibition following castration, estrogen or antiandrogen treatment. Most prostatic cancers in humans respond to androgen deprivation (castration or estrogen therapy), but it is generally concluded that hormonal therapy is not curative, and subsequent relapse occurs in essentially all cases to a hormone-insensitive state. There are very few exceptions and, therefore, this feature should be one of the most important requirements of an appropriate animal model for prostatic cancer, since a model should mimic the most consistent and important clinical response seen with the human cancer [14]. At present the treatment of prostatic cancer is limited severely by the hormonally insensitive state that almost invariably follows favorable response to hormonal treatment. At present we have no insight into the mechanism of induction of hormone insensitivity in humans. The mechanism of the development of this hormonal insensitivity appears to have been resolved for the first time for prostatic cancer in an animal model [14, 15]. The mechanism appears to be a phenomenon of preexisting resistant cell selection (clone selection) as opposed to a conversion or induction of hormone-sensitive cells to an insensitive state. There is some reason to believe that human prostatic cancer may also be multifocal in nature [16].

Immunologic Parameters

Tumor immunology is increasing as an important consideration in cancer biology, etiology, and immunotherapy. Although many expectations for immunotherapy of cancer have not been realized, there is still great potential for immunologic approaches as we increase our basic understanding of immunology. Tumor-associated antigens have been detected in membrane extracts from human prostatic cancer [17, 18]. Similar tumor membrane antigens have also been detected in the Dunning R-3327 rat prostatic adenocarcinoma [19]. These findings emphasize the need for further immunologic studies in prostatic cancer, and immunology can best be studied in tumor models in syngeneic animals. Syngeneic animals are essentially immunologically identical and will accept transplants between animals of the group.

It is important to remember that many of the transplantable animal tumors might have picked up viral particles or foreign elements during the years of continuous transplantation. These foreign factors could complicate immunologic studies, since they may appear as tumor-associated antigens not common to the host.

Growth Rate and Cell Kinetics

Human prostatic cancer is known to be a relatively slow-growing tumor, although the time for one cell to double has not been determined. It is estimated that the tumor doubling time may be greater than one month, which is not uncommon for many human solid tumor adenocarcinomas. Preliminary DNA labeling studies indicate a low ^{3}H-thymidine labeling index, which indicates a small fraction of the prostate cancer cells in active DNA synthesis. One individual tumor cell must divide or double approximately 30 times to grow one billion (10^9) tumor cells, which is a total tumor volume of 1 cc and is about the minimal size for early clincial detection. For example, a single original tumor cell doubling each month would require a minimum of two and one-half years to grow to a tumor volume of 1 ce [1 month/division (30 divisions) = 30 months]. These cell kinetic considerations have been discussed for prostatic cancer [20].

Most animal tumors are rapidly growing, with division times of hours or days. These systems would not mimic the very slow growing human prostatic cancer. The Dunning R-3327 rat prostatic adenocarinoma is the only slow-growing model available and has a tumor doubling time of 20 days [3].

Although slow-growing animal tumor models may be more similar to the human situation, they nevertheless limit the number of investigations because they require long periods for the inoculated tumors to grow to detectable sizes and another long period before the cancers result in death of the animals. This limitation requires maintenance of large colonies of animals under study for an extended time.

Availability

Canine prostatic cancer would probably be an excellent animal model, but unfortunately the low incidence makes it difficult to obtain sufficient numbers of animals for statistical study. The Dunning rat prostatic tumor (R-3327) has been made available to interested investigators through the National Prostatic Cancer Project. Other models such as the Pollard tumor are being distributed on an individual basis but must be carried in a Lobund-Wistar rat line in order to propagate properly. Unfortunately the Fortner hamster tumor has been lost and is not available. Individual centers have the aged A X C rat tumor, as well as the mastomy tumors under study (see Table III).

In order to preserve many valuable prostatic tumor lines, the National Prostatic Cancer Project has established a tissue bank at the University of Miami School of Medicine under the direction of Dr. Theodore I. Malinin. This bank will serve as a safe depository for these animal tumors and not as a distribution center. It is important to note that cryopreserved tumor samples require several cycles of transplantation before they stabilize their properties.

SUMMARY

Numerous contributions to our understanding of the human prostate have been obtained from previous animal studies. The use of newly available animal models of prostatic adenocarcinoma described in this paper should provide the means for further developing new concepts that can be tested in the human disease. In so doing, each animal model must first be characterized and demonstrated as being an appropriate model for a particular form of the human tumor. In this regard this review has discussed several important considerations.

ACKNOWLEDGMENTS

These investigations were supported by grant CA-15416, awarded by the National Prostatic Cancer Project of the National Cancer Institute, DHEW.

REFERENCES

1. Handlesman H: The limitations of model systems in prostatic cancer. Oncology 34: 96–99, 1977.
2. Leav J, Ling GV: Adenocarcinoma of the canine prostate. Cancer 22:1325–1345, 1968.
3. Smolev J, Heston W, Scott W, Coffey DS: Characterization of the Dunning R-3327–H prostatic adenocarcinoma: An appropriate animal model for prostatic cancer. Cancer Treat Rep 61:273–287, 1977.
4. Catalona WJ, Scott WW: Carcinoma of the prostate. In Harrison JH, Gittes RF, Perlmutter A, Stamey TA, Walsh PC (eds): "Campbell's Urology," vol 2: Philadelphia: W.B. Saunders Co., 1979, pp 1085–1124.
5. Dunning WF: Prostatic cancer in the rat. Natl Cancer Inst Monogr 12:351–370, 1963.
6. Pollard M: Spontaneous prostate adenocarcinoma in aged germfree Wistar rats. J Natl Cancer Inst 51:1235–1241, 1973.
7. Pollard M, Luckert PH: Transplantable metastasized prostate adenocarcinoma in rats. J Natl Cancer Inst 54:643–649, 1975.
8. Pollard M, Chang CF, Luckert PH: Investigations on prostatic adenocarcinomas in rats. Oncology 34:129–132, 1977.
9. Shain S, McCullough B, Segaloff A: Spontaneous adenocarcinomas of the ventral prostate of aged A × C rats. J Natl Cancer Inst 55:177–180, 1975.
10. Shain S, McCullough B, Nitchek W, Boesel R: Prostate carcinogenesis in the A × C rat. Oncology 34:114–122, 1977.
11. Coffey DS, Isaacs JT, Weissman RM: Animal models for the study of prostatic cancer. In Murphy GP (ed): "Prostatic Cancer." Littleton, Massachusetts: PSG Publishing Co., 1979, pp 89–109.
12. Rivenson A, Silverman J: The prostatic carcinoma in laboratory animals: A bibliographic survey from 1900 to 1977. Invest Urol 16: 468–472, 1979.

13. Fidler IJ: Tumor heterogeneity and the biology of cancer invasion and metastasis. Cancer Res 2651–2660, 1978.

14. Smolev JK, Coffey DS, Scott WW: Experimental models for the study of prostatic adenocarcinoma. J Urol 118:216–220, 1977.

15. Isaacs JT, Heston WDW, Weissman RM, Coffey DS: Animal models of the hormone-sensitive and insensitive prostatic adenocarcinomas, Dunning R-3327-H, R-3327-HI, and R-3327-AT. Cancer Res 38:4353–4359, 1978.

16. Byar D, Mostofi F: Carcinoma of the prostate: Prognostic evaluation of certain pathologic features in 208 radical prostatectomies. Examination of the step-section technique. Cancer 30:5–13, 1972.

17. Brannen G, Gomolka D, Coffey DS: Specificity of cell membrane antigens in prostatic cancer. Cancer Chemother Rep 59:127–130, 1975.

18. Brannen G, Coffey DS: Tumor-specific immunity in patients with prostatic adenocarcinoma or benign prostatic hyperplasia. Cancer Treat Rep 61:211–216, 1977.

19. Claflin AJ, McKinney FC, Fletcher MA: The Dunning R-3327 prostate adenocarcionma in the Fisher-Copenhagen F_1 rat; a useful model for immunological studies. Oncology 34:105–109, 1977.

20. Weissman RM, Coffey DS, Scott WW: Cell kinetic studies of prostatic cancer: Adjuvant therapy in animal models. Oncology 34:133–137, 1977.

Summary

R. F. GITTES

This last session has offered a glimpse of the potential uses of animal models in prostate cancer. Without recapitulating the extensive work reported, we can generalize by pointing out that in the case of Dr. Coffey's group, we have seen the model used for a dissection of the kinetics of a hormone-dependent tumor which is remarkably familiar to the clinician in terms of temporary responses to hormonal manipulation. Dr. Coffey's group has elegantly demonstrated in rats the coexistence of histologically indistinguishable clones of hormone-dependent and hormone-independent cells in a given tumor passage. The parallel to the human clinical experience is obvious. The inhibition of the hormone-dependent clones does give temporary dramatic results but does not prevent the eventual outgrowth of the hormone-independent clone. The important questions as to what therapeutic tactics will be most desirable for the human case can be explored in various sublines of these tumors in rats. For instance, does early or late castration make any difference in the survival time of an individual with prostate cancer? This is readily subject to experiments in their model and they have given us a glimpse of that by showing that castration after 120 days of tumor growth did improve the group's mean survival time.

Other pertinent questions to be asked include whether such late castration offers any advantage over earlier castration, as in a clinical situation, and whether the tumor regression that occurs after castration interferes with coincident chemotherapy aimed at the residual hormone-independent clone. With much work to be done, we can be satisfied that we now have a better conceptual understanding of what is probably going on in the clinical case of cancer of the prostate. We can manipulate the animal models in a way which is clearly impossible in the clinical situation.

The enormous amount of work carried out by Dr. Drago and his group in the testing of chemotherapeutic agents, using another model of prostate cancer, is a good example of another use for the available models. While it may be said that any individual tumor in a rat is unlikely to be representative of the average human tumor, a collection of tumors such as those induced in rats by the techniques of

Models for Prostate Cancer, pages 393–394

Dr. Noble offer a variety of hormone-dependent and -independent tumors that permit the testing of panels of simple chemotherapeutic agents and of their combination. To those who would minimize the significance of this effort, it must be pointed out that in past years drugs which were widely tested and found to be useful by the National Prostatic Cancer Project, such as cytoxan and 5FU, were selected on an even flimsier thread of evidence using the response of DNA synthesis in normal prostatic tissue to androgens after prior orchiectomy. Surely, this extensive effort applied to the various models now available and those to come will give us a much more rational selection of therapeutic regimens for the patients who need it.

The immunological studies of Dr. Claflin and her colleagues are an example of the type of serious investigation of the immunological corollaries of prostate tumor growth in animal models. Using the Dunning tumor, they have been disappointed in its lack of immunogenicity. With sophisticated biochemical probes, they have elicited some differences in the immunological properties of sublines of the tumor. Although the initial enthusiasm for a role of the immunological response of the host in the natural history of prostate cancer has been greatly dampened, as it has in the study of most other organ sites, the careful quantitative work demonstrated in Dr. Claflin's study puts such an immunological investigation on a firm scientific basis and allows it to become the technological yardstick for corresponding studies of human tumors, both in the extraction of potential antigens and the detection of specific antibodies. The field of immunological investigation in prostate cancer has been clouded with premature and irreproducible results. The new animal models are allowing several laboratories to do first-class work that should give us reliable conclusions.

In a feeling shared by most of us, we are pleasantly surprised at the amount of good scientific work that has been made possible by the nurture of the few animal models available to us. The future looks brighter than it did when this organ site program was started.

Index